HOW TO BE A
PERFECT 10

Women's Guidebook to Increasing Attractiveness

DIANA POLSKA

Editors: Rob Tilley, Gina Melissa Fusco, Gail Lennon
Cover Design: Heidi Sutherlin
Cover Image: Shutterstock, Ana Canales
Interior Design: Velin Saramov
Interior Images: Arimac Lanka (Pvt) Ltd.

Publisher's Cataloging-in-Publication
Polska, Diana.
    How to be a perfect 10 : women's guidebook to
    increasing attractiveness / Diana Polska.
    p. cm.
    Includes bibliographical references and index.
    LCCN 2012949667
    ISBN 978-0-9916903-0-5

    1. Beauty, Personal. 2. Women—Health and hygiene. I. Title.

RA778.P65 2012   613'.04244
                  QBI12-600198

DISCLAIMER

Dedication

This book is dedicated to my mother (1961-2010),
who inspired me with her breathtaking beauty.

I also dedicate this book to every single woman
who wants to become a magnificent piece of artwork.

Contents

Preface

I know what women want. They want to be beautiful.
- Valentino Garavani, Italian fashion designer

*W*omen desire to be beautiful more than anything else. Beauty is a global industry worth US$160 billion per year. Women spend a great deal of time and money on their looks. The problem is that not all women "get it right." This book is designed to help all women "get it right." Many of the guidelines within this book are research-based.

For the purpose of this book, generalizations are made about what the majority of people find attractive, since all the research studies in this book favor the opinions of the majority over the minority. No one woman can be attractive to everyone, but she can be attractive to the majority.

Many of the opinions throughout the book are those of men, since women value beauty mainly for the reason of attracting them. It's fairly common knowledge that men in many cultures rate women on a scale of 1 to 10. A "perfect 10" woman commands nearly all male attention, while a woman with a score of 5 or below receives very little attention.

The secret to looking good is first to know what looks good. As Antoine Pierre Berryer, a French advocate, once said, "There are no ugly women; there are only women who do not know how to look pretty." Any woman with a desire to be beautiful can achieve her desire by learning the art of observation, analysis, and application.

There is a template for beauty. Studies reveal that we all have an innate template of what a woman "should" look like, which we automatically use for every single woman we encounter as we assess their physical beauty in a nanosecond. Canadian artist Agnes Martin said, "In our minds there is awareness of perfection." Studies confirm that the fashion doll is the ideal beauty template and all the physical traits of the fashion doll are considered very attractive traits in a real woman.

> "There are no ugly women; there are only women who do not know how to look pretty."
> - Antoine Pierre Berryer

This book can be life changing if you lack the physical beauty that attracts people at first glance. You will learn to "charm them with your presence as soon as they look at you," as Polish beauty, Anna Held, once said. The often denied but very true fact is: being physically beautiful commands respect and attracts friendship and love.

This book is also for women with physical beauty who lack the inner beauty required to hold people's long-term attention. Physical beauty may capture instant attention, but inner beauty will capture long-term attention and admiration. American model Christy Turlington said, "I sincerely feel that beauty largely comes from within."

A "perfect 10" beauty score is a combination of inner and outer beauty. French actress Emmanuelle Beart said, "Usually, when people say you are beautiful, it is when there is a harmony between the inside and the outside."

Physical beauty is highly valued in today's society, but it is not a new phenomenon. Past cultures placed a very high emphasis on physical beauty, but they had slightly different standards of beauty. The ideal standards of beauty change over time. What was considered beautiful in the past may not always apply to-day. Changes are always made in hairstyles, makeup application techniques, fashion, and ideal weight. As German fashion designer Karl Lagerfeld said, "Beauty is also submitted to the taste of time, so a beautiful woman from the Belle Epoch is not exactly the perfect beauty of today, so beauty is something that changes with time." However, there are certain timeless and universal standards of beauty that apply regardless of the day and age, and these standards are found within this book.

Products and services are rarely mentioned in this book. Trends, techniques, and technologies are constantly changing. This book is an outline only, so fill in the details with beauty and health magazines for the latest and greatest products or services. Only truly exceptional products or services will be mentioned.

Some sections of this book suggest cosmetic procedures. It is important to keep in mind that the basis for cosmetic procedures should be improvement and near perfection, but not idealist perfection. Swedish musician Agnetha Fältskog said, "There is a danger of changing too much in the search for perfection." With that said, cosmetic procedures are essentially artistry and are better called artistic terms such as chiseling or sculpting. Cosmetic procedures are only "plastic" when overdone or when unnatural augmentation fillers are used.

Many wise quotes are used within this book because collective wisdom is the greatest wisdom. A few wise words are much more powerful than volumes of information. English singer Jonathan King said, "A good quote is worth a thousand words."

What is beauty? Plato defined beauty as "proper measure and proper size of parts that fit harmoniously into a seamless whole." Aristotle defined beauty as "order and symmetry and definiteness." A dictionary defines it as the quality that gives pleasure to the sight, evokes a high degree of attraction, and is associated with such properties as harmony of color, form, proportion, and excellence of artistry. From these definitions, we grasp that female beauty is a form of art that attracts admiration.

Female beauty, like art, can be created or enhanced. American writer Ralph Waldo Emerson once said, "Love of beauty is taste, the creation of beauty is art." This book shows you that you can create or enhance your inner and outer beauty and become a "perfect 10" because every single woman should be a magnificent piece of artwork.

Introduction

Personal beauty is a greater
recommendation than any letter of reference.
- Aristotle, Greek philosopher

*B*eing beautiful comes with many advantages. Many women can be successful in life mainly because of their beauty. Psychology professor Ingrid Olson, PhD, says, "Research has demonstrated time and again that there are tremendous social and economic benefits to being attractive." The disadvantages of being attractive are few and tolerable, such as jealousy from the same sex or being accused for using physical beauty for wrong motives.

Beauty is a very valuable commodity for a woman to possess. American author Alex Comfort said, "A woman's greatest asset is her beauty." African-American journalist Jill Nelson said, "We learn as girls that in ways both subtle and obvious, personal and political, our value as females is largely determined by how we look." Some women realize, as did American actress Jorja Fox that "beauty is everything."

"A woman's greatest asset
is her beauty."
- Alex Comfort

Initially, a woman with physical beauty will receive respect and admiration. American actress Pauline Frederick said, "When a man gets up to speak, people listen, then look. When

5

a woman gets up people look; then, if they like what they see, they listen."

A woman's beauty holds magnetic power over many, especially over men. Chanakya, an Indian diplomat and one of the greatest figures of wisdom in Indian history, said, "The world's biggest power is the youth and beauty of a woman."

Lookism is a term used to refer to discrimination against people based on their physical appearance. Lookism is pervasive. Research proves that it exists and impacts every sector of life.

Dr. Mona Phillips, a professor of sociology, says that beautiful people are treated differently because culture places a high value on physical appearance. Dr. Frederick Work, a plastic and reconstructive surgeon, agrees that attractive people get better treatment than others. Dr. Work says, "Our society is very much fixated on physical appearance. Attractive people do receive special treatment, and there are more opportunities available to them." Gordon L. Patzer is a writer and researcher on physical attractiveness as well as the author of *Looks: Why They Matter More Than You Ever Imagined.* According to Dr. Patzer, "Good-looking men and women are generally judged to be more talented, kind, honest and intelligent than their less attractive counterparts." Dr. Patzer adds, "Controlled studies show people go out of their way to help attractive people—of the same and opposite sex—because they want to be liked and accepted by good-looking people."

Several studies show that physically attractive people receive lighter jail sentences when found guilty of a crime. Those rated as less attractive were perceived to be prone to committing future violent crimes, suggesting that unattractive people are more likely to be branded as criminals.[1] A study found that attractive people received shorter sentences than unattractive people accused of a similar crime. Defendants who were perceived as attractive, clean, neat, and well-dressed were treated with greater leniency.[2] Another study also found that physically attractive people received shorter sentences.[3] Unattractive defendants are 22 percent more likely to be convicted and tend to get hit with longer, harsher sentences than attractive defendants.[4] "You will judge a person on looks the less you have to go on," said psychiatrist Christos Ballas, MD. He states, "The more you have to go on, the more you'll judge them differently. The default for human beings is to judge on appearance."

Studies show attractive people are more likely to be hired than less attractive individuals.[5] Hiring preferences were shown for attractive applicants.[6] Less attractive female applicants were routinely at a disadvantage.[7]

"Attractive people earn 12 to 16 percent more than unattractive people," says Steven M. Jeffes in his book, *Appearance Is Everything*. Management professor Timothy Judge did separate studies of 11,253 Germans and 12,686 American residents and found that very thin women earned an average $15,572 a year more than women of normal weight. Women experienced an income loss as their weight increased. A woman who gained twenty-five pounds above the normal weight earned an average of $13,847 less than women of normal weight.[8]

We expect physically attractive people to be better at things and have a better life than physically unattractive people. Research shows that we believe "what is beautiful is good." Researcher Alan Feingold analyzed research data from more than one hundred studies on the sociological and psychological effects of beauty. He found that physically attractive people were perceived as more mentally healthy, intelligent, and socially skilled than physically unattractive people.[9] Evidence shows that beautiful women are perceived as having more desirable personality traits and having more successful jobs and relationships than unattractive women.[10]

We use the "halo effect," in which we judge a person to have positive qualities in one area, such as good looks, and make a similar positive assumption in other categories, such as personality. Psychologist Edward Thorndike was the first to support the "halo effect" with research. We also use the "horn effect" wherein one negative aspect is known about a person, other negative qualities are assumed.

Beauty is not in the eye of the beholder. Studies show that there is strong agreement across cultures about who is and who isn't attractive. This suggests that people everywhere are using the same, or at least similar, criteria in their judgments of physical beauty.[11] Therefore, all people have the same or similar beauty template of what a woman should look like.

We are born with a love and appreciation for beauty. Psychology researcher Judith Langlois has discovered that at even six months of age, infants gaze longer at attractive and symmetrical faces than at unattractive and asymmetrical faces.[12] Babies haven't learned what our culture considers attractive, but they still respond to physical beauty. Even two- to three-month-olds looked longer at attractive faces.[13]

Psychologists have found that infants prefer brightly colored faces and also prefer what most adults consider a beautiful face. In infancy, they also begin to discriminate as to whom they are like and whom they do not like.[14] A study found that newborns show a preference for beautiful faces that are judged as attractive by adults. In this study, one hundred newborns were shown two images side-by-side, one showing an attractive face and the other a less attractive one. Approximately 80 percent of the time, the babies looked exclusively at the more beautiful face. "Attractiveness is not simply in the eye of the beholder; it is in the brains of newborn infants, right from the moment of birth and possibly prior to birth," says Dr. Alan Slater, a developmental psychologist who conducted the study.[15]

As we grow older, we are programmed to give favorable assumptions and expectations to physically attractive people. The media portrays ugliness as badness and beauty as goodness.

Disney movies usually portray physically attractive characters with mild tempers and kind personalities.

The best way to explain the importance of beauty is to look at the way we were created. We have been biologically programmed by God to seek partners who will guarantee reproductive success. God's purpose was to fill the whole earth with humans (Genesis 1:28). Reproductive success was required to fulfill that purpose. A man is programmed to want a beautiful woman because beauty indicates that a woman is able to pass on a man's genes.[16] Leslie Zebrowitz's well-researched book *Facial Attractiveness* states, "Attractive traits signal aspects of mate quality, such as fertility, youthfulness, or health."

Brazilian novelist Paulo Coelho said, "Beauty is the greatest seducer of man." Men place the highest priority on physical beauty when selecting a mate.[17] A study found that when people were on a first date, the only factor that determined how much someone was liked and wanted for future dates was physical beauty.[18]

Beauty is important in the animal kingdom as well. Animals rely on external traits, such as size, shape, and color, to attract mates.[19] The animals with the biggest horns, the shiniest coat, or the most brightly colored feathers will find partners much more easily because they appear healthier. Biologists discovered that mother birds will feed the most brightly colored of their offspring first so she does not spend her energy on a less healthy offspring that may not survive. According to anthropologist Laura Betzig, like animals, humans are programmed to recognize health through beauty.

In women, glowing skin, shiny hair, good facial features, and a toned body are all indications of health and fertility. "These inbuilt preferences seem to be aimed at ensuring males find suitably fertile females who are healthy enough to reproduce and in turn produce healthy children," says evolutionary anthropologist Sean McBride. "Facial neoteny, or the continuation of juvenile traits into adulthood, is appealing to males because it signifies youth. We unconsciously associate large eyes, a small nose and chin, and full red lips with fertility," he says. Researcher Dr. Craig Roberts found that a woman's face is most beautiful during ovulation, exactly when she is at the peak of her fertility.[20]

Polish researcher Krzysztof Kościński discovered that facial attractiveness is a reliable cue to the biological quality of a woman. Women who have beautiful faces have better parasite resistance, longevity, higher intelligence, better mental health, and higher reproductive success than unattractive individuals.[21]

A study found that facial attractiveness is a sign of physical fitness.[22] Evidence shows that facially attractive people may be physically healthier than unattractive people.[23] Researchers measured the facial features of around four hundred young people and analyzed their health records over three years. Features measured included chin length, jaw width, lip width, eye width, and eye height. They found that those with more symmetrical faces were healthier and more disease resistant.[24] A woman's physical attractiveness in face and body honestly signals hormonal and developmental health.[25]

One study across thirty-five cultures showed men desire, on average, a woman two years younger than themselves as a wife. As men age, they also desire an even larger age gap.[26] Anthropologists Martin Fieder and Susanne Huber discovered that men prefer young women due to their high fertility and reproductive capability. They found that couples that had the most children were in a relationship in which the man was four to six years older than the woman.

Men desire beautiful women not just for reproductive reasons but also for the ego boost it provides in social settings. A man that is seen with a beautiful woman has increased social status with both men and women. One study found that when people are shown pictures of a man with a very attractive woman, they view the man more favorably.[27]

Besides biological and social reasons for desiring beauty, admiring beauty gives feelings of pleasure and happiness. American sociologist Lewis Mumford said, "A day spent without the sight or sound of beauty, the contemplation of mystery, or the search of truth or perfection is a poverty-stricken day; and a succession of such days is fatal to human life."

God created us to admire and appreciate beauty. American poet Ralph Waldo Emerson said, "Never lose an opportunity of seeing anything beautiful, for beauty is God's handwriting." French playwright Jean Anouilh said, "Beauty is one of the rare things which does not lead to doubt of God."

God created only beauty. Nature is filled with striking beauty: brilliantly colored butterflies, parrots, flowers, rainbows, coral reefs, sunsets, mountainous regions, and the list goes on. Admiring and appreciating the beauty that God created through nature can definitely bring us closer to God. The enjoyment of beauty can be a spiritual experience and give a sense of transcendence.[28] A poem written by Ella Wheeler Wilcox says of beauty, "The search for beauty is the search for God...he who seeks shall find." Saint Augustine said, "Beauty is indeed a good gift of God."

Chapter 1: Face

*T*he face is the physical feature nearly all people notice at first and is the most important defining factor of beauty since it provides so much information. The face is a means of identification in much the same way as a fingerprint. It tells others about a person's health and age. The face also displays emotions and attitudes that are apparent to others. French physician and philosopher La Mettrie said, "A person's face tells much about their character and feelings."

Men who are seeking a long-term relationship value a beautiful face much more than a beautiful body in a woman. American businesswoman and socialite Paris Hilton said, "If you have a beautiful face you don't need fake boobs to get anyone's attention." Scientists discern that men looking for a long-term relationship prefer a beautiful face since it provides signs of a woman's long-term reproductive potential.[1]

A face that is feminine in appearance is particularly attractive and indicates high fertility.[2][3] There are common differences between male and female faces. In males, the forehead is often higher than in females. Men have more brow bossing (the ridge above the eyes). The distance between the brows and the hairline for women on average is 5 cm; for men it is 7 cm. Another difference is the shape of the hairline. Men have an M-shape or rectangular shape while women have an inverted U-shape hairline. Women have larger lips and smaller noses and chins than men.

Any woman can achieve a "perfect 10" face. As Irish writer Oscar Wilde said, "A woman's face is her work of fiction." Cindy Jackson is a woman who underwent a complete transformation and proved that the shape, proportion, and features of the face can be completely transformed with specific cosmetic procedures. Women can also wear makeup to enhance their facial beauty.

SHAPE

Facial width and length, as well as the shape of the jawline and chin, determine the face shape. Every "perfect 10" woman will have either a heart-shaped or oval-shaped face. Many beauty experts and scientists agree that these two face shapes are considered the most attractive and feminine of all face shapes.

Fashion dolls have an oval-shaped face. The oval face shape is very well balanced and can have any hairstyle, eyebrow shape, makeup technique, or sunglasses style.

The heart-shaped face is oval from the forehead to the edge of the jawline. Then, it will taper into a triangular shape to a slightly rounded, small chin. Psychobiologist Victor Johnston believes that the heart-shaped face is particularly desirable to men. A small lower face conveys the impression of youth.[4] Anthropologist Donald Symons says that a thin, pointed jaw and a small lower face are the results of high levels of estrogen, and an indicator of fertility.

A round face shape is fairly short with a wide forehead, often with full cheeks and a rounded chin. It is the least attractive face shape since it gives the face a chubby appearance.

A long face shape has a high forehead, flat cheekbones, and a high chin that causes the face to appear very long. A very long face shape is unattractive since facial features tend to look unbalanced. Barely visible, flat cheekbones are masculine and elongate a face. They give the face a more serious appearance.

A square face shape is wide and tends to drop down in a straight line from the ear toward the jawline and then turn at a sharp angle toward the chin, giving the face a square appearance. The square face shape is very masculine and particularly unattractive for a woman.

A triangular/pear face shape is narrow at the forehead and eye line, broadening to the jawline. The triangular/pear face shape is unbalanced and masculine.

A rectangular face is longer than it is wide and has a square jawline and a square hairline. A rectangular face is commonly found in men and is particularly unattractive for women.

A very round face can be corrected by a chin augmentation to lengthen the face. For chubby cheeks, a buccal excision removes the excess fat from the cheeks and leaves a more contoured midface and defined, model-like cheekbones. Jaw reduction will slim the lower face. Facial liposuction removes excess fat along the jawline or neck.

The best way to shorten a very long face is to perform a chin reduction to reduce the height of the chin. Hairline lowering involves removing a section of the skin on the forehead and pulling the scalp forward, effectively shortening a high forehead. To shorten a long midface you can undergo a cheek augmentation with hyaluronic acid injections to give your midface more volume.

A square face can be corrected by a jaw reduction procedure to slim the lower face. It softens and contours the face shape and can make a dramatic difference. Jaw angle reduction surgery will reduce the square corners near the back of the jawbone. Cheek and lip augmentation will make a square-shaped face appear much more feminine.

A triangular/pear face shape can be corrected with jaw reduction to slim the lower face. Cheek augmentation will help create more facial balance. A chin reduction may be considered if you need to reduce a large chin. If your face is more triangular than it is pear-shaped, then jaw angle reduction will reduce the squareness near the back of the jawbone.

A rectangular face can be corrected with jaw reduction to slim the lower face. A chin reduction will shorten the height of the chin. Repositioning the scalp hairline forward will shorten a long forehead. Lip and cheek augmentation will make the face appear more feminine.

DISCOVER YOUR FACE SHAPE

Measure your face with a tape measure using the following directions:

1. Measure your face across the top of your cheekbones. Write down the measurement on a piece of paper.

2. Measure across your jawline from the widest point to the widest point. Write down the measurement.

3. Measure across your forehead at the widest point. Generally, the widest point will be somewhere about halfway between your eyebrows and your hairline. Write down the measurement.

4. Measure from the tip of your hairline to the bottom of your chin.

Oval: Length equal to one and a half times width.
Heart: Narrow at jawline, wide at cheekbones and forehead.

Diamond: Widest at cheekbones, narrow forehead and jawline of approximately equal widths.

Oblong: Longer than it is wide.

Round: Wide as it is long. This may vary a little, but generally the measurement is close.

Square: Wide as it is long, with a square jawline.

Triangular/Pear: Forehead and cheekbones are narrow and jawline is wide. If your jawline is rounded, rather than square, the face is pear-shaped.

Rectangular: Longer than it is wide with a square jawline and a square hairline.

Researcher Kang Lee says changing a woman's hairstyle is one way in which the beauty of the face can be manipulated. His study on ideal female facial dimensions was published in the journal Vision Research. "Our study explains why sometimes an attractive person looks unattractive or vice versa after a haircut," says Kang Lee. Hairdresser Robert Ari explains: "If your hair is wrong for your face shape, it will accentuate features you may want to minimize and hide those you may want to show off."

PROPER HAIRSTYLE FOR YOUR FACE SHAPE

OVAL
An oval face shape can have almost any hairstyle because it is so well balanced. You can experiment with different hairstyles.

HEART
Your chin tends to be the focal point of your face. Draw attention to your eyes and cheekbones with bangs. Half-up hairstyles look flattering. Avoid hairstyles that add width to the upper face.

DIAMOND

The diamond can experiment with a variety of styles. However, if you are a dramatic diamond shape, you need to follow the same rules as the heart-shaped face.

OBLONG

You will want to shorten and widen your face. Bangs are vital for oblong face shapes. Volume, curls, and waves will add width to your long face. Avoid middle parts, height, and very long hair because it will only make your face look longer. If you desire very long hair, consider a V-shaped style where your hair is longer in the back with shorter length in the front.

ROUND

You will want to add height and length to reduce the roundness of your face. Long, straight hair looks best. The most flattering hairstyles are those with fullness and height at the crown. Off-center parts help reduce roundness. Avoid waves or curls. When you do style your hair with waves or curls, add them to the bottom part of your hair only. Long layers of hair kept close to the sides of the face at the cheekbone reduce and hide some of the roundness.

SQUARE

You will want to downplay your strong, angular jaw. Waved or curled hair will bring balance to your face. Height at the crown looks flattering. Ask your hairstylist to cut layers that start at the jawline and continue downward. You can soften your face with wispy bangs. Avoid straight-across bangs or center parts. Avoid straight bobs and short hair; these hairstyles intensify the squareness.

TRIANGULAR/PEAR
You must narrow your chin and widen your forehead. Hair that is cut and layered around the face is more flattering than straight cuts.

RECTANGULAR
Your goal is to create the illusion of a shorter, wider face and to soften your jawline. Side-swept bangs are highly recommended. Hair volume and waves will round out your face. Avoid long, straight hair that is all the same length.

Visibility and definition of the face shape is vital to beauty. If you are overweight you will have fatty layers covering your face and neck, making your face very round with no visible jawline. Top models have very well-defined facial features because they are thin. Losing weight will slim and define the face by removing the fatty layer covering the cheekbones, jawline, and neck.

Weight loss is usually effective for women looking to lose weight in their face. However, for women who have a hard time removing excessive fat in their face despite proper diet and exercise, then cosmetic procedures are an option.

Facial liposuction removes excessive fat in the face. Facial liposculpture is an alternative, minimally invasive form of liposuction and recommended for younger women. Rather than using large incisions to remove fat from the body, liposculpture uses a small suction mechanism to target specific fat deposits under the skin.

"Turkey neck" is caused by loose skin. A neck lift will provide significant improvement by tightening very loose neck skin. A neck lift will restore a tight, youthful appearance to skin and muscles under the chin and neck area. Neck liposuction is for women who have good neck elasticity and only excess fat to remove.

A face-lift involves fairly extensive surgery and works best for older women with loose, wrinkled, saggy skin. A woman can look at least ten years younger with a face-lift.

Some women have the appearance of chubby cheeks, or a "chipmunk" look, that can be corrected with buccal fat excision. Removal of cheek fat achieves a sculptural, high-fashion, defined look of the cheekbones. However, as some women age, they lose the fat in their face through atrophy, and buccal fat removal can eventually result in a hollow, prematurely old look. Therefore, if a woman feels she really needs this procedure, it is best if she does a partial buccal fat removal.

HOW TO CHOOSE THE BEST COSMETIC SURGEON

1. Make sure your cosmetic surgeon is board certified.
2. Pick a surgeon who specializes in specific surgical procedures.
3. Examine before and after pictures, and see if you like their work.
4. Find out how long they have practiced and how many operations they have performed in the last five years—the more, the better.
5. Ask them if they perform conservative or dramatic cosmetic surgery. Some women who had procedures done by a conservative cosmetic surgeon ended up with little or no improvement.
6. Find out if your chosen surgeon uses the Stephen Marquardt beauty mask or would be open to using it.
7. Interview the surgeon and follow your instincts.

PROPORTION

The right proportions are fundamental to facial beauty. Irregularities in proportion reduce facial beauty. Proportion refers to ratio and symmetry. Proper proportions can be seen in all things of beauty, whether in nature, architecture, or female faces.

Kang Lee discovered the exact ratio of the most attractive female face in his research. He says the key to the ideal arrangement of female facial features is the measurements between the eyes, mouth, and ears. The most attractive face is formed when the vertical distance between the eyes and the mouth is 36 percent of the length of the face, and the horizontal distance between the eyes is 46 percent of the width of the face. However, the study looked only at Caucasians, and the findings could not be applied to other ethnic groups.[5]

The Greeks said that all beauty is in mathematics. The golden ratio seems to recur in beautiful things. Twelfth-century Italian mathematician Leonardo Fibonacci discovered that the golden ratio is 1:1.618. The number 1.618 is called phi. This ratio of 1:1.618 is known by several names, including the divine proportion, the golden mean, and the golden ratio. This proportion is said to be the most attractive to the human eye.[6] Artists such as Michelangelo and Da Vinci used the golden ratio extensively in their artwork to achieve balance and harmony.

Former plastic surgeon Dr. Stephen Marquardt created a beauty mask that is based on the golden ratio. If an individual's face conforms to the beauty mask then the face will be beautiful, regardless of race, age, or nationality. Beautiful faces throughout the ages fit within this mask, including legendary Egyptian beauty Queen Nefertiti (ca. 1370 BC – ca. 1330 BC), and Hollywood actresses Marlene Dietrich and Marilyn Monroe. This proves that the standard of facial beauty is timeless.

You can use the Stephen Marquardt beauty mask to measure your level of facial beauty or to plan cosmetic procedures. You'll have to take a picture especially for this experiment because it's important to make sure your head is tilted to match the grid of the mask.

MARQUARDT'S BEAUTY MASK

1. WHAT YOU NEED
(a) A camera, and a friend to take your picture.
(b) Access to a copy machine that can resize pictures.
(c) Sheets of clear acetate (A4 or Letter) to make copies of the mask.
(d) A ruler to measure your face.
(e) A print of the mask, available from www.beautyanalysis. com.

2. TAKING THE PHOTO OF YOUR FACE
Face directly into the camera so that your face isn't turned even slightly right or left. Place the tips of your index fingers gently against the holes in your ears, keeping your fingers straight and horizontal. Do not put your fingers into your ears. Now, tilt your head up or down until the bottoms of your right and left irises (the round, colored part of your eye) are aligned on the top of an imaginary line connecting the tops of your index fingers, as seen through the camera viewfinder. Let the person taking the picture tell you when you're in the right position. With a relaxed face and without smiling, place your back teeth together so that they barely touch and bring your lips together until they touch gently. Your head will seem to be tilted slightly down.

3. DEVELOPING THE PHOTO
The photo size should ideally be as large as 13 X 18 cm or 20 X 26 cm (5" X 7" or 8" X 10").

4. CREATING THE CORRECT SIZE MASK FOR YOUR PHOTO

(a) On the photo of your face: Create a line connecting the center of your right and left pupils (the round, black, center part of your eyes). This is your pupil line.

(b) Create a second line connecting the right and left corners of your mouth. This is your lip line.

(c) Create a third line connecting the middle (or center) of your pupil line with the middle (or center) of your lip line. This is your facial vertical line.

(d) Take your copy of the mask and enlarge or shrink it on a copy machine until the facial vertical line (the vertical distance from the lip line to the pupil line) on the mask is the same as that distance on your face photo. Copy the final, correctly sized mask image onto a sheet of clear acetate.

5. APPLYING THE MASK TO THE PHOTO

Place the clear acetate mask over your face photo and match up the pupil line, the lip line, and the facial vertical line of the mask with the pupil line, the lip line, and the facial vertical line of the photo of your face.

Biostatistics expert Kendra Schmid, PhD, says there is a formula for the "perfect" face. She uses specific measurements to determine a person's facial beauty on a scale of one to ten.

Schmid says that most people score between four and six. She has never come across a "perfect 10." Dr. Schmid says the ratio of the length of the face to the width of the face should be 1.6:1. Whose face is the most perfect? Brad Pitt scored a 9.3. The closer the physical ratio is to the golden ratio, the more beautiful it becomes.

"PERFECT 10" FACIAL CALCULATION

1. First, Dr. Schmid measures the length and width of the face. Then, she divides the length by the width. The ideal result—as defined by the golden ratio—is roughly 1.6:1, which means a beautiful person's face is about one and a half times longer than it is wide.

2. Next, Dr. Schmid measures three segments of the face—from the forehead hairline to a spot between the eyes, from between the eyes to the bottom of the nose, and from the bottom of the nose to the bottom of the chin. If the numbers are equal, a person is considered more beautiful.

3. Finally, Dr. Schmid measures other facial features to determine symmetry and proportion. On a perfect face, Dr. Schmid says, the length of an ear is equal to the length of the nose, and the width of an eye is equal to the distance between the eyes.

Facial symmetry refers to having one side of the face exactly match the other side of the face. Research shows that women who are more symmetrical have higher levels of estrogen than less symmetrical women. Higher estrogen levels in women mean higher fertility and a higher chance of getting pregnant.[7] Symmetry also advertises immune system strength. Humans have the natural inclination to favor fertile individuals with strong immune systems.[8]

Symmetry is simply a way for animals or humans to advertise their genetic health. Numerous studies have proven that symmetrical features are a good indicator of health and the health of future offspring. Asymmetrical features give clues to underlying genetic problems, leading to less healthy offspring.[9] Biologists Randy Thornhill and Anders Møller have discovered that asymmetrical animals have lower survival rates and less successful reproduction. Environmental stressors such as parasites, radiation, pollution, and extreme temperatures can interfere with the precise expression of developmental design during the growth of animals and humans.

Women's symmetry changes during their menstrual cycle. They are more symmetrical and attractive right before or during ovulation. Women might find they attract more attention from men during ovulation. Biologist John Manning found that asymmetrical features actually decrease by 30 percent in the twenty-four hours before ovulation.[10]

Taking a whole food supplement and eating a healthy diet is vital to developing symmetry during puberty. If you are past puberty you can still subtly influence your symmetry through a strong immune system and high estrogen levels. Test for parasites living in your body. Test your hormone levels and correct estrogen deficiency or androgen excess.

FEATURES

Studies show that a face with a combination of feminine and childlike features is the most attractive.[11] Childlike features include a small nose, small chin, and large eyes. Feminine features include full lips, narrow jawline, arched eyebrows, small forehead, and prominent, high cheekbones.

In various studies conducted by psychologists Victor Johnston and David Perrett, men consistently showed a preference for women with large eyes, full lips, small nose, and a short chin. Men even predicted a woman's personality based on her facial features.[12]

French plastic surgeon Pierre F. Fournier believes childlike facial features are vital for beauty. His theory is that to elicit a protective desire, an adult's face must display childlike traits or expressions, called beauty. Everyone is instinctively attracted to a child's face. The sight of a child's face immediately causes us to feel a desire to protect. All babies have small noses and chins, so a small nose and chin signals extreme youthfulness in an adult woman.

As a woman gets older, her lower face lengthens and becomes less defined. Cartilage is deposited on ears and nose, making them bigger and longer. Facial muscles atrophy and volume decreases, causing cheekbones and facial structure to degenerate. Lips tend to get thinner as collagen production decreases.[13] A woman with small eyes, thin lips, and a large nose will look older and less attractive. Therefore, feminine facial features are a signal of youth.[14]

Feminine facial features also reflect high estrogen levels and low testosterone levels.[15] Studies have found that women with the highest beauty score ratings have the highest estrogen levels.[16,17] High estrogen levels result in enlargement of the lips and upper cheek area by fat deposition, similar to estrogen causing fat deposition in the thighs, buttocks, and breasts.[18] Among women in the same age group, high estrogen levels are associated with a higher chance of getting pregnant.[19]

Evolutionary biologist Randy Thornhill found that a feminine face signals hormonal and developmental health. Estrogen's by-products are toxic in the body. Feminine facial features may reliably signal an immune system of such high quality that it can deal with the handicap of high estrogen.[20]

A woman who is going through puberty can enhance her chance of growing into a beautiful woman by ensuring she has balanced hormone levels. Hormone testing should be conducted annually during puberty to measure estrogen and progesterone levels. John R. Lee, MD, an expert in natural hormone replacement therapy, says that progesterone and estrogen balance each other in the body. There are health risks associated with excess estrogen or excess progesterone.

Women who are going through menopause can extend their youth and beauty with natural hormone replacement. Dr. John R. Lee recommends supplementing with natural estriol cream. If you are using estriol cream, you may also want to take natural progesterone for balance. *Pueraria mirifica* is the most powerful natural estrogen source available and is also useful for menopausal women. Take all-natural hormone supplements under the supervision of a naturopath doctor who will monitor your hormone levels.

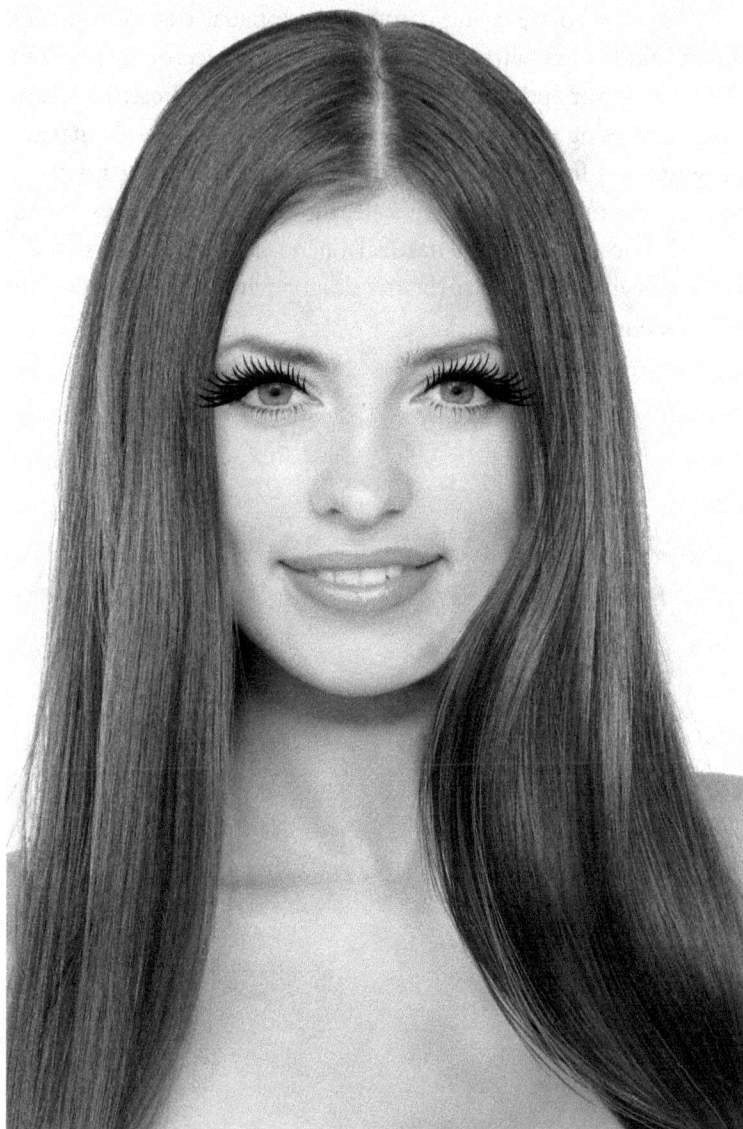

Figure 1 - Study this "perfect 10" face. Notice the combination of childlike and feminine facial features which include a small nose, small chin, large eyes, full lips, narrow jawline, arched eyebrows, small forehead, and prominent, high cheekbones.

COSMETIC PROCEDURES FOR FACIAL FEATURES

FOREHEAD

Forehead recontouring will correct a prominent brow bone (brow bossing). It is a procedure that involves brow shaving and surgically altering the bone. Hairline lowering will shorten a high forehead.

NOSE

A woman should make sure the surgeon does not do "natural noses" or subtle surgery. Many times a nose can look natural but still appear too large. A woman should compare photographs of her nose to photographs of her ideal nose to help her decide what to change in terms of shape, height, length, and width. She can then bring those photographs to her chosen cosmetic surgeon.

CHIN

A chin reduction will reduce the height, shape, or size of a chin. Trimming the chin bone will change the shape and size. Sliding genioplasty changes the height and projection of the chin.

JAWLINE

A jawline reduction procedure reduces the size of the lower face; the bone is filed down, and a part of the muscle is removed. This reduction will only reduce the fullness and will not affect the function. The final result of jawline reduction will be a more oval-shaped jawline that has a smoother and softer angle.

CHEEKS

Cheek augmentation is recommended for women with long faces, women with no definition in the cheeks, or women with sagging cheeks. Cheek augmentation is best done with hyaluronic acid filler. Hyaluronic acid is a substance that is naturally present in the human body. For chubby cheeks, a buccal excision removes the excess fat from the cheeks and leaves a more contoured-looking midface and more defined model cheekbones.

LIPS

Hyaluronic acid filler stimulates the body to produce more collagen, which is why so many women get extended results with this particular filler for their lips. Cindy Jackson, beauty and cosmetic surgery expert, says *Perlane* injections last the longest compared to any other filler. The upper lip may get longer as a woman gets older; an upper-lip lift decreases the distance between the nose and upper lip.

EYES

Eyes can be made to appear larger with an eyelid lift. An eyelid lift will remove the excess skin from the upper eyelid. Sagging eyebrows can be corrected with a brow lift.

Research shows that people wearing glasses are judged to be less attractive.[21] Glasses lessen facial discriminability.[22] A study at the London Vision Clinic found that people who wear glasses are perceived to be approximately three years older. Respondents said that those who wear glasses appear more "geeky" than people who do not wear them. The perceived image was even worse for people who were forty-five years and older, as they appeared to be five years older than they really were. Psychologist Dr. Glenn Wilson, who analyzed the results, said, "In addition to glasses making you look older, it seems we still make the unconscious assertion that people who wear glasses are weaker and less confident." Even young children consider glasses unattractive. A quarter of those surveyed revealed they were teased as children for wearing glasses.

If you choose to wear glasses, pick frames that complement your face shape; otherwise, improve your vision with natural vision correction methods.

Vision therapy, also known as behavioral optometry, is a progressive program of supervised in-office vision exercises designed to improve myopic (nearsighted), hyperoptic (farsighted), or presbyopic vision.

The Tibetan Eye Chart was developed by Tibetan monks to correct vision. Vision is improved with daily exercise performed with the Tibetan Eye Chart. Even if vision is perfect, having a daily routine of eye exercises helps to preserve eyesight.

The Bates Method is a natural method of vision correction designed by ophthalmologist Dr. William Horatio Bates (1860–1931). Dr. Bates noticed that when he prescribed eyeglasses, his patients' vision worsened. He realized that eyeglasses were relieving symptoms but not correcting the causes of poor vision. He determined that eyeglasses make eyesight worse over time. His techniques were all designed to achieve "central fixation," which leads to perfect eyesight.

Pinhole glasses are an alternative to glasses and may actually improve vision over time instead of worsening it. They improve myopia, astigmatism, hyperopia, and presbyopia by improving "central fixation".

Orthoculogy (Ortho C) is a method of correcting nearsightedness by wearing a slightly flat plain contact lens that gradually reshapes the eyes permanently. Developed by Canadian optometrist John William Yee, these contact lenses can reverse mild to moderate myopia. The advantage of Ortho C over laser surgery is the absence of any side effects such as halo effect, decrease in night vision, teary eyes, scarring, undercorrection, overcorrection, progressive visual acuity deterioration, or risk of rupture.

Facial ornaments do nothing to increase facial beauty. Studies show that women with facial piercings were rated as less physically attractive and intelligent than those without piercings. Multiple piercings were given the most negative beauty ratings.[23]

A brilliant iris color and defined lips as seen on fashion dolls are highly attractive. Most people direct their attention mainly to the eyes and lips.[24] Studies show that women were rated more attractive when the contrast and luminance of the eyes and lips were increased as compared with the rest of the facial skin.[25 26]

In Caucasians, blue eyes are considered highly attractive.[27] In particular, men with blue eyes are more attracted to women with blue eyes.[28] Almost all Caucasian babies are born with blue eyes. Therefore, blue eyes are considered to be a very youthful physical trait. If you have a dull eye color such as blue-gray, or green-gray, consider brilliantly colored contacts. If you have dark eyes you need to consider hair and skin color before wearing colored contacts to avoid looking unnatural. Dark-colored eyes are highly attractive in dark-skinned women.

Iridology is the science of reading the iris (colored part of the eye). The iris maps the condition of the body, mind, and emotions in a comprehensive manner. Iridology can reveal malfunctioning and toxic organs in the body. Many of those born with blue eyes that darkened to brown in adulthood reported a return to the original blue color after detoxification of the organ revealed as toxic by iridology.

Some people have reported they were able to change their eye color progressively over a period of one to three years with methylsulfonylmethane (MSM) eye drops. MSM eye drops are sold as a remedy for softening the leathery membranes of the eye, normalizing eye pressure, and clearing red spots and broken blood vessels in the eyes.

There have been a few reports of eyes being lightened by taking iodine internally. Iodine is an essential trace mineral. People in Japan consume about 12 milligrams of iodine or more per day. The recommended dose for eye lightening is 2.5 milligrams of iodine or more daily.

Eyebrows are an important part of the face. Studies show that the ideal arch peak of the eyebrow should be halfway between the edge of the pupil (lateral limbus) and the edge of the eye (lateral canthus).[29][30] Another study found that the ideal arch peak is different for younger women than it is for older women. The study found that the most desirable eyebrow peak was the edge of the eyes for younger women and the edge of the pupil for older women.[31] The best way to get perfect eyebrows is to go to an eyebrow-shaping salon.

To make eyebrows and eyelashes thicker, look for eyelash products with prostaglandin analogues. Studies show application of bimatoprost 0.03 percent to the upper lash line results in longer, thicker, and darker eyelashes within four months.[32] Bimatoprost is a safe method for growing the eyelashes.[33] Latanoprost, a prostaglandin analog, has been shown to induce the hair growth phase and cause eyelashes to grow thicker and longer.[34] Travoprost can also be used for eyelash growth. The least desirable possible side effect of prostaglandin analogues is permanent darkening of the iris to brown. Be very careful if you have bright blue or bright green eyes.

HOW TO GROW EYELASHES AND EYEBROWS

Apply bimatoprost, travoprost, latanoprost, or castor oil to the eyebrows or lash line with a very fine artist's-type paintbrush. Apply every day before falling asleep. Disinfect paintbrush with hydrogen peroxide before and after use.

An alternative to using prostaglandin analogues is to use castor oil. Castor oil has been used for centuries for hair and eyelash growth. Castor oil should be applied at night before falling asleep and left on eyelashes and eyebrows overnight.

A study found that men rate a woman more attractive when she smiles because happy expressions give the appearance of femininity and low dominance. Women are rated as the least attractive when they look proud.[35] Research shows that by frequently practicing to smile, you can increase the attractiveness of your smile.[36]

An attractive smile has white-colored teeth versus yellow-colored teeth. A study found that teeth that are darker in shade were rated as very unattractive in Caucausians.[37] However, `very bright, white teeth was rated as "too bright" against dark skin. This could be because of the greater contrast between skin color and tooth shade. Therefore, darker-skinned women do not need to concern themselves with excessive tooth whitening.

Teeth-whitening procedures can be performed on your own or at the dentist's office. However, be careful of tooth-whitening products with a low pH as they can damage tooth enamel. Be sure to avoid acid-etching techniques as they are known to damage tooth enamel.

To make your own natural tooth-whitening paste, add two or three teaspoons of hydrogen peroxide to baking soda. Be sure it is the same consistency as toothpaste. If you wish, you can add a bit of mint flavoring or a small amount of toothpaste. This treatment can be done weekly or monthly. Do not brush with this mixture more than once per week.

A study reveals that the most important factor in the attractiveness of teeth is the crown shape.[38] Consider tooth shaping if you have uneven and asymmetrical teeth. Tooth shaping can shorten long teeth, round off pointed teeth, and help create a pleasing smile that gently follows the contour of the lower lip.

For women with crooked teeth, ALF (Alternative Lightwire Functionals) is a method to align teeth and improve the bite without braces (orthodontic treatment). It is barely visible from the outside and more gentle and comfortable than braces.

Healthy teeth are a result of a healthy diet. Dr. Weston Price, a prominent dentist, conducted several field studies and found there were people immune to tooth decay despite not using a toothbrush or going to the dentist. He found that those who were

100 percent immune to tooth decay had a sufficient amount of minerals and fat-soluble activators. He concluded that the main cause of tooth cavities is a deficiency in nutrients.

Dr. Price created a protocol that cured and prevented tooth decay and remineralized teeth with a 90 percent success rate. The diet consists mainly of freshly ground, soaked and fermented whole grains; grass-fed bone marrow; rare-cooked, organic, grass-fed meat; organic, grass-fed organ meats; raw eggs; wild, uncooked fish; fish eggs; seafood; nuts; seaweed; olive oil; grass-fed yellow butter; grass-fed cream; tomatoes; raw/unpasteurized organic milk from grass-fed cows; and green vegetable juices. Green vegetables to use for the juice can include parsley, cilantro, zucchini, and cucumber. The raw eggs can be made into a smoothie by combining one cup raw milk or kefir with two to four ounces raw cream and two raw eggs along with some stevia for sweetness. In addition, half a teaspoon of fermented cod-liver oil is taken with a quarter teaspoon "high-vitamin butter oil" two to three times daily with meals. The diet must be free of white flour, breakfast cereal, packaged foods, sugar, salt, vegetable oils, pasteurized milk, coffee, fruit juice, soft drinks, soy milk, protein powder, tofu, alcohol, and non-organic foods.[39]

Vegans and vegetarians have a very hard time healing tooth decay since they can't acquire the trace minerals, phosphorous, and fat-soluble vitamins available in animal foods. Due to the depletion of the soil, it is difficult to obtain adequate nutrients from plant foods only. Certain people in India are immune to tooth decay despite being vegetarian, but the vegetables grown in many parts of India are superior to the vegetables in North America because the quality of the soil is much higher. They also consume high-quality milk and ghee from grass-fed cows.

Many people have healed gum disease with white oak bark powder or myrrh gum powder. These herbal powders strengthen the teeth and ligaments holding the teeth in place.

To heal a tooth infection, you can place a few drops of echinacea tincture on the tooth. You can also place wild plantain leaf directly on the infected area.

Checking for cavities should be done annually. The laser cavity detection device is an accurate cavity detection tool used in dentistry. Visit a biological or holistic dentist because they use procedures that are less toxic than conventional dentists.

Toothbrushes must be kept meticulously clean. In his book, *Why Your Toothbrush May Be Killing You Slowly*, biochemist James Song suggests that a range of serious health problems, including heart disease, stroke, arthritis, and chronic infections, could be linked to unhygienic toothbrushes. Scientists have found that a single toothbrush can be the breeding ground for millions of bacteria. An ozone toothbrush sterilizer will eliminate nearly all bacteria on toothbrushes. Changing toothbrushes frequently is also important.

The best way to cleanse teeth is to use herbal tooth powder, which is available from the health food store or can be made on your own. Add licorice root (*glycyrrhiza glabra*) to the tooth powder. It contains anticavity compounds and has an antibacterial effect.[40]

You can use an electric toothbrush or an oral irrigator. An oral irrigator is an at-home device that uses a stream of pulsating water to remove plaque and food debris effectively between teeth and below the gum line.

NATURAL TOOTH POWDER RECIPE

2 tablespoons pure sodium bicarbonate

1 teaspoon licorice root powder

1 teaspoon finely ground sea salt

5 drops organic peppermint or tea tree essential oil

Facial hair in women is rated as very unattractive.[41] A completely hair-free face indicates fertility since high estrogen levels discourage hair growth on the face. A hair-free face also signals youth since as a woman gets older, facial hair typically increases.[42]

Threading is an effective method of facial hair removal. Electrolysis is effective for hair removal and will stop hair growth permanently. Laser hair removal and intense pulse light (IPL) will reduce the growth of hair but may not permanently stop hair growth.

Some women suffer from a condition known as hirsutism, which causes excessive hair growth on the face. Hirsutism develops when hair follicles become overstimulated by androgens. The herb saw palmetto or spearmint tea taken internally may be helpful since they have antiandrogen effects. The recommended dosage of saw palmetto is 160 milligrams twice daily. The suggested dose of spearmint is one cup three times daily.

Having a beautiful quality that no other woman possesses can be very attractive. Coco Chanel said, "In order to be irreplaceable one must always be different." Throughout the centuries, women have always strived to mimic a certain look that was considered beautiful at the time. Today, we see this "follow the crowd" attitude when many young women look almost the same. It is the quality of being unique that can make a woman stand out from the crowd, especially a beautiful crowd of women. A good example of unique beauty is the American model Cindy Crawford, who was known for her trademark mole just above her lip. Many women were penciling on a mole in an effort to copy her look. If you have a special feature—differently colored eyes, dimples, or moles—flaunt it! German fashion designer Karl Lagerfeld once said, "There is no beauty without strangeness." If you don't have a unique facial feature, you can always create a signature look. By always being seen with a certain look, you make it your own. Celebrities change their look constantly, but many stick with one or two signature looks.

MAKEUP

The application of makeup is an age-old ritual. It is very important in adding to a woman's appeal. Just like a peacock attracts a mate with its display of brightly colored feathers, men are attracted to a more colorful female face. Research shows that men give a higher beauty rating to women wearing makeup than women without makeup.[43][44]

Makeup increases a woman's attractiveness and femininity.[45] Evolutionary psychologist Miriam Law Smith says, "Women are effectively advertising their general fertility with their faces. Makeup can improve appearance across the board, but it will obviously help people who are less attractive more."

A study found that foundation and eye makeup have the most impact on increasing attractiveness. In the study, female volunteers were made up under the following five cosmetics conditions: (i) no makeup, (ii) foundation only, (iii) eye makeup only, (iv) lip makeup only, and (v) full facial makeup. Participants were asked to view photographs of the women and rank each set from most attractive to least attractive. Faces with full makeup were judged more attractive than the same faces with no makeup. Men rated eye makeup and then foundation as having the most impact on enhancing a woman's attractiveness. Lipstick on its own did not appear to contribute to attractiveness.[46]

Balance is the key to physical beauty. Too much makeup can look very unattractive and be a big turnoff for men. In every single poll or survey conducted by various women's beauty and fashion magazines, men revealed that they strongly prefer "a natural makeup look." Many of the men disliked heavily applied makeup.

A survey conducted by skin care expert St. Ives revealed that one in five men wish their partner would tone down their makeup. The study found that men's biggest turnoffs were thick foundation, too much blush, clumpy mascara, bright lipstick, bright blue eye shadow, and penciled-in brows. "Men don't like anything that looks fake," says renowned biological anthropologist Helen Fisher, PhD, author of *Why We Love*. She says, "It's distracting, and they want to see the real you." In the book *How to Be a Hottie*, Romy Miller states that if you wish to attract men like crazy, go with a very natural makeup look.

The best rule to follow when applying makeup is to create a "no makeup" look. Polish cosmetics industrialist Helena Rubinstein once said, "Whether you are sixteen or over sixty, remember, understatement is the rule of a fine makeup artist."

Makeup should always be used to enhance, not disguise. Iconic makeup artist Kevyn Aucoin once said, "Beauty is about perception,

> "Whether you are 16 or over 60, remember, understatement is the rule of a fine makeup artist."
> - Helena Rubinstein

not about makeup. I think the beginning of all beauty is knowing and liking oneself. You can't put on makeup, or dress yourself, or do your hair with any sort of fun or joy if you're doing it from a position of correction."

Focus on defining features with neutral or flesh tones. The least effective way to pick a blush, lip, or eye color is to pick a color that looks good in the package. Heavily pigmented and bright colors look good in the tube but do not look natural when applied to the face.

The most attractive lip color is one to three shades redder than your natural lip color. Research suggests that red is the most attractive lip color. The scientific theory is that red lips signal good blood circulation and sexual excitement.[47] A red lip color could be a good indicator of high estrogen levels, sexual arousal, and health.[48] Sheer lip gloss or sheer lipstick is the best option for a more natural look. Apply a silicone-based lip color primer before applying lip color to make the lips appear very smooth and for lip color to stay on better.

HOW TO CONTOUR AND HIGHLIGHT YOUR CHEEKS

STEP 1

Apply bronzing powder two shades darker than your natural skin color right under your cheekbones. You can suck in your cheeks by making a pouty face, and then apply the color to the hollow part of your face. Start close to your ear and continue to extend the color down until you reach the middle of your cheek. Blend the color well with a blending brush to remove any harsh lines.

STEP 2

Apply a peachy nude or a flesh-toned blush right on your cheekbones.

STEP 3

Apply an illuminator on top of your cheekbones.

Fashion dolls are a great example of perfect makeup application. In Western societies, the cultural icon of the fashion doll as a symbol of female beauty seems to have some biological grounding.[49]

Fashion dolls have eye makeup that is designed to make the eyes look larger. To create the appearance of large eyes, start by applying white eye shadow on your eyelids. Then define your eyes with a very thin line of black, liquid eyeliner on your top lash line and brown eyeliner on your bottom lash line. Applying black eyeliner all the way around the eyes can make the eyes appear smaller in some women. Apply a dark brown in your eye crease with an eye shadow stick. Then apply a neutral or flesh-toned eye shadow on your brow bone with an eye shadow stick. The brow bone is the best place to experiment with other eye shadow colors if you so decide. Finally, apply a black lengthening and thickening mascara on your top lashes, and brown mascara on your bottom lashes.

Very thick and long eyelashes (as seen on fashion dolls) are extremely feminine. Most fashion dolls only have eight or nine extremely thick and long eyelashes. Mascaras create eyelashes that do not have much impact. To create the dramatically feminine doll eyelash effect, you can use "spike false eyelashes" that contain very thick false eyelashes.

Fashion dolls have blush that is very subtle and flesh-toned. Use flesh-toned blush that is one to three shades darker than your natural skin color. Blush should always be the least heavily applied makeup. Heavily applied blush tends to be a top complaint of many men.

Lip color can vary among fashion dolls, but tends to be a subtle, muted pink, peach, purple, or red. These lip colors are the best choices because other colors tend to look unnatural.

Chapter 2: Skin

Everyone wants to have flawless skin.
- Kristin Baker, American artist

*S*kin has a large impact on beauty-score ratings. The quality of the skin has a great influence on the perceived health and age of a woman since it is more changeable than any other physical feature. As British journalist Nigella Lawson said, "What makes people look youthful is the quality of their skin." German research scientist Dr. Bernhard Fink said, "Whether a woman is seventeen or seventy, the contrast of skin tone plays a significant role in the way her age, beauty, and health is perceived. Skin tone homogeneity can give visual clues about a person's health and reproductive capability, so an even skin tone is considered most desirable."

Men strongly prefer women with a clear complexion, as well as smooth and youthful looking skin. Skin color in women is darker during pregnancy and lighter around the time of ovulation. Therefore, men tend to prefer lighter skin. However, the preference within a culture is for skin that is lighter for that culture and not the lightest possible skin color. In Western societies, there is a preference for tanned skin.[1]

Skin color is used to identify ethnicity and has been a source of discrimination in many parts of the world. *Colorism* is a term used to describe discrimination in which people determine social status or personality based on skin color and ethnicity. However, as Ghanian diplomat Kofi Annan said, "We may have different religions, different languages, different colored skin, but we all belong to one human race." American author Mark Twain wisely said, "One of my theories is that the hearts of men are about alike, no matter what their skin color." The key to overcoming prejudgment based on skin color is getting to know someone. Mexican actor Ricardo Montalban said, "After a few weeks, you're not aware of skin color differences. You see the color; you're not blind, but it doesn't matter. You see the human being first."

FLAWLESS

Flawless skin is smooth, blemish-free, even toned, and without visible pores. Flawless skin is best achieved with the right skin care products, diet, and supplements. Women who meticulously care for their health and skin rarely need to wear foundation makeup.

For women with less than perfect skin, a quick and easy way to get perfect skin is proper makeup application. Some women are not sure whether to use foundation or concealer first. Makeup artist and beauty expert Cynde Watson says, "If your face feels naked without foundation, apply it first. Then dot concealer only where you need extra coverage."

Select a well-reviewed primer, liquid foundation, concealer, finishing powder, and illuminator. Begin by applying a primer all over your face. Liquid foundation is best applied in a patting motion using a stippling brush to achieve flawless-looking, airbrushed skin. Liquid foundation can also be applied with fingers. All the great makeup artists agree that clean fingers are a good way to apply liquid foundation. Apply liquid foundation on your face all the way into your hairline and on your neck so there is no "mask" of foundation. Then apply a concealer on areas with visible skin imperfections. You can then apply a bronzer on your face to give a tanned appearance or to contour your face. To add a glow to your face, apply an illuminator on the tops of your cheekbones and brow bone. Complete your look with finishing powder lightly dusted on your face. Then, to set your powder, apply a light mist of thermal water facial spray.

For all skin care products, the general holistic rule is that if it can't be eaten then it shouldn't be applied on the skin. The chemicals contained in skin products get absorbed into the body. Once inside the body they get stored and build up over time to toxic levels, resulting in health issues such as cancer. To reiterate, the Organic Consumers Association says, "In just twenty-six seconds after any exposure to chemicals on your skin or in your lungs, traces of these chemicals can be found in every organ of your body. When you put these chemicals on your skin, up to 60 percent will end up in your body and much of it will stay as residuals." Studies have revealed that preservatives such as parabens found in skin care products and cosmetics have been found in breast cancer tissue samples.[2]

Flip over all your skin care products and carefully examine the ingredients. Ingredients should be vitamins, minerals, or plant extracts. If you don't understand what the ingredient is, most likely it is toxic. Many preservatives and chemicals are very harmful to general health. The two most common health-hazardous ingredients are sodium lauryl sulfate (SLS) and propylene glycol.

SLS is found mainly in shampoos and soaps. SLS has a very dehydrating effect on the skin.[3] It has a degenerative effect on the cell membranes because of its protein-denaturing properties. Low levels of skin penetration may occur at high-use concentration.[4] When combined with other chemicals, SLS can be transformed into nitrosamines, which are carcinogens (cancer-causing).

Propylene glycol is found in deodorants and skin products. The Material Safety Data Sheets (MSDS) warns against skin contact with propylene glycol because of possible brain, liver, and kidney abnormalities. The Environmental Protection Agency considers propylene glycol so toxic that it requires workers to wear protective gloves, clothing, and goggles.

Besides watching out for toxic ingredients, you may also want to avoid fragrance, alcohol, and glycerin in skin care products. Fragrance is a major skin irritant. Many women have found that over time, both glycerin and alcohol have led to dehydrated skin that constantly needs moisturizing.

The only two options for achieving flawless skin are preparing homemade skin care products or buying 100 percent certified organic and natural skin products from reputable companies.

Homemade skin care products are superior to commercially prepared skin care products because you can be 100 percent sure where the ingredients come from. You also know how fresh they are, how safe they are, and you can control what ingredients are added. The ingredients for homemade skin care products can be bought from cosmetic ingredients suppliers online.

For women with little time, commercially prepared organic skin products are a good option but only if well selected. Even some organic and natural skin care products can sometimes contain toxic ingredients.

Natural oils can replace the use of commercially prepared moisturizers and can reverse many skin problems. They are also useful for body massages performed at spas.

Grape seed oil protects the skin from premature aging and is effective in fighting acne. Scientific studies have shown that the antioxidant power of proanthocyanidins from grape seeds are twenty times greater than vitamin E and fifty times greater than vitamin C.[5] Grape seed oil is easily absorbed into the skin, instead of sitting on top of the skin.

Squalene is naturally present in skin but the amount drops rapidly after age twenty-five, leading to dry, aging skin. Squalene reduces free radical oxidative damage to the skin.[6] It stimulates the skin's natural ability to regenerate, nourish, and hydrate tissue. Shark liver oil is considered the richest source, with smaller amounts found in olive oil. Squalene oil is quickly absorbed into the skin without leaving an oily residue.

Rosehip seed oil prevents and reverses photoaging. Rosehip seed oil is high in essential unsaturated fatty acids, specifically oleic, linoleic, and linolenic. It is also high in vitamin A and retinoic acid, a natural constituent similar to tretinoin. In a two-year study, rosehip seed oil was applied to patients with scars, as well as to a group suffering from premature aging of the skin. The results were remarkable. Continuous application of rosehip seed oil effectively reduced scars, wrinkles, and brown spots.[7]

Jojoba oil is a powerful moisturizer. It has a composition very similar to human skin oil (sebum). Applying jojoba oil balances oil production in the skin since it may trick the skin into thinking it is producing enough oil. Jojoba oil has anti-inflammatory properties.[8] It is helpful for acne, oily skin, and rosacea.

Borage seed oil contains a high percentage of gamma-linoleic acid (GLA), a natural fatty acid that maintains healthy skin and repairs tissue damage. A study found borage seed oil was able to restore the softness and moisture of scaly, dry skin.[9]

Avocado oil is perfect for sensitive and dry skin since it is rich in nutrients such as vitamins A, D, and E. It is helpful for eczema and psoriasis. Avocado oil penetrates the skin easily.[10]

Sea buckthorn oil is rich in nutrients such as vitamins A, C, E, and carotenoids. It prevents premature skin aging. A study found that it promotes wound healing.[11]

Acne is one of the most common skin imperfections, especially during puberty. For every woman, the cause of acne is different. Chinese face reading can be helpful when trying to determine the cause of acne. It is a method of observing the face, eyes, skin, and other parts of the body to determine the state of a person's health.

CHINESE FACE READING FOR ACNE

The forehead: Toxic intestines
Above eyebrows: Toxic liver
Between eyes: Spleen
Cheeks: Toxic lungs
Tip of nose or on ears: Heart
Creases at base of nostrils: Brain
Upper lip: Stomach
Lower lip: Toxic intestine
Corners of mouth: Fallopian tubes
Chin: Uterus
Jawline: Female reproductive organs
Chest: Toxic lungs
Back: Toxic intestines

Studies show that acne is related to diet.[12] In one study, patients were discouraged from eating excessive amounts of carbohydrates and high-sugar foods. Their diet during the study consisted of foods low on the glycemic index. After twelve weeks, the patients showed a 50 percent reduction of acne. The study suggests that changes in acne may be closely related to changes in insulin sensitivity.[13] The role of insulin in acne development is also supported by the high prevalence of acne in women with polycystic ovary syndrome (PCOS), a condition associated with insulin resistance, hyperinsulinemia, and hyperandrogenism.[14]

Acne can be a result of hormone imbalance. To determine this, undergo testing for androgen levels or PCOS. If high androgen levels or PCOS are the main cause of acne, then antiandrogenic herbs may be helpful. Glycyrrhizic acid from licorice root is effective in the reduction of androgen levels; specifically serum testosterone levels.[15] Saw palmetto is also an effective antiandrogenic herb.[16]

If acne appears before menstruation, then chasteberry (Vitex agnus-castus) may be helpful. German research found that chasteberry contributes to the clearing of premenstrual acne, possibly by regulating hormonal influences on acne.[17]

Low stomach acid, also known as hypochlorhydria, is common in those who have acne.[18] A naturopath can diagnose and treat low stomach acid with betaine hydrochloride or other suitable remedies.

Many naturopaths believe that acne may be a result of candida infection. A German study found that people with candida had more acne lesions than people without candida infection.[19] A naturopath can diagnose and treat candida infection with a low dose of nystatin along with oil of wild oregano (*Origanum vulgare*) or other suitable remedies.

Tea tree essential oil can be used as a spot treatment on pimples. A study found that 5 percent tea tree oil is an effective treatment for mild to moderate acne.[20] Fewer side effects were experienced by those treated with tea tree oil than other topical acne treatments.[21]

Tretinoin has been shown to be an effective topical treatment for acne.[22] However, a study found that adapalene gel 0.1 percent applied once daily was significantly more effective in reducing acne lesions and was better tolerated than tretinoin gel 0.025 percent.[23]

Many commercially prepared soaps and face washes leave the skin tight and dry. Each time the oil is stripped away, the skin overcompensates for the lack of moisture by creating more oil. An organic face wash with white willow bark extract is best for acne-prone skin. White willow bark extract is a natural source of salicylic acid. It provides natural beta hydroxy acid without skin irritation commonly associated with synthetic salicylic acid.

Witch hazel is an effective skin toner to be used after cleansing acne-prone skin. It works to reduce oil, redness, and acne marks, and tightens pores. However, it shouldn't be used long term since it can be quite drying to the skin.

A strawberry and Greek yogurt facial mask is very effective for reducing acne if used daily. Strawberries are a natural source of salicylic acid, and Greek yogurt contains lactic acid, an alpha hydroxy acid that brightens and evens out the skin tone.

An aspirin-honey mask used once a week is very helpful for reducing acne. The aspirin-honey mask effectively unclogs the pores and exfoliates the skin. Salicylic acid products available commercially are priced higher than a bottle of aspirin, which contains salicylic acid. It is best to use organic manuka honey in the aspirin-honey mask. Manuka honey is antibacterial, antioxidant, and anti-inflammatory. Look for manuka honey that is at least UMF 16+ to guarantee antibacterial potency.

ASPIRIN-HONEY FACE MASK RECIPE

INGREDIENTS
6 uncoated aspirin tablets
Organic manuka honey, UMF 16+

DIRECTIONS
Place a few drops of water on six uncoated aspirins to create a paste. Uncoated aspirin will take a few seconds to turn into a powder once water is added. Add a few drops of organic manuka honey to the aspirin paste. Leave the aspirin mask on for twenty minutes then rinse it off while rubbing the skin very gently in a circular motion.

The most common skin imperfections in women past puberty are dark circles under the eyes, large pores, brown spots, melasma, eczema, psoriasis, rosacea, stretch marks, visible veins, cellulite, vitiligo, and scars. Most skin imperfections can be corrected with the appropriate skin care products, proper diet, and supplements. However, serious skin imperfections are best corrected with the help of an experienced cosmetic dermatologist.

STRAWBERRY YOGURT FACE MASK RECIPE

INGREDIENTS
1 tablespoon minced strawberry
1 tablespoon organic, full-fat Greek yogurt

DIRECTIONS
Blend ingredients in a food processor until smooth. Apply to the entire face or only on problem areas. Leave on for twenty minutes for the best results.

CHINESE FACE READING

PSORIASIS
Cause: Toxic or weak liver or gallbladder.
Solution: Perform a liver/gallbladder flush and herbal liver cleanses. Take milk thistle capsules daily.

DARK UNDER-EYE CIRCLES
Cause: Lack of rest, allergies, weak or toxic liver, bowels, or kidneys.
Solution: Remove common food allergens such as wheat and dairy from the diet. Eat a high-fiber diet. Perform herbal liver, kidney, and bowel cleanses. Take milk thistle capsules daily.

ENLARGED PORES

Cause: Long-term consumption of sugar and foods high on the glycemic index.

Solution: Completely avoid foods high on the glycemic index and take chromium picolinate capsules, which control sugar cravings.

OILY T-ZONE

Cause: Excessive milk and saturated fat consumption or cholesterol buildup in arteries.

Solution: Cut out milk products and use monounsaturated fats such as olive oil. Take chickweed capsules daily.

PALE COMPLEXION

Cause: Iron and chlorophyll deficiency.

Solution: Take a whole food supplement and colloidal minerals.

UNDER-EYE BAGS

Cause: Lack of rest, kidney problems, or kidneys needing to be flushed out.

Solution: Drink plenty of water. Cut out all coffee, tea, and soda. Take hydrangea capsules daily. Perform herbal kidney cleanses.

CROW'S-FEET

Cause: Excessive intake of tannic acid from coffee, tea, and soda.

Solution: Cut out coffee, tea, and soda.

FROWN/SMILE LINES

Cause: Improper assimilation of fatty acids and poor food combining.

Solution: Follow proper food combining rules. Remove saturated fat from the diet. Take chickweed capsules daily.

SWOLLEN EYELIDS
Cause: Improper ratio of potassium and sodium, gallstones, kidney stones, high blood pressure.
Solution: Take a potassium supplement daily.

EARLOBE CREASES
Cause: Heart problems and high cholesterol.
Solution: Take gingko, hawthorn, and vitamin E daily.

LINES ON NECK
Cause: Improper assimilation of fatty acids, or thyroid problems.
Solution: Take kelp tablets or thyroid extract daily.

MOLES
Cause: Toxic or weak liver.
Solution: Perform a liver/gallbladder flush and herbal liver cleanses. Take milk thistle capsules daily.

Scars and stretch marks are common and can be difficult to remove. Dermabrasion or chemical peels can be effective in reducing scars. A microneedle roller device can be effective for scars, stretch marks, and pockmarks. Squalene oil, tamanu oil, vitamin E, rose hip oil, and cocoa butter are helpful. Treatment with 0.05 percent tretinoin and a serum of 10 percent L-ascorbic or 20 percent glycolic acid can also be effective. Silicone sheets or silicone creams are helpful for scars with a raised appearance. Many women have found that DMSO cream combined with castor oil works well in softening scar tissue.

Varicose veins and spider veins are usually caused by venous insufficiency. Sclerotherapy is a nonsurgical alternative to surgery for treating all types of varicose veins and spider veins. Nutritional vein-support supplements that contain horse chestnuts, diosmin, hesperidin, gotu kola, and butcher's broom are reported to be effective. Grape seed extract and pine bark extract both contain oligomeric proanthocyanidin complexes (OPCs), which are antioxidants that strengthen the connective-tissue structure of blood vessels and reduce inflammation.

Cellulite is caused by poor elimination of waste by-products through the lymphatic system, the body's filtration system. A treatment plan should be composed of a variety of therapies, including change in diet, massage, spa treatments, exercise, and herbs. Eliminate carbohydrates, animal fat, and sugar from the diet. Lymphatic drainage, a gentle form of massage that stimulates the lymphatic system, is helpful for treating cellulite. Seaweed body wraps are also helpful if used regularly. Rebounding exercise is an excellent way to stimulate the lymphatic system and eliminate cellulite. Dry skin brushing will improve the texture and appearance of the skin. It involves the use of a natural-bristle brush that is used to gently scrub the skin of the entire body in gentle circular motions to stimulate the lymph system. It should be performed daily for at least five minutes and ideally be followed by a bath. The herbs gotu kola, horse chestnut, and grape seed extract taken internally have been reported effective for cellulite.

Vitiligo is a condition that causes depigmentation of patches of skin. It occurs when melanocytes, the cells responsible for skin pigmentation, die or are unable to function. Some women have had success in treating their vitiligo with ginger root. It triggers the melanocytes that are not working under the skin to react and mimic their neighboring cells. It's a slow process and may take six weeks for blending to start visibly occurring. Ginger root is also effective for the treatment of white scars. You can add ginger root tincture to a skin cream and apply it to the skin or purchase a commercially prepared skin cream with ginger root.

Dark circles and bags under the eyes are very common. Chrysin, vitamin K, retinol, and Haloxyl are helpful for reducing dark circles under the eyes. Dark circles may be caused by a deficiency of vitamin K in the body. Daily vegetable juicing of kale is very beneficial since kale is a very rich source of vitamin K. You can talk to a cosmetic dermatologist about options, such as dermal injections and lasers for lightening dark circles. Bags under the eyes can be treated with lecithin cream, left on overnight. Lower eyelid blepharoplasty will permanently correct bags under the eyes.

Brown spots on the skin are generally the result of excessive sun exposure. Q-switched laser and intense pulsed light (IPL) are effective at removing brown spots. Trichloroacetic acid (TCA) peels can be done on your own or by a dermatologist and are very effective. Start at 12.5 percent for three months, moved up to 20 percent for six months, and then move up to 30 percent. Do not go higher than 30 percent for a TCA peel. Perform one TCA peel every five weeks until brown spots fade. Hydroquinone 4 percent or 6 percent is effective for treating browns spots, but it takes at least six months to see results.

Melasma is a patchy brown discoloration of the skin. Hydroquinone 4 percent or 6 percent may be effective for treating melasma in the short-term, but permanent treatment requires addressing the cause. Melasma can be caused by candida overgrowth, copper toxicity, adrenal fatigue, and leaky gut syndrome. Going to a naturopath to determine the cause is the best way to treat melasma.

Eczema and psoriasis are both chronic, red, scaly skin conditions. Essential fatty acids (EFAs) deficiency is a common cause of eczema and psoriasis. A study found that supplementation with hemp seed oil improved symptoms of eczema.[24] Evening primrose oil was also helpful.[25] Food allergies are also a cause of eczema and psoriasis. Get food allergy testing done and avoid the most common allergens, which include shellfish, nuts, eggs, soy, milk, and gluten. Topical application of 2 percent licorice gel has been shown to be effective at reducing redness, swelling, and itching.[26]

Rosacea is characterized by facial redness. B vitamin deficiencies are common in women with rosacea. Supplementing with B complex has been reported effective for some women. A deficiency of hydrochloric acid (HCl) or pancreatic enzymes may also be a cause of rosacea. Supplementation with HCl capsules (taken after meals) or pancreatic enzymes may bring relief in some cases. Going to a naturopath to determine the specific cause is the best way to treat rosacea.

Large pores are common in those with oily skin. Chemical peels and dermabrasion are helpful for reducing large pores. Vitamin B3 serum has been reported to be effective for reducing large pores.

Queen Cleopatra, the last Pharaoh of Egypt, was known for her flawless skin. Her secret was that she bathed in fresh milk. Milk contains lactic acid, an alpha hydroxy acid that is extremely hydrating and exfoliates the skin. Research have shown that it increases collagen production and reverses photoaging.[27][28] Lactic acid lotion is very beneficial for relieving and preventing dry skin. Lactic acid lotion is made in small batches since it expires quickly. To make lactic acid lotion, add two and a half teaspoons of 88 percent lactic acid to two teaspoons of any lotion.

VITAMIN B3 SERUM RECIPE

INGREDIENTS

¼ teaspoon vitamin B3 (niacinamide)

½ teaspoon NAG (N-acetyl D-glucosamine)

5 teaspoons distilled water

DIRECTIONS

Mix all the ingredients together and store in an airtight container or bottle. Apply the vitamin B3 serum after washing your face at night. Wait at least thirty minutes before applying any other skin care products.

Feet need special skin care since the bottom of the feet tend to get very rough and dry. Apply a lactic acid lotion and special "moisturizing socks" every night before bed. Mafura butter is great for applying to the feet during the day since it's not greasy and is very emollient.

A callus file or rough stone helps to exfoliate the feet but usually leaves a rough skin surface. Using a Dremel Moto-Tool to reduce the calluses and corns on a weekly basis is the easiest and most effective treatment. You can do it on your own or go to a podiatrist to get it done. A podiatrist will also help resolve feet issues such as athlete's foot, bunions, heel pain, or ingrown toenails. For at-home treatment of the feet, the best choice is a battery-type Dremel drill with a medium-grit sandpaper attachment. This can be found at any hardware store.

Besides proper skin care, good nutrition is vital for flawless skin. Mariska Hargitay, a former beauty queen and American actress, said, "You know how you wake up in the morning, and sometimes you look gorgeous and other times you look like you got hit by a Mack truck? I realized that my Mack truck is food. If I have no sugar, yeast, or wine, I have no under-eye bags, and my skin is perfect."

Studies show that nutritional deficiencies cause negative changes in the condition of the skin.[29] Many women report an improvement in the appearance of their skin when taking a whole food supplement, eating well, and taking specific supplements designed to improve the condition of the skin.

A study found that the skin of those with a higher intake of vegetables, olive oil, fish, and legumes, and a lower intake of milk, sugar, butter, and margarine had a much better appearance. A higher intake of meat, dairy, sugar, and butter appeared to give the skin a less attractive appearance.[30]

Women have reported a dramatic difference in their skin when they increased their daily intake of vegetable juices. Juicing of vegetables eliminates the fiber, leaving only the nutrients in a concentrated liquid. Eating twenty carrots every day would not typically be possible, but juicing twenty carrots a day makes it easy to consume a high level of nutrients. Vegetable juices can be made from beets, carrots, cucumbers, bell peppers, ginger, and parsnips.

Ideally, food should be organic to nourish the skin. Organic produce is grown in nutrient-rich, fertile soil. Thus, organic foods are higher in nutrients. In a review of four hundred published papers comparing organic and non-organic foods, Soil Association Certification Ltd. determined that organic crops are higher in essential nutrients. Organic foods are also free of pesticides, herbicides, fungicides, and insecticides.

Herbalists and naturopaths agree that eliminating toxins is an effective way to correct various skin problems. Linda Page, PhD, naturopath and author, says that if you have acne, brown spots, wrinkles, or other skin problems, you need a body cleanse.[31] Chinese herbalists say moles and brown spots are caused by poor circulation and poor liver function. Detoxification of the colon, liver, and kidneys is very important since these organs collect toxins from the environment, food, and water. Colon, liver, and kidney herbal cleanses are available commercially.

The body needs adequate levels of oxygen for the skin to appear healthy. A study found that increased blood oxygenation enhances the healthy appearance of the facial skin. Active oxygen supplementation gives the skin a healthy appearance.[32]

A woman needs adequate rest and relaxation for her skin to look its best. Research has provided scientific evidence that people who get a good night's sleep look more attractive. Scientists took two sets of photos of twenty-three men and women once after the subjects had eight hours of sleep, and once after they'd spent thirty-one continuous hours awake. The subjects were asked to maintain the same facial expression, the same distance from the camera, and to refrain from wearing makeup while being photographed. These photos were later observed and rated based on how healthy and attractive the subjects appeared. Sleep-deprived people were rated as less healthy and less attractive than those who'd had a normal night's sleep.[33]

YOUTHFUL

The main aspect of youthful skin is that it is very tight and has an even tone. Fat redistribution and loss of collagen in the skin are factors that cause the appearance of aging.

An anti-aging skin care routine should be started at twenty-five years of age. However, the prevention of photoaging should begin from birth. Photoaging is the result of excessive UV exposure. It leads to wrinkles, brown spots, and sagging skin. Dermatologists warn that up to 90 percent of skin aging is caused by UV exposure.

Photoaging is prevented by the meticulous daily application of sunscreen of at least SPF 30. It can even cause a reversal of photoaging.[34] A study found that women who look young for their age avoid sun exposure.[35] Therefore, sunscreen should be treated like the most precious beauty product and youth preserver. However, the selection of the right sunscreen makes all the difference.

Chemical sunscreens can be harmful. Chemical sunscreens work by absorbing UV rays. The penetration of sunscreen ingredients into the lower layers of the skin increases the amount of free radicals and reactive oxygen species (ROS). The generation of ROS is thought to play a major role in skin aging. ROS generation leads to increased collagen breakdown.[36] A study found that after sixty minutes, the amount of ROS was higher in sunscreen-treated skin than in untreated skin.[37]

Titanium dioxide as a sunscreen ingredient is not recommended because it is photocatalytic. It reacts with UV light to form free radicals on the skin, and damages fibroblasts and RNA.[38]

Zinc oxide is the most effective sunscreen ingredient available. It is a mineral that sits on the skin, absorbing and scattering damaging UVA, UVB, and even UVC rays. Zinc oxide sunscreen should be free of nanoparticles to prevent deep absorption of zinc oxide into the skin. Reapply zinc oxide sunscreen every two hours for optimal protection against the sun.

Along with wearing sunscreen, take extra precautions to prevent photoaging. Stay out of the sun when it is at its strongest, which is between 10:00 AM and 2:00 PM. Wear UV-protective clothing instead of regular clothing.[39]

The most powerful tools for preventing and reversing skin aging, besides zinc oxide sunscreen, are tretinoin and vitamin C serum.[40] After at least one full year of daily use, they were found to reverse skin aging dramatically. There are many reports of women who are in their sixties who look like they are in their thirties because they use these two products meticulously along with sunscreen. Collagen degradation doesn't generally start until the mid-twenties, so it's best to start using tretinoin and vitamin C serum in one's mid-twenties.

Collagen is a major structural protein in the skin. Collagen and elastin provide strength, resilience, and flexibility to the skin. Increased breakdown and decreased production of collagen lead to wrinkles and sagging skin. Studies have shown that collagen production is stimulated by the use of tretinoin[41] and vitamin C.[42]

Topical tretinoin is especially powerful in reversing skin aging. Some women call tretinoin an anti-aging "miracle cream." Tretinoin is a retinoid, a derivative of vitamin A. In studies, topical tretinoin increased collagen formation in photoaged skin.[43] A study evaluated the changes occurring in skin after daily application of 0.05 percent tretinoin cream for a period of twelve months. After this time, formation of new collagen fibers was observed.[44]

There are more studies on tretinoin than on any other topical skincare product. It is the only skin care product on the market that has been proven to reduce fine lines and wrinkles. Many skin products claim to improve the appearance of photoaged skin. In general, however, substantive evidence is not available. In contrast, a large number of controlled clinical studies have been published demonstrating that topical application of 0.025 percent to 0.1 percent all-trans retinoic acid (ATRA) improves the appearance of photoaged skin.[45] Improvements in the appearance of the skin are best seen after six to twelve months of daily use.[46]

Tretinoin is safe for long-term use. No systemic side effects of long-term treatment with tretinoin have been observed.[47] Tretinoin is best used for a lifetime. Long-term tretinoin treatment continues to improve photoaged skin.[48]

TRETINOIN TESTIMONIALS

"I have been using tretinoin for twenty-one years. I started with the 0.5 percent cream but have used the 1 percent cream the majority of the time. I am fifty-seven years old and have extraordinary skin for my age. My jawline is firm and my skin is smooth and soft. I have been using sunscreen religiously since my twenties. I stop using the tretinoin every now and then to give my skin a rest but start up again after a month. I truly believe this is a miraculous product."

"I have been using tretinoin since age forty. I am currently fifty-eight and have no wrinkles. My skin is even and clear. I have no age spots on my face. Using tretinoin is so much better than buying expensive creams that have no long-term effects. When you begin using tretinoin, you may have some irritation, but stick with it. The flaking and redness will disappear eventually. I have very sensitive skin, and tretinoin really works for me."

There is a difference between retinols and retinoids. Retinoids are much more powerful and effective for preventing and reversing skin aging. Retinols are also proven effective[49] and are an option for women who can't tolerate tretinoin. In a study of participants in their eighties, 0.4 percent retinol lotion applied three times a week for twenty-four weeks resulted in significant reduction of wrinkles.[50]

There are three types of retinoids: adapalene, tretinoin, and tazorac. In general, adapalene is the mildest, tretinoin is in the middle, and tazorac is the most intense. Women who have sensitive skin can start with adapalene and graduate to tretinoin over time.

To start using tretinoin, use the 0.025 percent strength for a few months. Apply once every three days for the first one or two weeks. After the skin adjusts to the product, use it up to once every two nights for another few weeks. Then, use it every other night for another week and finally nightly. You can eventually graduate to the 0.05 percent strength and use it every day for one full year. After one year, you can graduate to the 0.1 percent strength and use it two to four times per week. Many dermatologists advise that using the 0.1 percent strength two to three times a week is plenty. Some women choose to use it only once a week.

You can cause severe skin irritation from foolish initial use of tretinoin. A strict protocol must be followed in the initial use of tretinoin, until the skin adjusts to it. Wait twenty minutes after washing your face before applying tretinoin, in order to reduce irritation. When you wash your skin, you disturb your skin's natural barrier, and waiting a bit before applying a powerful product will give your skin more time to recover. Applying tretinoin onto damp skin will cause it to absorb faster, increasing the chances of irritation. Apply only a pea-sized amount of tretinoin to the entire face. Always wear sunscreen during the day, and apply tretinoin at night before bed since tretinoin makes your skin more sensitive to the sun.

When you begin using tretinoin, you may experience some skin irritation, but stick with it since the skin will adjust to it over time. If the skin irritation continues, reduce the frequency of application or switch to a lower percentage of tretinoin. You can also add 1 percent hydrocortisone cream to the tretinoin formulation.

Most women buffer tretinoin when they first start using it and then use it full strength after their skin adjusts. To buffer tretinoin, put on moisturizer, and then apply tretinoin or apply tretinoin, then apply moisturizer shortly afterward. You can also mix tretinoin with a moisturizer or serum and then apply it. Some women have to go through different types of retinoids before finding one that works. For women who can't use tretinoin regardless of anything, they can use a rosehip serum or retinol serum at night.

The use of tretinoin can leave the skin dry. Therefore, a moisturizer can be applied after tretinoin application. You must wait one hour after applying tretinoin to apply moisturizer so you do not diminish the effects of the tretinoin.

The best anti-aging moisturizer contains both peptides and ceramides. Ceramides help keep moisture in the skin while peptides increase collagen production. You can also add lactic acid to the moisturizer to treat very dry skin. Add two and a half teaspoons of 88 percent lactic acid to two teaspoons of moisturizer.

To increase the effectiveness of retinols or retinoids, you can use them with other scientifically proven ingredients such as glycolic acid, vitamin C, vitamin E, kinetin, niacinamide, and idebenone.

Glycolic acid serum can be used on days when tretinoin is not used. A study found that using glycolic acid as well as tretinoin improves the appearance of the skin better than tretinoin alone.[51]

A controlled clinical trial found that retinol (0.3 percent) and hydroquinone (4 percent) effectively diminished hyperpigmentation better than 0.05 percent tretinoin cream alone.[52] However, hydroquinone should only be used for short-term treatment of hyperpigmentation because it hasn't been proven safe for long-term use.

A study found that the application of retinol and vitamin C could reverse skin aging caused by both chronological aging and photoaging.[53] Topical vitamin C on its own increases collagen synthesis.[54] Vitamin C combined with vitamin E is even more effective and has been found to reduce hyperpigmentation.[55] In a double-blind study, a topical vitamin C complex was applied to one half of the face. There was a significant improvement in hydration, increased collagen formation, and reduction in wrinkles when used for twelve weeks.[56] Topical vitamin C improved skin firmness, smoothness, and hydration.[57]

Topical vitamin C is most effective for preventing and reversing aging at 15 to 20 percent. Vitamin C skin injections are a very effective method of delivery and can be used once per month.

Vitamin C shows promise as a broad-spectrum photoprotectant.[58] Therefore, vitamin C serum is best used in the morning for protection from the sun during the day. Apply vitamin C serum, then wait at least twenty minutes and apply zinc oxide sunscreen.

The addition of ferulic acid into a topical solution of 15 percent L-ascorbic acid and vitamin E skin product improved chemical stability of the vitamins (C plus E) and doubled photoprotection of skin from fourfold to approximately eightfold.[59]

Kinetin/NAG/niacinamide serum is a great addition to an anti-aging skin care regimen and can be used on days when tretinoin is not used. A study found that kinetin and niacinamide exert a synergistic anti-aging effect. A reduction in spots, pores, wrinkles, and evenness was seen at weeks eight and twelve. A

C+E, FERULIC ACID SKIN SERUM RECIPE

INGREDIENTS
1 teaspoon L-ascorbic acid

3 teaspoons distilled water

1 teaspoon SKB (sea kelp bioferment)

¼ teaspoon ferulic acid

¼ teaspoon food-grade DMSO

¼ SOD (superoxide dismutase)

⅛ teaspoon vitamin E or rose hip oil

½ teaspoon hyaluronic acid serum

DIRECTIONS
To prepare, use two little glasses. In glass one, put the water, DMSO, L-ascorbic acid, and ferulic acid. Stir frequently. It can take up to thirty minutes to fully dissolve. Mix the remaining ingredients in glass two. When the contents of glass one have fully dissolved, combine both glasses, stir well, and put in a one ounce bottle. Store in the fridge or in a cool, dark place and always shake before use. Vitamin C serum has to have a pH of 3.5 or below to penetrate the cells. The serum should be white. If it turns yellow it has oxidized and should be thrown out.

significant increase in hydration was also seen at twelve weeks.[60] Topical kinetin lotions are effective in partially reversing the clinical signs of photodamaged facial skin.[61] Idebenone can be used in place of the kinetin in the NAG/niacinamide serum. Idebenone is a synthetic analog of coenzyme Q10, with potent antioxidant activity. It reduces skin roughness, increases skin hydration, reduces fine lines, and improves the appearance of photoaged skin.[62]

KINETIN/NAG/NIACINAMIDE SKIN SERUM RECIPE

INGREDIENTS

Kinetin 0.04 grams

NaOH 0.39 grams

Niacinamide 1.75 grams

NAG (N-acetyl D-glucosamine) 0.7 grams

Citric acid 0.04 grams

Sea emollient 10.5 grams

Distilled water 8.75 grams

Borage oil or oil of choice 10.5 grams

Lecithin powder 2.2 grams

Vitamin E 0.35 grams

Polysorbate 80 0.25 grams

Preservative 0.18 grams

DIRECTIONS

Place 0.39 grams of NaOH in a glass container and add 10 milliliters of distilled water. Measure 0.04 grams of kinetin into a small glass. Then from the solution you prepared before, add 0.5 milliliters to the kinetin. Stir until dissolved. Combine 1.75 grams of niacinamide, 8.75 grams of distilled water, and 0.7 grams of NAG. Stir until dissolved. Add sea emollient and citric acid to the niacinamide and NAG, and stir until the citric acid crystals are dissolved. Add your chosen preservative and blend. Mix 10.5 grams of your oil of choice and 2.2 grams of lecithin, and heat in a double boiler until all is smooth, then add vitamin E. Mix all the ingredients together. Add the polysorbate 80 to the serum and pour into a sterilized container.

Skin naturally sheds billions of skin cells each day. When this natural shedding slows or stops, the results are dull, dry, or

66

flaky skin, clogged pores, blemishes, and uneven skin tone. Exfoliating the skin helps to gently get rid of built-up skin cells, and improvements can be seen in fine lines, wrinkles, skin discolorations, and skin texture.

Scrubs are not the best choice for exfoliating skin. Scrubs deal only with the very top, superficial, layer of skin. Many scrubs have a rough, coarse, uneven texture that can cause skin damage by tearing into the skin, causing tiny tears that damage the skin's barrier. If you do want to use a manual scrub, you can simply use a microfiber cloth with your daily cleanser to exfoliate the skin gently.

A cleanser that contains alpha hydroxy acids (AHA) is a good way to exfoliate dead skin cells daily and reverse skin aging. A study found that AHAs reverse skin aging by stimulating the synthesis of collagen and elastin fibers.[63]

Homemade fruit enzyme facial masks are great for exfoliating the skin every week. They are also wonderful for giving the skin a glow before a special event.

Organic, full-fat Greek yogurt is one of the most beneficial ingredients to use in any homemade facial mask recipe. Yogurt contains lactic acid, an

FRUIT ENZYME MASK RECIPE

INGREDIENTS

1 teaspoon minced papaya

1 teaspoon minced pineapple

1 teaspoon minced carrot

1 teaspoon organic, full-fat Greek yogurt

1 teaspoon organic manuka honey, UMF 16+

½ teaspoon juice squeezed from a lemon

DIRECTIONS

Blend all the ingredients in a food processor. Apply onto the skin. Leave on for twenty minutes for the best results.

alpha hydroxy acid that brightens and evens out the skin tone. Other beneficial ingredients to add to a facial mask are papaya, pineapple, lemon, and carrot. Organic papaya and pineapple contains high levels of fruit enzymes that help dissolve dead skin cells. Lemon is a rich source of vitamin C while carrot is a rich source of vitamin A. Use organic fruits in a facial mask whenever possible.

A good way to exfoliate the skin is to use chemical peels. Doing chemical peels on your own is convenient and cost effective. Each chemical peel is categorized by the concentration and the resulting depth of the peel on the skin, which can range from superficial (also known as micro or light peels) to medium or deep peels. Results are closely linked to the depth of peel performed. Superficial peels (AHA or BHA) offer less dramatic improvement than medium or deep peels (Jessner's or TCA). However, several mild- to medium-depth peels can achieve similar results to one deep-peel treatment, with less post-procedure risk and a shorter recovery time.

CHEMICAL PEELS GUIDE

WEAKEST TO STRONGEST PEELS

Pumpkin: Pumpkin peels at 30 percent can be used every week and are well tolerated by sensitive skin. They contain a high concentration of beta-carotene and vitamins A and C, which encourage the production of collagen and elastin. Pumpkin also possesses nutrients like zinc and potassium that nourish the skin, while natural AHAs and enzymes exfoliate.

Mandelic: Mandelic acid is a gentle acid that exfoliates the skin with very little topical discomfort and can be used at 25 percent every week. It is helpful for inhibiting the formation of brown spots and hyperpigmentation. It helps treat melasma, sun damage, large pores, wrinkles, and dull and sallow skin.

Salicylic: A salicylic acid peel can be superior for many skin types because irritation and inflammation are kept to a minimum.

Lactic: Lactic acid is useful for correcting hyperpigmentation and uneven skin tones. Lactic acid pulls moisture into the cells and exfoliates surface cells, which helps to perfect the skin's surface and restore the skin's natural glow.

Glycolic: Glycolic acid stimulates collagen growth more effectively than any of the other chemical peels. Its small molecule allows it to slip beneath the epidermis to reach the collagen fibers below. Glycolic acid peels are best used every month at 70 percent to prevent and reverse skin aging. Begin by using 30 percent and work your way up slowly to using a 70 percent glycolic acid peel.

Jessner's: Jessner's peel is a medium peel containing 14 percent salicylic acid, 14 percent lactic acid, and 14 percent resorcinol. It is used to treat severe skin discoloration and aging.

Retinoic: Retinoic acid is chemically similar to tretinoin and has a very similar effect on collagen-producing skin cells. The peel is used to treat aging on mature skin types. It effectively removes scars, wrinkles, and hyperpigmentation.

TCA: Trichloroacetic acid (TCA) peels in concentrations up to 30 percent are medium peels. It is excellent for "spot" peeling of specific areas. TCA peels are effective for reducing lines, wrinkles, hyperpigmentation, sun damage, lip lines, and age spots. Start at 12.5 percent for three months, move up to 20 percent for six months, and then move up to 30 percent. Do not go higher than 30 percent for a TCA peel. You can perform one TCA peel every five weeks until skin imperfections fade and then perform a TCA peel once a year.

Tanaka massage is a very effective method of massage for preventing and reversing facial aging. Many women have reported amazing results by doing the Tanaka massage while applying moisturizer. Tanaka massage how-to videos are widely available.

At-home electronic devices such as the microneedle roller, LED light therapy, microcurrent, or ultrasonic waves have been shown to be effective for many women in reducing the signs of skin aging.

The microneedle roller uses skin needling to increase the levels of collagen and elastin in the skin. It combines ancient Chinese acupuncture techniques with mesotherapy. The microneedle roller helps reduce fine lines and wrinkles and increases the penetration of products applied on the skin. A study found individuals with wrinkles, scars, and stretch marks saw a 60 to 80 percent improvement in the appearance of their skin.[64]

To begin using a microneedle roller, start with a 0.5mm twice a week. Within a few months you can try using a 1.5mm once every three weeks. You can use a 2.0mm on skin scars every five weeks. Many women apply a serum with copper peptides and hyaluronic acid during each microneedle roller session.

LED light therapy is the use of light to increase the production of collagen and elastin in the skin. Various studies have shown that LED light therapy reduces the signs of aging effectively.[65][66]

Microcurrent technology is used at cosmetics clinics, but the at-home, handheld microcurrent devices are just as effective and affordable. At-home microcurrent devices help reduce wrinkles and tighten the skin by strengthening the underlying muscles in a way similar to facial exercises. The companies selling these devices tend to offer conductive gels to be used with their devices that are full of chemicals and preservatives. You can purchase organic galvanic gel with natural ingredients separately.

Ultrasonic machines use sound wave technology to penetrate deep below the surface of the skin to smooth out fine lines and wrinkles, tighten sagging skin, shrink enlarged pores, relieve puffy eyes, fade dark eye circles and brown spots. Ultrasound may be used on most parts of the body, including the face, neck, arms, breasts, stomach, waist, hips, buttocks, and legs. The most important thing to know about ultrasound is that the lower the frequency, the deeper the sound waves will penetrate.

ANTI-AGING SKIN CARE ROUTINE

MORNING
Microneedle roller
C/E/ferulic serum
Eye serum
Wait twenty minutes
Non-nano zinc oxide sunscreen

NIGHT
AHA face wash
Wait twenty minutes
Tretinoin or preferred skin serum
Wait one hour
Ceramide and peptide moisturizer
Tanaka massage
At-home electronic devices

ONCE A WEEK
Fruit enzyme mask
Pumpkin peel 30 percent
Mandelic acid peel 25 percent

ONCE A MONTH
Glycolic acid peel 30-70 percent
Vitamin C skin injections

ONCE A YEAR
TCA peel

The most publicly exposed areas of the body should receive the same skin care routine as the face. Tretinoin, serums, masks, peels, and electronic devices can be used on the hands, shoulders, arms, neck, and below the neck. The rest of the body such as the legs, stomach, breasts, and back can be treated with glycolic acid or lactic acid lotion at night and vitamin C cream in the morning along with zinc oxide sunscreen.

Facials are a great addition to your skin care routine. However, selecting the right facial treatment makes all the difference. Facials can actually do more harm than good. Facial steaming, especially with abnormally hot steam, can worsen redness and potentially result in broken capillaries that show up as thin, spider-like lines. Being too aggressive with extractions for acne or blackheads can make clogged pores worse and push acne lesions deeper into your skin. Oxygen facials have no credible evidence to confirm long-term benefits. Oxygen is best delivered in a hyperbaric (pressurized) booth.

A good facial should include exfoliation with alpha hydroxy acid (glycolic or lactic acid), beta hydroxy acid (salicylic acid), microdermabrasion, or chemical peeling.

In a youthful face, fat is distributed evenly. In an aging face, fat is unevenly distributed. Correcting the distribution of fat throughout the face to mimic the facial structure present in youth can help restore a youthful appearance.[67][68]

Hyaluronic acid is a substance naturally made by the body that can correct the distribution of fat throughout the face. Older skin has much lower levels of hyaluronic acid than younger skin.

Hyaluronic acid does not penetrate the skin upon topical application from skin care products. However, hyaluronic acid is used successfully as a temporary filling agent for the skin.[69] Areas with wrinkles or lacking fat can be filled in with injections of hyaluronic acid.[70]

Studies found that hyaluronic acid fillers stimulate collagen production while also interfering with collagen breakdown.[71] So not only do you get a filling effect, but you also have an actual increase in natural collagen production.

Botox (botulinum toxin type A) works to relax the contraction of muscles by blocking nerve impulses. The result is muscles that can no longer contract, and so the wrinkles relax and soften. The effects tend to last from four to six months. Most patients require periodic reinjections to remove wrinkles and lines as they begin to reappear, but after each injection the wrinkles return less severely as the muscles are trained to relax. Botulinum toxin is very effective for women with frown lines, forehead creases, crow's feet, and platysmal bands on the neck.

THE BEST SPA FACIALS

- Alpha hydroxy acid (glycolic or lactic acid)
- Beta hydroxy acid (salicylic acid)
- Microdermabrasion
- Chemical peel
- Photofacial
- Microcurrent facial
- Ultrasonic facial

Botox can be addictive. Doctors have reported that some women use Botox excessively, to the point where their faces look frozen. These women are referred to as having "wrinklerexia". They are obsessed with having wrinkle-free skin and see lines where there are none.

A face-lift is a surgical cosmetic procedure meant to tighten and lift sagging skin on the face. A face-lift can only lift the muscles, not fill them out, which is why face-lift surgery doesn't look natural in some cases. Doing daily facial exercise can help a woman look younger without a face-lift. Daily facial exercises actually lift up sagging facial muscles, which give the face a fuller and firmer appearance. In addition, facial exercises bring more oxygen to the cells of the skin, which results in skin that has a luminous glow and healthy color. Many women have reported a dramatic difference in the appearance of their facial skin after doing facial exercises for at least six months.

ANTI-AGING FACIAL EXERCISES

EYEBROW LIFT

Take three fingers of each hand and place them directly under your eyebrows. Push the eyebrows upward and hold, then try to contract the eyebrows downward. Hold for a count of ten, then let go and relax. Repeat for three sets.

LOWER EYELID LIFT

With eyes open, place three fingers of each hand on the top of each cheekbone and put your head all the way back. Now try to close or squint your eyelids lower, while keeping the fingers in place. Hold for a count of ten, then let go and relax. Repeat for three sets.

CHEEK LIFT

Place the palms of your hands on top of each cheekbone. Smile as wide and hard as you can. You will feel your cheek muscles and your hands rise up a bit. Using your palms, try to push your cheek muscles down. Hold for a count of ten, then let go and relax. Repeat for three sets.

JOWL LIFT

Place your thumb and forefinger on either side of your chin, feeling your jaw bone. With a closed mouth, make a smile, drawing the corners of your mouth out toward your ears. Using your thumb and forefinger, try to hold the muscles in place—creating resistance—as if to stop the smile. Hold for a count of ten, then let go and relax. Repeat for three sets.

> **NECK LIFT**
> Press your tongue up into the roof of your mouth. Tilt your
> head back as far as you can, keeping your tongue firmly pressed
> to the roof of your mouth. Now, lower your head and bring
> your chin down toward your chest, remembering to keep your
> tongue against the roof of your mouth. Hold for a count of ten,
> then let go and relax. Repeat for three sets.

Specific supplements and superfoods are very beneficial for
preventing skin aging. Vitamin C, Pycnogenol, evening primrose oil, MSM, carnosine, milk thistle, astaxanthin, pearl powder, and certain Chinese remedies have helped many women
look younger for longer.

A study found that supplementing vitamin C, Pycnogenol,
and evening primrose oil prevents wrinkle formation.[72] The body
does not naturally synthesize vitamin C, and thus adequate dietary intake is required.[73]

Methylsulfonylmethane (MSM) is referred to as "the beauty
mineral" because it is necessary for collagen synthesis. Many
women reported an improvement in the appearance of their
skin after MSM supplementation.

Carnosine is an amino acid and antioxidant that may extend
the life span of humans.[74] Studies show that carnosine is effective
against cross-linking and the formation of advanced glycation
end products (AGE).[75] Advanced glycation end products cause
rapid skin aging. By taking at least 1,000 milligrams a day of
carnosine, you will reap anti-aging skin benefits.

The herb milk thistle prevents damage to the liver by acting as an antioxidant. Herbalists suggest that, taken daily, it
flushes out the toxins in the liver and cleanses the body, resulting in younger-looking skin.

Zeatin has been reported to have several in vitro anti-aging
effects on human skin fibroblasts.[76] Zeatin was discovered to be
the primary active ingredient in coconut milk. Coconut water

is the richest natural source of cytokinins. Cells exposed to cytokinins do not undergo the severe degenerative changes that occur with normal aging.

Carotenoids and flavonoids contribute to protection against harmful UV radiation.[77] A study found that beta-carotene supplementation protects against sunburn. However, a minimum of ten weeks of supplementation is required before protection is provided. Time is required for the supplement to take effect.[78] Beta-carotene taken at a dose of 30 milligrams per day was shown to prevent and repair photoaging.[79]

Polypodium leucotomos extract is a natural fern extract that protects the skin from sun damage and photoaging.[80] It also slows the absorption of harmful UV rays and prevents DNA damage.[81][82]

Astaxanthin is a sun-protective agent that blocks the damaging effects of UV radiation.[83] In one study, astaxanthin was shown to increase moisture levels as well as reduce wrinkles after four weeks.[84] In another study, astaxanthin reduced wrinkles, freckles, and dark rings around the eyes.[85] Still another study showed that astaxanthin improved fine lines, wrinkles, and elasticity in skin.[86]

Collagen hydrolysate can effectively reduce fine lines and wrinkles by increasing skin collagen expression.[87] Collagen hydrolysate was shown to inhibit collagen loss and collagen fragmentation in aging skin.[88]

The use of pearl powder can be traced back to China in AD 320. The empress, Wu Zetian (AD 625–705), regularly took pearl powder as a supplement and used pearl cream on her skin. When she ascended the throne at sixty-five years of age, her beauty had become legendary. Her skin was said to be as radiant as that of a young woman. According to *Bencao Gangmu*, a Chinese medical book, pearl powder can stimulate new skin growth, release toxins, and remove age spots. Pearl powder increases glutathione peroxidase.[89] Glutathione peroxidase is an enzyme that is responsible for protecting cells from free radical damage. The level of glutathione in the body begins to decline at the rate of about 10 percent every decade as we age past twenty-five. Pearl powder is a beneficial source of calcium for adults and nanonization improves calcium bioavailability.[90] The recommended dose is 1200 to 1500 milligrams per day.

Edible bird's nest is the nest of the swift and is constructed with salivary glue. Edible bird's nest contains carbohydrates, amino acids, mineral salts, and glycoproteins. The Chinese have considered edible bird's nest to be one of the most important items of food for thousands of years. In China, it is known to prevent skin aging and improve the appearance of the skin. It also has immune-boosting capabilities. A study found that edible bird's nest is helpful in the prevention of influenza viruses.[91]

He Shou Wu is widely used in Chinese herbal medicine as a tonic to prevent skin aging. He Shou Wu cleanses the blood by directly strengthening the functioning of the liver and the kidneys.

Jiaogulan is very useful in preventing skin aging by increasing superoxide dismutase (SOD) in the body. In China, this herb is called "the longevity herb."

Goji berries are considered a superfood. They are a very rich source of vitamin C and carotenoids. Goji berries have the highest antioxidant content of all foods. Eating goji berries is twenty times more beneficial than drinking goji juice. Taking the liquid extract is about five times as powerful as eating the berries.

In China, it is said that those who take schizandra regularly will remain youthful in appearance. All women who start taking schizandra see their skin improve dramatically.

The most beautiful woman in the history of China, Yang Kuei-Fei, ate longan fruit every day. Longan fruit contains several vitamins and minerals, including iron, magnesium, phosphorus, and potassium, and large amounts of vitamins A and C. In China, longan fruit is known to help prevent skin aging.

In Chinese herb shops, the longan fruit is available in a formula or as dried fruit.

Estrogen influences the amount of collagen synthesized and increases the synthesis of hyaluronic acid. Most estrogen receptors are found on the facial skin.[93] Estrogen deficiency can lead to premature wrinkles. According to Chinese face reading, vertical wrinkle lines on the upper lip signal estrogen deficiency.

Hormone replacement therapy (HRT) has been shown to prolong the look of youthful skin. Women who are long-term HRT users have more elastic skin and less severe wrinkling.[92] Get all your hormones tested annually after age forty, and use natural hormone replacement therapy.

Topical estriol cream applied on the face could reverse the signs of skin aging. In one study, the effects of the topical application of 0.01 percent estradiol and 0.3 percent estriol were evaluated. After treatment for six months, elasticity and firmness of the skin had improved and the wrinkle depth and pore sizes had decreased by 61 to 100 percent in both groups. Both estrogen compounds were found to be highly effective in preventing or treating skin aging in perimenopausal women.[94]

Progesterone cream is an effective treatment for delaying skin aging in women after menopause. A study found that 2 percent progesterone cream reduced wrinkles and increased elasticity and firmness of the skin. Progesterone is well absorbed into the body through the skin.[95]

Levels of human growth hormone (HGH) start to decrease with age after peaking in the late teens. Dr. Daniel Rudman found that the effects of six months of HGH injections on skin thickness were equivalent to ten to twenty years of reversed aging. Skin thickness increased by 7.1 percent on subjects in the study.[96]

There are a few natural options for raising HGH levels in the body. Deer velvet extract is a source of growth factors. Mucuna pruriens (velvet bean) is one of the best natural substances for raising HGH levels. It contains L-dopa, which is a precursor for dopamine. Dopamine increases the production of HGH within the body. L-glutamine is an amino acid that raises HGH levels. Take a gram of L-glutamine in the morning and another gram in the evening. Gamma-aminobutyric acid (GABA) is helpful for women over the age of thirty. Take 1,500 milligrams every night before bedtime.

Drinking rooibos tea daily is very beneficial for maintaining healthy skin. Studies have shown that rooibos tea possesses significant antioxidant and free radical scavenging properties due to substances that mimic the activity of superoxide dismutase (SOD).[97][98] The superoxide dismutase enzymes remove free radicals. The antioxidant and free radical scavenging activity of rooibos has been compared with that of green, black, and oolong teas.[99] Rooibos extracts were found to be stronger free radical inhibitors than either black or oolong teas but slightly weaker than green tea. Green tea is also very beneficial for the prevention of photoaging.[100]

ANTI-AGING SKIN SUPPLEMENTS

- Whole food vitamin C 1,000 milligrams
- Pycnogenol (Pine bark extract) 100 milligrams
- Evening primrose oil 1300 milligrams
- MSM 1,000 milligrams
- Carnosine 1,000 milligrams
- Milk thistle 300 milligrams
- Astaxanthin 8 milligrams
- Pearl powder 1,200–1,500 milligrams

Diet can have an impact on the rate of skin aging. A study found that higher vitamin C intake in the diet was associated with a lower likelihood of wrinkles. Higher linoleic acid intake was associated with a lower likelihood of dry, damaged skin. A

17-gram increase in fat and a 50-gram increase in carbohydrate intake increased the likelihood of wrinkles and skin damage. These associations were independent of age, race, education, sunlight exposure, income, menopausal status, body mass index, supplement use, physical activity, and energy intake.[101]

Studies show that sugar causes wrinkles and accelerates the aging of the skin.[102] Sugar causes the skin to age by changing the structure of collagen.[103] Internally, simple sugars attach themselves to proteins in collagen fibers, and it is this damaging process that is known as glycation. The resulting cross-linked collagen fibers lose their flexibility and strength, resulting in looseness of skin.[104] Scientists now believe that reducing glycation is a means of slowing the aging process. Advanced glycation end products are known as AGE. The more sugar you eat, the more AGEs you develop.

The most comprehensive study on the effects of diet on skin aging was published in the *Journal of the American College of Nutrition* in 2001. The researchers analyzed the diets of over four hundred people (aged seventy years and over from Australia, Greece, and Sweden) to determine the correlation, if any, between the consumption of certain types of foods and skin wrinkling. In the study, more skin wrinkling in the elderly was associated with higher intakes of saturated fat, meat (especially fatty, processed meats), full-fat dairy products (especially unfermented products and ice cream), soft drinks, sugar, potatoes, butter, and margarine. The overall conclusion was that a low-glycemic diet high in varied fruits, vegetables, nuts, legumes, and fish was associated with less skin wrinkling.[105]

Alcohol and cigarettes are very aging since they promote the generation of reactive oxygen species (ROS).[106][107] ROS are small, highly reactive, oxygen-containing molecules that damage DNA and cause skin aging.

Smokers look older than nonsmokers of the same age.[108] There is a very strong correlation between cigarette smoking and skin wrinkling.[109] In one study, twins with the same amount of sun exposure were monitored for skin aging. Both led the same life-style and had the same type of job. However, one smoked (fifty-two packs a year) and the other didn't. The twin who smoked had more severe skin aging than the nonsmoking twin.[110] When excessive sun exposure and heavy smoking occur together, the risk for developing wrinkles is eleven times higher than for nonsmokers and those with less sun exposure at the same age.[111]

In the book *Ancient Secret of the Fountain of Youth*, Peter Kelder reveals exercises that he calls the Five Tibetan Rites, which are over twenty-five hundred years old and are known to prevent and reverse physical aging. After practicing these exercises daily for a few years, many have reported younger-looking skin. Five Tibetan Rites how-to videos are widely available.

ANTI-AGING SKIN DIET

- Monounsaturated fat
- Olive oil and olives
- Fish (especially fatty fish, such as sardines)
- Reduced-fat milk and milk products, such as yogurt
- Nuts and legumes (especially lima and broad beans)
- Vegetables (especially leafy greens, spinach, eggplant, asparagus, celery, onions, leeks, and garlic)
- Whole-grain cereals
- Fruit and fruit products (especially prunes, cherries, apples, and jams)
- Zinc (seafood, lean meat, milk, and nuts)

TANNED

Skin coloring reflects the internal health of a woman. A very ill woman tends to be very pale. Caucasian women have the problem of looking pale if they are avoiding UV exposure to prevent skin aging.

One scientific study examined the importance of overall skin color. The study found that skin redness and yellowness enhanced the perception of health.[112]

Before the 1920s, tanned skin was regarded as an indicator of lower class status, since the lower class did a lot of outdoor work. Starting in the 1920s, tanned skin became very attractive. Coco Chanel accidentally got sunburnt while visiting the French Riviera. Suddenly, it was fashionable to be tanned. Tanned skin came to be viewed as attractive and a sign of wealth in Caucasian women. Wealth allows a woman to enjoy frequent traveling to warm and sunny destinations, with a tan to prove it.[113]

Sunless tanning with dihydroxyacetone (DHA) is an option for having tanned skin without the sun. However, most commercial sunless tanning solutions contain toxic ingredients. Instead, use an organic DHA sunless tanning solution that contains 100 percent natural ingredients.

A sunless tanning solution must have ingredients that are pH balanced since DHA is a pH-sensitive ingredient. The pH level is the single factor that determines how brown or orange you will be. The pH scale runs from one to fourteen. In order for DHA to produce a golden tan color, the pH must fall no lower than three and no higher than six. A pH over six results in skin developing an orange color. Stearic acid, triethanolamine, and mineral oil have a naturally high pH, over six. Skin treated with DHA at a pH level of five to 5.5 develops a perfect golden tan color. Fragrance amplifies the developing odor of DHA so be sure to get a fragrance-free sunless tanning solution to prevent the smell of DHA on the skin and clothes.

You can make your very own sunless tanning lotion with DHA. DHA is available in a powder form made up of tiny grains. Approximately 12 granules combined with distilled water is all that is needed for the face.

DHA may be of some concern. "A proportion of the ingredients, however, may penetrate deeper, reaching living epidermis layers and the dermis, and there promote protein glycation, one of the principal aging mechanisms."[114] However, until a better ingredient for sunless tanning gets developed, DHA is most likely still better than UV exposure.

If you are naturally very pale, then check that you are not iron deficient. Iron supplementation will restore healthy coloring to your face. Juicing of iron-rich vegetables is also an option. Take a handful of spinach, a handful of chard, and a few large beets and put them through a vegetable juicer. Drink one to two cups every day.

A study found that nutrients play a role in the pigmentation of skin. One group in the study took 13 milligrams of beta-carotene, 2 milligrams of lycopene, 5 milligrams of vitamin E, and 30 milligrams of vitamin C. Another another group took only 3 milligrams of beta-carotene. An increase of skin coloring was seen in eight weeks in the group that took 13 milligrams of beta-carotene.[115] Therefore, taking 13 milligrams of beta-carotene every day results in healthy skin coloring.

SUNLESS TANNING LOTION RECIPE

INGREDIENTS

1 teaspoon distilled water
Pinch of hyaluronic acid
12 granules of DHA

DIRECTIONS

Mix together a teaspoon of distilled water with a pinch of hyaluronic acid and 12 granules of DHA. Stir until the DHA powder is dissolved. This amount is enough for your face. You can substitute the teaspoon of water with a teaspoon of a water-based moisturizing lotion.

Chapter 3: Hair

Gorgeous hair is the best revenge.
- Ivana Trump, Socialite and Model

*H*air frames the face and is nearly as important as facial beauty in contributing to a woman's overall beauty score. "The hair is the richest ornament of women," said German monk Martin Luther. It is a physical feature nearly all people notice at first, in much the same way as the face.

Like the face, hair is a sign of a woman's health and age. The appearance of the hair is affected by diet, stress, hormonal changes; and illness.

In one study, long hair increased a woman's beauty score ratings. The women with the highest beauty scores had long hair along with an attractive face.[1]

"Perfect 10" hair looks a certain way. "Violet will be a good color for hair at just about the same time that brunette becomes a good color for flowers," said American author Fran Lebowitz. The most attractive hair colors are blonde, brunette, and dark red.

Hair colors have been stereotyped and used to prejudge a woman's personality. Some women even take on the personality that they believe to be associated with their hair color. Blondes become playful, brunettes become mysterious, and redheads become the center of attention.

A woman's overall appearance can be dramatically changed with a different haircut, style, or color. "If I want to knock a story off the front page, I just change my hairstyle," said First Lady of the United States Hillary Clinton. American actress Emma Stone said, "A different hair color changes everything!"

British fashion designer Vivienne Westwood said, "I think dress, hairstyle, and makeup are the crucial factors in projecting an attractive persona and give one the chance to enhance one's best physical features."

COLOR

High-impact, vibrant hair colors such as light blonde, jet black, dark brown, or dark red are the most noticeable. The most desirable female celebrities and models of all time tend to have either light blonde hair or dark brunette hair. According to various polls, men indicated that they like light blonde hair or dark brunette hair the most.

Dull colors do not catch the eye. Although extremely beautiful faces could pull off any hair color, dull hair colors such as mousy brown and dirty blonde do not enhance a woman's beauty. The *Urban Dictionary* defines mousy hair as a "drab, pale brown hair color" on a woman that "ruins her face." A woman with a dull hair color can increase her beauty score by dramatically lightening or darkening her hair.

Bright colors or streaks such as red, bright yellow, orange, or pink look unnatural and unattractive, since no woman is ever born with such hair colors. Bright red is an exception, because some Irish women have naturally bright red hair. However, it is so uncommon a hair color that it is not considered attractive by the majority of people.

Women should not stray too far from their ethnic hair color. Kathy Ireland, an American model, once said, "Beauty comes in all ages, colors, shapes, and forms. God never makes junk."

Asian or very dark-skinned women should not go blonde, because it looks very artificial. Many European or North American women have the most freedom to experiment with various hair colors because of their neutral skin tone and facial features.

THE PERFECT HAIR COLOR

In the book *Gentlemen Really Prefer Blondes?* Jena Pincott states that hair colors are more desirable when they're uncommon. In countries where blondes are uncommon, men tend to be attracted to blonde women. In countries dominated by women with lighter hair, darker-haired women are considered attractive and exotic. In Scandinavia, various surveys reveal most men prefer brunettes because brunettes are uncommon in that area.

Besides culture, there are definite media trends when it comes to ideal beauty. Marilyn Monroe was the most popular blonde of all time and started a trend for blonde hair. In the 1990s, a Caucasian blonde was considered highly desirable. Beginning in 2007, there was an increasing trend to prefer brunettes. Every few years, a different look is "in," made popular by the desirable celebrities and models of the time. A lot of men eventually get tired of the "popular look."

Men's preference for hair color is based mainly based on what hair color is considered uncommon in their country and what look is in at the moment. Some men are not easily influenced by culture and media, and have a certain preference based simply on personal taste.

Black or brunette hair is the most common hair color and is found in the vast majority of the world's population. Natural blonde hair tends to darken with age, resulting in dark-haired women with light-colored eyes.

Dark hair looks stunning on women with darker skin tones. Dark hair defines the facial features in the same way black eyeliner defines the eyes. Dark hair can give a woman a mysterious and sultry appearance. In some parts of North America or parts of Europe, dark-haired women are considered exotic. Looking exotic means looking strikingly different from the majority of people in a specific country.

Jet-black or dark, chocolate brown are the most attractive brunette shades. Dark brown with medium brown or auburn highlights looks very attractive as well. Dark hair looks its best when it is very shiny since it is a shade lacking light. Glimmering, shiny, dark hair will stand out among a brunette crowd.

Red hair is noticeable because of its rarity. It is found in less than 4 percent of world's population. The majority of redheads are found along the edges of both eastern and western Europe, mostly in Scotland, England, and Ireland. The rarity of red is due to its genetic makeup: the chromosome for red hair color is a recessive gene, meaning that an individual must inherit the gene from both parents in order to have red hair.

Not all women look good with red hair, but the ones that do look very beautiful. Red hair can give a woman a very radiant, daring, and striking look. Red hair suits women with a cool or pinkish skin tone, and may not look good on women with golden or olive skin.

Red hair looks its best when it is a darker shade and not too bright or orangey. Bright red hair looks unnatural in the same way bright orange, pink, or blue hair looks unnatural. The best red shade is deep ruby red.

Blonde hair is most common in Europe, particularly in Scandinavia and other northern regions. Blonde hair indicates youth since women who are born with light blonde hair tend to have their hair darken with age. After a blonde woman becomes pregnant, her hair tends to darken even further. Therefore, men who prefer blonde women are unconsciously attempting to partner up with a younger woman.

ARE BLONDES UNINTELLIGENT?

Speaking roughly, the blonder the country, the more Nobel Prizes it wins per capita. The blonder nations of Europe such as Sweden, the Netherlands, England, Germany, Austria, and Poland scored higher on IQ tests than the darker nations of southern Europe, Italy being the exception. The stereotype that "blondes are dumb" may have developed because lighter hair signals youth. In the past, before women discovered methods for coloring their hair, they could not conceal their natural hair color. The average age of a lighter-haired woman in the past would be around fifteen. The age of a darker-haired woman would be thirty-five. A fifteen-year-old woman is bound to be more naive and less intelligent than a thirty-five-year-old woman, no matter what her hair color. It's not that blonde women are less intelligent than brunette women; it's that younger women are less intelligent than older women. Therefore, in the past, before the invention of hair dyes, blonde hair was an honest, reliable signal of youth.

Studies are not conclusive about whether men prefer blondes but suggest that blonde hair makes women look younger. In a Polish study, pictures of blonde-haired women were generally rated as younger than the others.[2]

Jena Pincott says, "The human eye is attracted to light, bright colors, and blondes stand out more than brunettes and even redheads." Blonde hair is more noticeable than dark hair color because it reflects more light.

Blonde hair may attract higher tips. In a survey of waitresses, blondes earned higher tips than brunettes.[3] Another study showed that blondes induce more households to contribute to fund-raising efforts and receive higher donations than women with other hair colors.[4]

Light blonde is the most attractive shade of blonde. Medium blonde with light blonde highlights can look attractive and will stand out among a light blonde crowd.

All expert hair colorists advise that hair color must be properly matched with skin tone. Therefore, consult an experienced hair colorist to determine the ideal hair color to wear.

The chemicals in hair dyes are extremely damaging to hair and harmful to health. Organic, natural, and non-damaging hair dyes are the best choice. Organic hair salons specialize in natural and safe hair-coloring services.

HOW TO COLOR HAIR

BLONDE

The best option is to get your hair professionally colored in a high-end salon that specializes in blonde hair. To do it yourself, you will need to select a natural-looking blonde shade. After conditioning, you can apply a hair toner. Do not bleach your hair since the same degree of lightness can be achieved with a hair toner. Toner deposits color to cancel out yellow tones, orange tones, and brassiness.

BRUNETTE

Dark hair looks its best when it is shimmery and shiny. Pick a brand of hair color that gives super shiny results. At a salon, you can get a glossing treatment. You may need to use a color-enhancing shampoo and conditioner to avoiding fading. Avoid the sunlight, or spray on a hair sunscreen to avoid color fading.

RED

It is best to get red hair done professionally in a high-end salon that knows how to get the perfect shade of red. The best brand of red hair color is fade resistant and vibrant. Red hair color fades the fastest of any other hair color. Always use a color-enhancing shampoo and conditioner. Avoid the sunlight at all costs, or spray on a hair sunscreen to avoid color fading.

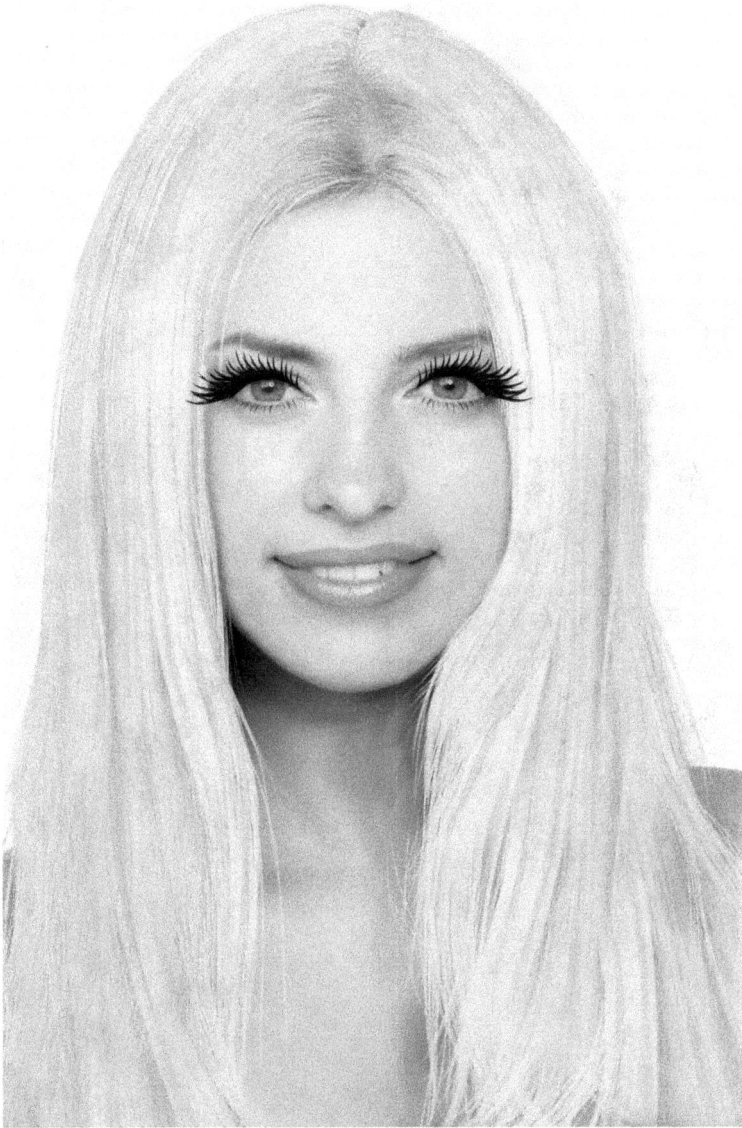

Figure 2 - Very light blonde hair color with extra-light platinum hair toner to cancel out yellow tones, orange tones, and brassiness.

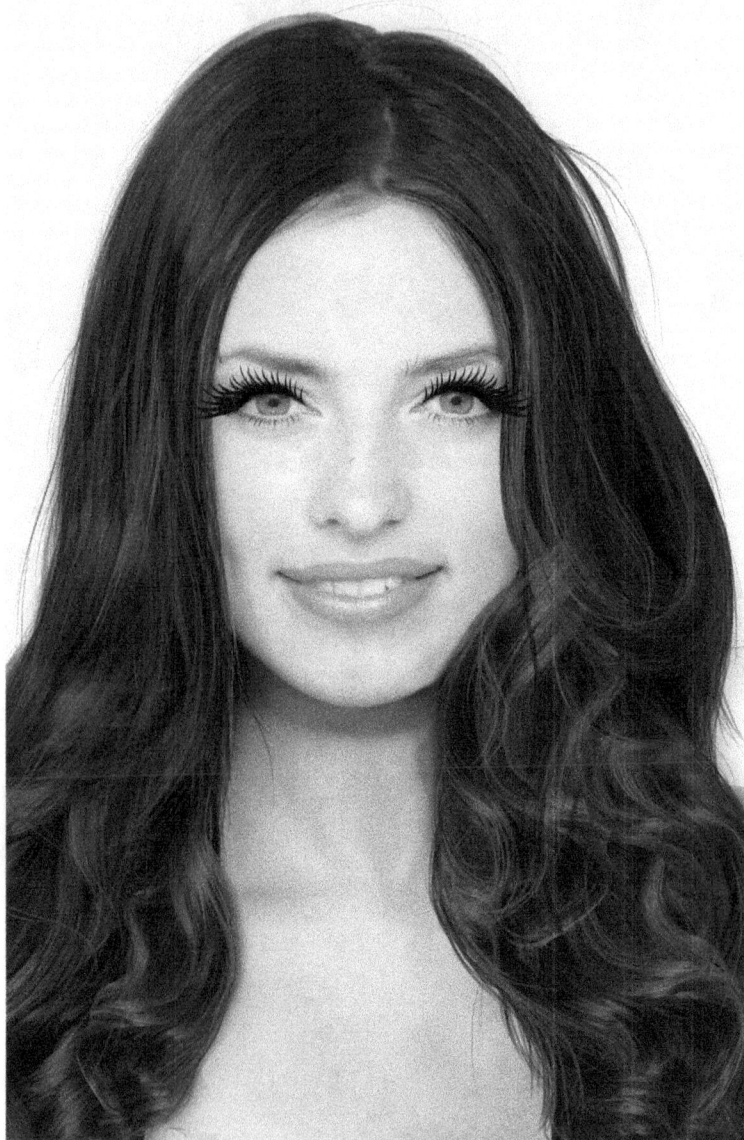

Figure 3 - Dark, chocolate brown shade with a glossing treatment to deliver super shiny results.

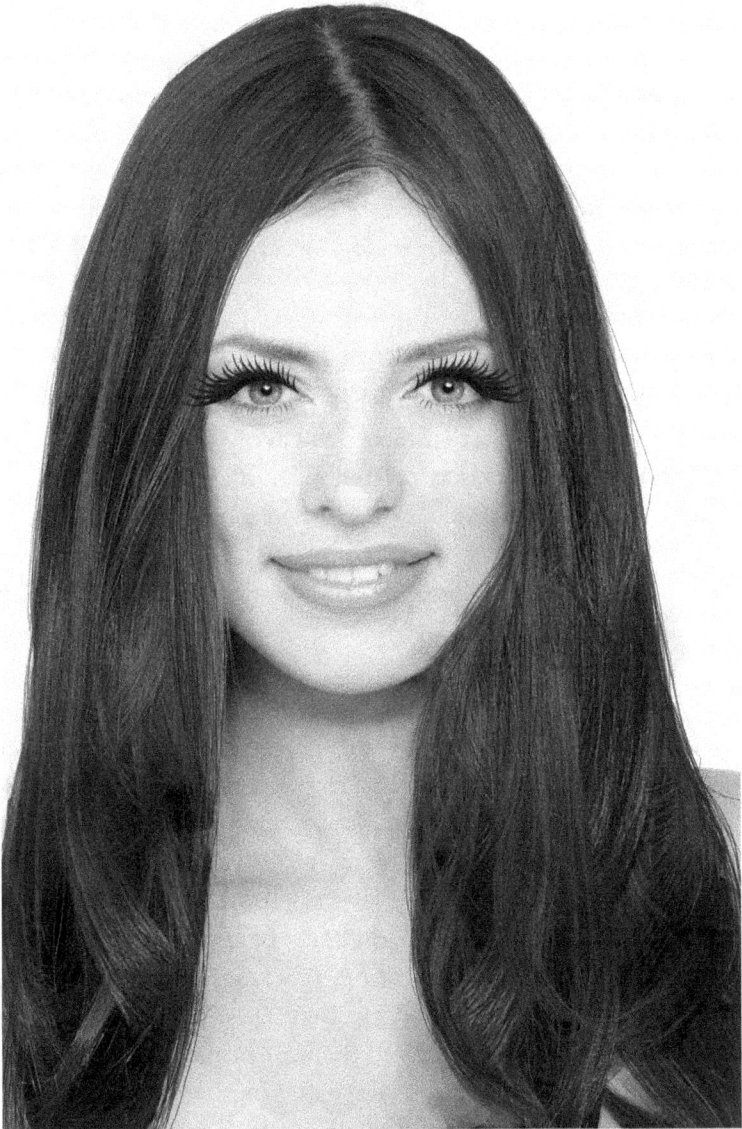

Figure 4 - Deep ruby red, with no bright or orangey tones.

LENGTH

Long hair is very feminine and will always be considered attractive. A study found that long hair, worn down, enhanced the femininity of women. Women with their hair tied up in a bun were rated as looking older.[5] The wisdom of the Bible confirms that "it is a woman's pride to wear her hair long" (GWT, 1 Corinthians 11:15).

Ask almost any man and he will tell you he prefers long hair on women. In the book, *The Hard Truth About What Men Want*, Brad Whitman found that the number one reason for complaint among married men was having a wife who cut her hair short. Short hair is associated with masculinity. American actress Ashley Scott said, "When I had long hair, you kind of got male attention from everything. But when you had short hair, it was a different kind of man that was attracted to you or I found coming up."

Tamás Bereczkei, professor of psychology, performed a study in which men rated the attractiveness of women who were depicted in six different photographs. Three of the photos were of the same young woman who had the same facial expression, but her hair was altered with a computer program to short, medium, and long. Long was at least eight inches below the shoulders. Men found the long hair to be "overwhelmingly" more attractive than the short or medium-length hair. "Longer hair had a significant, positive effect on the ratings of a woman's attractiveness; shorter styles did not," stated Dr. Bereczkei. The study showed that the women who were rated the least beautiful significantly improved their beauty score when wearing long hair.

Hair length and quality signal a woman's youth, health, and reproductive potential.[6] Each strand of hair has its own blood supply and can reflect a woman's internal state. Asian medicine views hair as an outgrowth of blood and bone marrow. "Hair is a track record of your health," says Jena Pincott. She explains:

"It's an honest record of the food you've eaten, the drugs you've taken, the seasons you've weathered, the stresses and sicknesses you've endured, and the grooming you've given it." If a woman's hair is shoulder length or longer, it shows she's been healthy for at least two years. The longer her hair is, the healthier she appears.

The perfect length is midback; any longer and it looks disorderly. According to various polls, midback hair length is the most preferred by the majority of men.

"Longer hair had a significant positive effect on the ratings of a woman's attractiveness; shorter styles did not."
- Tamás Bereczkei

Everyone's hair growth rate is a little bit different, but, on average, hair grows about half an inch per month and about six inches per year. Hair goes through three phases of growth: the anagen, the catagen, and the telogen. The anagen is the growth phase. The catagen is the transitional phase. The telogen is the resting phase. At any point in time, about 90 percent of the hair follicle is in its growing phase. The growing phase is genetically determined and is anywhere between two to six years. Therefore, hair growth rate depends on the length of the growing phase. For example, if a woman has a six-year growing phase, her hair will grow three times longer than a woman who has just a two-year growing phase.

Two hormones come into play when it comes to hair growth: estrogen and testosterone. Estrogen levels regulate how long the growing stage is, and testosterone levels regulate how fast hair grows while in the growing stage. The balance of thyroxin, androgens, dihydrotestosterone (DHT), and estrogen all work together to keep hair growing at the correct rate. When any one of these hormones becomes imbalanced, the rate at which hair grows can change, or the hair will fall out at a greater rate.

Pregnant women produce higher amounts of estrogen, resulting in faster hair growth. During pregnancy, the anagen (growing) phase is maintained for longer than normal, which allows hair to grow much longer. By increasing the body's estrogen levels, you can grow hair faster. Bovine ovary and *Pueraria mirifica*, typically used for breast enlargement, increases estrogen levels in the body and may cause the hair to grow faster.

Some women have reported their hair grew faster after taking prenatal vitamins. Prenatal vitamins contain higher concentrations of folic acid, calcium, and iron than regular multivitamins. These vitamins are beneficial for the growth of hair. However, they contain a high amount of iron, and excess iron can cause iron poisoning. Hence, it is best to take prenatal vitamins for hair growth only after consulting with a physician.

Besides prenatal vitamins, other nutrients are beneficial to the hair. Biotin is reported to help hair grow faster, although some women complain that it causes acne. MSM combined with vitamin C provides sulfur, which is known to promote hair growth. Fish oil contains omega-3 fatty acids, which nourishes the hair follicles.

Herbalists suggest horsetail extract and nettle for stimulating hair growth. Chinese herbalists recommend Fo-Ti, which is also known to prevent hair from becoming gray.

One of the best ways to promote faster hair growth is to apply oil on the hair regularly. The most effective oils for promoting hair growth are emu oil, amla oil, castor oil, and coconut oil.

Dr. Michael Holick conducted a study designed to find the effect of emu oil on hair growth. He discovered that 80 percent of hair follicles that had been asleep were awakened and began growing hair after emu oil was applied to the hair.[7] Researchers believe emu oil is very penetrating because it is almost 100 percent triglyceride lipid, containing no phospholipids.[8] The specific combination of rosemary, thyme, lavender, and cedarwood essential oils has been scientifically proven to grow hair in patients suffering from alopecia areata.[9] By combining the skin-penetrating properties of emu oil with the hair growth stimulating properties of essential oils of rosemary, thyme, lavender, and cedarwood, it is possible to promote hair growth successfully.

Massage the oil into the scalp once a day for at least three months, allowing it to penetrate the scalp overnight.

Indian women have used amla oil, also known as Indian gooseberry, for centuries to help their hair grow long. Amla is rich in vitamin C, tannins, and minerals.[10] Make sure you buy high-quality amla oil without mineral oil, petroleum, or artificial colors and fragrances added. You can prepare your own amla oil by boiling dry amla pieces in coconut oil.

Many women view castor oil as the elixir for growing hair faster. Women have reported that it helps their eyelashes grow longer. Ancient Egyptian women were known to use castor oil to encourage hair growth.

Coconut oil penetrates the hair shaft very easily, nourishing the hair and preventing breakage. Many women have reported their hair grew faster with regular application of coconut oil.

The most effective hair growth treatment would consist of an equal combination of emu oil, amla oil, castor oil, coconut oil, and essential oils. Apply the oil mixture to your hair and scalp, massage your scalp for five minutes, place a shower cap over your hair, and leave it in overnight. You can apply this oil treatment one to two times per week. For maximum benefit from the oils, they should be warmed before application to the hair. You can also apply the mixture to your hair and sit in a sauna.

Indian head massage (champissage) promotes hair growth and prevents hair loss. It facilitates the absorption of massage oils into the scalp. Indian women have used head massage along with massage oil to improve the condition of their hair.

Besides weekly hair oil treatments and head massage, washing your hair very infrequently will also help your hair grow faster. The best routine is to wash your hair every second or third day. Use a moisturizing conditioner each time you wash your hair and use a protein conditioner once a week.

Birth control pills used externally have helped some women grow their hair faster. Pick any brand of contraceptive pills containing estradiol. Take fifteen pills, put them in a plastic bag and crush them until they become a fine powder. Add the powder to your regular conditioner, mix it well, and let it stand for at least one day. Then use the conditioner as usual.

Studies show prostaglandin analogues such as bimatoprost, travoprost, or latanoprost could be effective for increasing hair growth and hair regrowth.[11] A study found that 500 mcg/ml of latanoprost daily over three months induced moderate hair regrowth.[12] You can mix bimatoprost, travoprost, or latanoprost with castor oil and leave it on the scalp overnight.

FAST GROWTH SUPPLEMENTS

SUPPLEMENTS
Prenatal Multivitamin
Suggested Dose: As directed on label

MSM (methylsulfonylmethane)
Suggested Dose: 1,500–3,000 milligrams daily

Whole Food Vitamin C
Suggested Dose: 1,000 milligrams daily

Biotin
Suggested Dose: 1,000 micrograms daily

Fish Oil/Flaxseed Oil
Suggested Dose: 1,000 milligrams, three times per day (3,000 milligrams per day)

Horsetail/Silicon
Suggested Dose: As directed on label

Nettle
Suggested Dose: 250 milligrams, three times per day

He Shou Wu
Suggested Dose: As directed on label

HAIR OIL TREATMENT
Equal parts emu oil, amla oil, castor oil, coconut oil, and essential oils (rosemary, thyme, lavender, and cedarwood) left in the hair overnight.

The secret to long hair is strong hair. Reducing hair damage will strengthen the hair. Apply a leave-in conditioner or jojoba oil to the ends of your hair daily to keep them strong.

Getting a trim to relieve split ends is a form of damage repair because split ends can weaken the hair. A split end will split the hair all the way up to the scalp, so get your hair trimmed whenever you see split ends. Some hair stylists believe in cutting the hair according to the moon phases. Cutting in the "full moon" is believed to make the hair grow thicker. Cutting in the "new moon" is believed to make it grow long faster.

Chemical hair color damages and weakens the hair, leading to split ends and breakage. Use natural, chemical-free hair products to minimize split ends and breakage.

Heat from hair appliances such as blow dryers, curling irons, flat irons, hot rollers, crimpers, and from perms can damage hair's protective cuticle, making strands susceptible to snapping off. When attempting to grow hair, it is important to stop using all heat appliances, or use them only once in a while and with thermal protection products.

Treat your hair gently, avoiding unnecessary brushing or handling. Never brush your hair while it is wet. When you brush wet hair it stretches and weakens. Wait until it is dry before brushing.

If you must remove tangles while it is still wet, use a comb that has widely spaced teeth.

Protect your hair from extreme weather by keeping it sheltered from the heat, sun, wind, and cold. Cover up your head when you go out in extreme weather, and use spray-in conditioner for extra protection if you will be outdoors for extended periods. Sleep with a silk or satin pillowcase, as it is much gentler on your hair than cotton.

A good way to speed up the growth of your hair is to use a shower filter. A shower filter will remove chlorine from the water and soften the water. Chlorine dries out and damages the hair, which will lead to poor hair growth. Do not swim in chlorinated water; it is not only bad for your hair and its growth, but also very bad for your health in general.

A boar-bristle brush is the best choice for brushing. It is excellent at distributing the oils from the scalp to the hair ends and increasing circulation in the scalp, which is important for helping the hair grow. For women who have thin, fine hair that takes forever to grow, they must choose a soft brush made specifically for sensitive hair.

Commercial shampoos are harsh on the hair. Sodium lauryl sulfate (SLS) slows down hair growth and causes hair shedding.[13] Many women report that after they stop using commercial shampoos, their hair stops shedding and grows faster. Switch to a natural, organic, chemical-free shampoo available at the health food store. To increase the speed of hair growth, look for natural shampoos that contain MSM, amino acids, B vitamins, He Shou Wu, *Russelia equisetiformis*,[14] and *Prunus persica* extract.

Hair is composed of the protein keratin, so a protein-rich diet will often result in improved hair growth. A diet that is too low in protein may cause thinning hair or slow the growth cycle. Fish and eggs are good sources of protein. Vegetarian sources of protein include beans, legumes, nuts, seeds, seaweed, and whole grains. Some nutritional experts suggest calf's liver, wheat germ, and two tablespoons of granulated lecithin daily to maximize hair growth.

Nutritional deficiencies and some disorders like hypothyroidism and hormone imbalances can also slow down hair growth or even lead to hair loss. Other things that slow down hair growth are stress, too much caffeine, alcohol, nicotine, and drugs.

SHINE

Many men express a strong preference for shiny hair. Shiny hair draws men in because it signals youth and good health. Health problems such as hypothyroidism can result in dull hair.

The best way to get hair its super shiniest is to get a "clear" glossing treatment at a salon or with at-home products. Glossing treatments give the hair a healthier look and completely eliminate frizz.

SHINE CONDITIONER RECIPE

INGREDIENTS
1 avocado
1 teaspoon honey
1 tablespoon coconut oil

DIRECTIONS
Mix all the ingredients together with a blender, apply to your hair, and rinse with ice-cold water after about twenty minutes.

You can also try hair-gloss spray or shine-serum products.

The smoother the hair cuticle, the shinier the hair will be because it will reflect light better. Always use a conditioner after shampooing. After conditioning use an acid hair rinse because the acidity helps close the hair cuticles and makes them smoother. Apple cider vinegar or lemon juice makes a good hair rinse. Many hairstylists recommend rinsing hair with very cold water or beer to leave it looking shiny.

SHINE RINSE RECIPE

INGREDIENTS
2 tablespoons apple cider vinegar
¼ cup ice-cold beer

DIRECTIONS
Mix all the ingredients together and use as a final rinse after conditioning.

Pure shea butter is effective for adding shine to the hair. To use pure shea butter, heat it up for a short time in the oven or microwave until it melts into oil, and then apply it to the hair. Once applied, put on a shower cap and leave it in overnight.

VOLUME

Many men clearly express a preference for hair with volume since it is a good signal of health. Health issues such as hyperthyroidism cause the hair to turn greasy and limp, which results in hair loss.

The biggest cause of hair thinning or hair loss is the production of dihydrotestosterone (DHT). A DHT blood test will determine if you need DHT blockers. You can use a synthetic or herbal DHT blocker to prevent hair loss. Saw palmetto, pygeum extract, stinging nettle, and pumpkin seed oil are effective natural DHT blockers. Emu oil contains a high level of linolenic acid, which is a DHT blocker. Emu oil applied to the hair is very helpful for preventing hair loss and adding volume to the hair. Swertia japonica extract is also a DHT blocker and can be mixed in with emu oil.

Besides DHT, other causes of hair loss include heat damage, iron deficiency, autoimmune disorder (alopecia areata), and extreme stress resulting in telogen effluvium. Consult with a medical professional to resolve a serious hair loss problem.

To help prevent shedding of hair, add 15 milliliters of bergamot oil to each 250-milliliter bottle of shampoo. Bergamot stimulates the root and encourages blood flow to the scalp, which in turn stimulates the hair follicle.

Look for organic and natural shampoos with *Russelia equisetiformis*, *Prunus persica* extract, *Swertia japonica* extract, licorice root extract, white peony root extract, rosemary extract, biotin, and panthenol, which help prevent hair loss. Hydrolyzed wheat protein is very effective at adding hair volume to limp hair. You can buy any one of these ingredients from bulk herbal stores or online herbal stores and add them into your regular shampoo or conditioner.

Sea kelp bioferment (SKB) has helped many women regain volume and prevent hair loss. Sea kelp bioferment is a natural kelp extract that has been derived by fermentation of sea kelp using lactobacillus.

The best way to style hair to give it volume is to use a volumizing mousse. Wash your hair with a volumizing shampoo and conditioner and then apply volumizing mousse to wet hair. Flip your head upside down and blow-dry your hair on a medium setting. For a final burst of hair volume, flip your head upside down again and lightly mist your hair with a light-hold hair spray. Bring your head right side up again

VOLUME CONDITIONER RECIPE

INGREDIENTS

1 cup beer
1 tablespoon hydrolyzed wheat protein
1 teaspoon *Russelia equisetiformis*
1 teaspoon *Prunus persica* extract

DIRECTIONS

Mix all the ingredients together in a blender, apply to your hair and rinse with water after about twenty minutes.

VOLUME LEAVE-IN CONDITIONER RECIPE

INGREDIENTS

15 percent sea kelp bioferment
15 percent sea emollient
5 percent goji berry extract
65 percent distilled water

DIRECTIONS

Place all the ingredients in a container, shake, and you're done. Apply to wet hair, massage into scalp, and gently pull through to ends.

and use your fingers to fix any stray hairs. Use a quarter-sized amount of hair pomade or styling wax to tame any frizzies.

STYLE

In polls conducted by various fashion and beauty magazines, men have expressed a strong preference for long and straight hair or long and wavy hair. Polls have revealed that most men prefer straight hair. Wavy hair comes in a close second. The polls reveal that curly hair is the least favored by men.

One of the reasons that men prefer straight hair is that straight hair reflects light more easily than curly hair and thus tends to be shinier. Curly hair tends to get frizzy and is less shiny since the cuticle layers don't lie perfectly flat, which means that light doesn't reflect off of it as much. Wavy hair is also favored since it gives the illusion of volume and thickness.

When asked, almost all men prefer women who wear their hair down most of the time. When you decide to put your hair

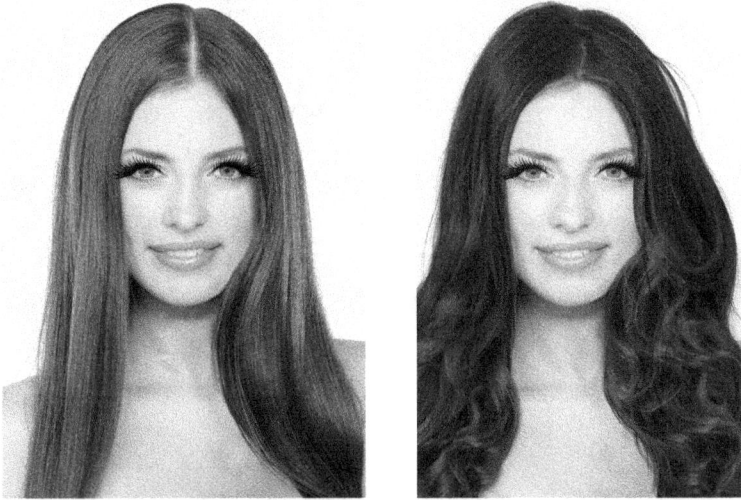

Figure 5 - Long and straight hair or long and wavy hair are
the most attractive hair styles.

up, go to a professional hairstylist so that your hair will look
as attractive as possible. Professional updos are very glamorous
and great for special events. They also dramatically show off a
gorgeous face shape, prominent cheekbones, and alluring features like neck and shoulders.

Perfectly straight hair can be achieved with a good straight-
ening iron. The best hair styling irons are expensive, but they
are an important "beauty investment." Many hair-care profes-
sionals prefer tourmaline irons. Wavy hair can be achieved by
using a curling iron or hot rollers along with hair spray. You
should always use a hair heat-protection spray when using hair
styling irons.

For haircuts, choose stylish cuts over fashionable cuts. French
fashion designer Yves Saint Laurent said, "Fashions fade, style is
eternal." A stylish haircut is about what makes you look your
best, while a fashionable haircut may not make you look your
best.

Classic and simple haircuts can look very sophisticated. Leonardo da Vinci said, "Simplicity is the ultimate sophistication."

"Simplicity is the ultimate sophistication."
- Leonardo da Vinci

Women with gorgeous faces and small foreheads look best with no bangs. For women with large foreheads and long faces, bangs are a must. Long side-swept bangs tend to look good on most women instead of straight-across, brow-skimming bangs.

Chapter 4: Body

A beautiful form is better than a beautiful face...
it gives a higher pleasure than statues or
pictures; it is the finest of the fine arts.
- Ralph Waldo Emerson, American writer

*T*he female body can be considered a work of art with its soft curves and fine structure. American film critic Richard Roeper said, "The female body is a beautiful work of art." Female bodies have been poetized, painted, sculpted, and photographed for centuries.

Much like the face, the body displays emotions and attitudes that are apparent to others through body language. "The body never lies," said American dancer Martha Graham.

Waist-to-hip ratio (WHR) and body mass index (BMI) are two factors that determine the attractiveness of the body. WHR indicates body shape while BMI indicates body size.

WHR is a reliable cue to a woman's fertility and health.[1] [2] Women with a low WHR are rated as being highly attractive, healthy, and young looking. Women with a high WHR are rated as looking older and less attractive.[3]

BMI was found to be the most important factor in rating the attractiveness of the body, even more so than either breast size or WHR.[4]

Research shows that men looking for short-term relationships are more interested in a beautiful body than a beautiful face since a woman's body conveys stronger cues to her current fertility and capability of conceiving. However, when asked to choose a long-term partner, men preferred a beautiful face.[5]

In most cases, the body reflects a person's lifestyle. "Our bodies are apt to be our autobiographies," said artist Frank Gelett Burgess. A woman must take care of her body through diet and exercise if she wants it to be in perfect form. "Revere the body and care for it, for it is a temple," said Indian guru Swami Muktananda.

WAIST-TO-HIP RATIO (WHR)

Waist-to-hip ratio (WHR) determines the amount of fat stored around the waist and hips. WHR is calculated by dividing the size of a woman's waist by the size of her hips. For example, if a woman's hips are thirty-two inches and her waist is twenty-four inches her WHR would be 0.75.

Devendra Singh, an evolutionary psychologist, conducted various experiments in different societies and found that men have a universal preference for women with a low WHR. In various experiments he found the ideal WHR to be 0.7. He found that *Playboy* models' WHR was between 0.71 and 0.68.[6]

The low WHR causes the torso to be V-shaped. The V-shaped torso has nearly always been favored throughout the ages. Being "beautiful" in Victorian times required wearing a corset to tighten and shrink the waist. An acceptable waist measured twenty inches but the ideal waist was sixteen inches or smaller.

The V-shaped torso as seen on the fashion doll is considered highly attractive in women.[7] "In Western societies, the cultural icon of {fashion dolls} as a symbol of female beauty seems to have some biological grounding," says Dr. Grazyna Jasienska, associate professor.

A low WHR is a signal that a woman is at the peak of her reproductive potential since hormone levels in the body determine body fat distribution.[8] Estrogen stimulates fat cells to accumulate in the buttocks and thighs and inhibits accumulation on the stomach. A small waist also indicates a woman's availability to reproduce since a woman who is already pregnant with another man's child cannot maintain a low WHR.[9]

A low WHR is a sign that a woman is reproductively capable. A study found that a woman with a WHR of 0.8 instead of the "ideal" WHR of 0.7 would have a 30 percent lower chance of becoming pregnant, regardless of age or total weight.[10] In studies conducted at fertility clinics, women with lower WHRs have higher success rates with in vitro fertilization programs.[11] Women's WHRs increase as they age, possibly due to reduction in estrogen levels.[12]

WHR may help men exclude women who are unhealthy.[15] Studies have found that a high WHR is associated with cardiovascular disease, premature death, stroke, type 2 diabetes, and certain cancers, even more so than is the total amount of body fat.[13][14]

Women with high levels of the male sex hormones (androgens) and low levels of estrogen have increased WHR.[16][17] Lowering androgen levels and increasing estrogen levels will help lower a woman's WHR.

Saw palmetto is an antiandrogen and is helpful for lowering androgen levels in the body. Saw palmetto can be combined with goat's rue (*Galega officinalis*) and black cumin seed (*Nigella sativa*), which are known to slim the waist. *Pueraria mirifica* has an estrogenic effect and is useful for perimenopausal women.[18]

Colon detoxification will flush out toxins from the colon and reduce the size of the waist. Colonics are effective for cleansing the colon. The colon can also be cleansed with the herbal combination of cape aloe leaf, rhubarb root, marshmallow root, and triphala churna. Non-addictive fiber supplements such as flax seeds and oat bran will keep the colon clean.

Cortisol is a hormone that is released in response to stress and tends to deposit fat around the waist. Lowering cortisol levels will reduce the size of the waist for women with stressful lifestyles. Holy basil (*Ocimum sanctum*) is an Indian herb that reduces elevated cortisol levels.[19]

Candida infection is a possible cause of an enlarged waist. Electrodermal screening can detect candida. Candida can be treated with oil of oregano, olive leaf, and grapefruit seed extract. A "candida diet" is also helpful. The candida diet consists of eliminating sugar, carbohydrates, vinegar, mushrooms, cheese, peanuts, and high-sugar fruits for up to one year.

Toning the abdominal muscles is a method of reducing the waist size to some degree. Many women have found that crunches tend to thicken the abs and fill out the muscles on the sides, making the waist boxy. Instead of crunches, perform twisting abdominal moves that don't involve lying down.

To reduce your waist temporarily, you can wear a corset. Corsets reduce the waist size by two to four inches. A satin or silk corset is the best option if you don't want anyone to see the lumps and bumps typically seen with lace corsets.

Corsets can be selected in either underbust or overbust, depending on preference. An underbust corset cinches the waist, while an overbust corset cinches the waist as well as supporting and lifting the breasts. The best corsets have steel boning (spring steel, which allows for bend but still gives a great deal of support).

To reduce the size of a number of body parts temporarily, you can wear a seamless full-body shaper. Full-body shapers will slim the thighs, shape the buttocks, and reduce the waist. You can choose extra firm, firm, medium, or light control.

Women who want to reduce their waist size permanently and get the perfect V-shaped waist can consider tightlacing, also called corset training or waist training. The female ribs are flexible, and continuous inward pressure on the ribs will force the bones gradually into a V-shape.

To begin tightlacing, acquire a custom-tailored training corset four or five inches smaller than the waist size. A zipper-closure corset is recommended since it is the fastest to put on. Start by wearing the training corset for a few hours each day and gradually increase the length of time you wear it until you are able to wear it twelve hours a day, every single day. Some women have worn a training corset for up to twenty-three hours a day. Once you achieve your desired waist size, you can wear the corset for only a few hours per day to maintain your shape.

The smallest waist recorded is that of Ethel Granger, who tightlaced for most of her life and slowly transformed from a twenty-four-inch waist to a thirteen-inch waist. Her husband, astronomer William Arnold Granger, loved small-waisted women and convinced her to wear a corset day and night.

Some women undergo surgical removal of floating ribs to reduce their waist size. This is unnecessary as the waist can be effectively reduced with tightlacing.

Abdominoplasty is a surgical option for women with excessive fat or sagging skin around their waist. It removes excess skin and fat from the abdomen and tightens the waist area.

Besides the size of the waist, the buttocks play a significant role in the attractiveness of the female body. The buttocks give the lower body a curvaceous shape that men find very attractive. English critic Kenneth Tynan said, "These pointless globes are as near as the human form can ever come to abstract art."

The ideal buttocks size varies among cultures. One study measured the actual WHR, which measures around the waist and hips/buttocks of women. The results of the study showed that American men prefer an actual WHR of 0.68. Hadza men in north-central Tanzania prefer a larger actual WHR of 0.78.[2]

"Most cultures have different ethnic ideals of buttocks shape," says Dr. Thomas L. Roberts, who specializes in buttocks augmentation. Caucasians generally want buttocks that are full but not extremely large. Hispanics want buttocks that are very full. Asians want buttocks that are small to moderate in size, but shapely. African-Americans and Caribbeans of African descent have a strong preference for very large buttocks, and several request a "shelf" (extreme prominence of the upper buttocks).

Thomas L. Roberts has determined the "perfect buttocks." These features are considered attractive by all ethnic groups: a smooth inward sweep of the low back area and waist, very feminine cleavage as the buttocks separate superiorly and inferiorly, maximum prominence in the mid to upper buttocks, and minimal crease below the buttocks, with no droop.

To enhance the buttocks temporarily, the padded panty will make up for lack of volume. Some padded panties also include hip enhancers and thigh control to increase the size of the hips and reduce the size of the thighs. A butt-lifter panty will lift up the buttocks for women who already have volume but lack firmness.

Many women have reported that taking the herb maca root (*Lepidium meyenii*) internally effectively increased the volume and projection of their buttocks. A strict schedule can be followed to achieve maximum results. Start by taking 1,000 milligrams per day for one week, and add 500 milligrams more every week until you reach week six. At week six you should take a break. At week seven start all over as in week one, taking 1,000 milligrams per day. Another option is to simply take 2,200 milligrams per day until you've achieved the desired results.

Some women have reported that rubbing fish oil directly on the skin of the buttocks has produced slight to moderate growth. Fish oil is rich in omega-3 fatty acids, which get absorbed and stored in the buttocks when applied topically. Taking fish oil orally won't make a difference.

Volufiline is a non-hormonal ingredient found in some butt and breast growth creams that increases the amount of fat cells in the area to which it is applied, leading to permanent volume.

For women with severely unattractive buttocks, cosmetic procedures are an option. When planning cosmetic procedures, keep in mind that projection and volume are the most important factors of beautiful buttocks.[21]

A buttocks lift will correct drooping buttocks associated with aging and weight gain. A buttocks augmentation will correct loss of volume. Skin on the insides of the legs lacks the elasticity of skin elsewhere on the body and may remain loose after major weight loss. In many women the only way to improve the appearance of this area is to remove the extra skin with a procedure called a medial thigh lift. Loss of skin elasticity in the back area of the thigh as well as dimpled appearance of the thigh can be corrected with a posterior thigh lift.

BODY MASS INDEX (BMI)

The body mass index (BMI) is a measure of body weight relative to height. The formula for calculating BMI is weight in kilograms divided by height in meters squared.

BMI is the most important factor in rating the attractiveness of the body.[22][23] Men rated the attractiveness of a woman's body based primarily on BMI rather than WHR.[24] Dr. Martin Tovee found that women with a BMI between eighteen and nineteen received the highest beauty ratings.[25][26] Dr. Tovee concludes that men use the BMI as a primary screening mechanism for selecting women from a wide range of possible partners and WHR helps the men further narrow down their selection.

A study found that a BMI of 19 is very closely correlated with health and fertility and that a higher BMI is responsible for infertility and health problems.[27] The lowest death rate for all disease was associated with a BMI close to 19. Women whose BMI was around 20 to 24.9 had a 20 percent increase in risk of death. There was a 33 percent increase in risk for a BMI of 25 to 26.9; 60 percent increase in risk for a BMI of 27 to 28.9; and an over 100 percent increase in risk for a BMI of 29 to 32.[28]

There are problems associated with a very high BMI and a very low BMI. A high BMI has a negative impact on fertility.[29] A BMI below 19 has a negative impact on both health and reproductive potential.[30] Evidence suggests that a woman must store a minimum amount of body fat in order to be able to reproduce.[31]

Studies confirm that men consider thinness an important physical trait in women.[32] However, women are sometimes not accurate when estimating the level of thinness that men find attractive. Anorexic and bulimic women are doing themselves a disfavor by thinking extreme thinness is attractive. In one study, women thought men would like women thinner than men reported they like.[33]

A study found that very thin women (BMI of less than 18) were not considered very attractive and desirable. Normal-weight women (BMI of 18.5 to 24.9) with a low WHR were rated the most attractive and desirable.[34]

Women who are naturally underweight may want to consider taking creatine supplements and appetite-stimulating herbs such as gentian, chen pi, ginger, or blessed thistle. If creatine and herbal appetite stimulants do not work, a naturopath can determine the cause of underweight.

Being overweight is a much more common problem than being underweight. One of the main causes of weight gain is an unhealthy diet consisting of packaged foods and refined carbohydrates.

Carbohydrates are a primary source of energy. They are converted to glycogen and stored in muscle or the liver for future use. However, some women consume an excessive amount of refined carbohydrates that significantly exceeds their storage capacity for glycogen, and when this happens, the sugar resulting from carbohydrate digestion is converted to body fat.

The glycemic index (GI) is a measure of the effects of carbohydrates on blood sugar levels. Foods with a low GI rating create a full feeling for longer, aiding weight loss and increasing energy. High GI-rated foods force the body to release large amounts of insulin into the blood, resulting in fatigue, sugar cravings, and mood swings.

Minimizing the consumption of refined carbohydrates and high GI-rated foods is truly one of the easiest ways to lose weight. However, many people are unwilling to give up the convenience and pleasure of eating processed foods or simply don't realize how much of a problem they are.

Going on "weight-loss diets" is very unhealthy and actually leads to increased weight over time. Weight cycling is the repeated loss and regain of body weight. Studies show that weight cycling is very much linked with an increased WHR.[35] Studies suggest that a stable weight over time is associated with the best health status.[36]

Many fad diets restrict or eliminate fruits, vegetables, dairy products, and whole grains. These foods are loaded with nutrients that the body needs. In addition, diets that are too high in protein may cause an increased risk of chronic disease, like heart disease, cancer, high blood pressure, and osteoporosis. Diets that are high in protein and low in carbohydrates often lead to the formation of uric acid and calcium oxalate, causing kidney stone formation and gout. A diet that is low in carbohydrates puts the body into ketosis, a condition that is unnatural. Ketosis most often occurs in starvation, but it can also occur if not enough carbohydrates are consumed.

The Mediterranean diet is the best way of eating to achieve a low BMI. It has been shown to reduce weight gain and slow down age-related weight gain.[37] It prevents the development of obesity.[38] Mireille Guiliano, author of *French Women Don't Get Fat*, believes the benefits of the Mediterranean diet are related to factors such as small portions and the emphasis on freshness and balance in food.

Foods with healthy fats that form part of a normal Mediterranean diet, such as olive oil and nuts, may actually be more effective at reducing weight than a low-fat diet. A study found that the Mediterranean diet was much more effective in weight reduction than a low-fat diet. The weight reductions among participants after two years were six to nine pounds for the low-fat group and nine to thirteen pounds for the Mediterranean-diet group.[39]

According to Dr. Demosthenes Panagiotakos and Christina-Maria Kastorini, MSc, PhD, the Mediterranean diet is not only the best way to lose weight but also the best way to prevent disease. The diet is associated with lower risk for cardiovascular disease, type 2 diabetes, obesity, and some types of cancer. A ten-year study found that following a Mediterranean diet and healthy lifestyle was associated with lowering early death rates by over 50 percent.[40]

Supplements are a beneficial addition to a proper diet in reducing weight. Research shows that chromium picolinate and 5-HTP effectively promote weight loss in women.[41] Herbal supplements may also be helpful for appetite control.

Chromium deficiency is common in North America and may increase cravings for sweets. Chromium is known to regulate blood sugar levels and reduce cravings for sweets.

5-HTP increases serotonin levels in the brain. Serotonin deficiency is associated with the brain's perception of starvation and hunger.

Hoodia gordonii is an appetite suppressant. A Dutch anthropologist studying the primitive San Bushmen of the Kalahari Desert noticed that they ate the stem of the hoodia plant to suppress hunger during long hunting trips. The active ingredient in hoodia is the appetite-suppressing molecule P57. Scientists found that P57 acts on the brain in a manner similar to glucose. It tricks the brain into thinking you are full even when you have not eaten, reduces interest in food, and delays the time before hunger sets in. Women with diabetes should not use hoodia.

Garcinia cambogia contains a component called hydroxycitric acid (HCA) that suppresses the appetite and reduces the body's ability to form fatty tissue.

Guarana works in much the same way coffee does due to high levels of caffeine. Caffeine impairs the appetite. A study found that guarana improved memory, mood, and alertness. The lower dose of 75 milligrams produced more positive cognitive effects than the higher doses.[42]

Ephedra sinica has thermogenic (fat burning) properties and is an excellent appetite suppressant. However, ephedra has some major safety concerns, including high blood pressure, tachycardia, CNS excitation, arrhythmia, heart attack, and stroke. It is not recommended unless under strict monitoring by a doctor.

Regardless of moods or weather, exercise is a must if you desire to lose weight. As the Irish poet William Butler Yeats once wrote, "To be born woman is to know—although they do not talk of it at school—that we must labor to be beautiful." Laziness is not an option for beautiful women. Helena Rubinstein once said, "There are no ugly women, only lazy ones."

The two most important types of exercise to perform for weight loss are cardio and strength training. Cardio burns calories, while strength training increases muscle mass, which increases metabolism. Cardio is effective for short-term weight-loss goals, while strength training is more beneficial for long-term weight-loss goals.

"There are no ugly women, only lazy ones."
- Helena Rubinstein

Perform five cardio workouts a week, with each lasting at least twenty to thirty minutes. Suggested workouts include walking, swimming, jogging, stair climbing, elliptical trainers, and group cardio classes. For strength training, perform two or three sessions weekly. Select two or three exercises per muscle group. Focus mostly on training the muscles of the legs, buttocks, chest, and back. However, keep in mind that too much muscle mass is very masculine, so don't overdo muscle training. Many men report being turned off by women with very defined muscles, especially on the arms, shoulders, and abs.

Besides improper diet and lack of exercise, another common cause of being overweight is eating out of boredom. Getting extremely busy and preoccupied is a good method of losing weight. Developing a passion for doing something will help take out the passion for eating.

Once you reach adulthood, the number of fat cells in your body is relatively fixed. Liposuction permanently removes fat cells and thus permanently changes where you will accumulate fat. Although no type of liposuction is a substitute for dieting and exercise, liposuction can remove stubborn areas of fat that don't respond to traditional weight-loss methods.

A wide range of factors, such as biochemical individuality, endocrine/hormonal imbalances, digestive problems, blood sugar fluctuations, candida, food allergies, organ dysfunction, psychological issues, and toxic load, can contribute to weight gain. A naturopath can determine and treat the cause of overweight if it remains a problem despite proper diet, supplements, exercise, and cosmetic procedures.

LIMBS

The length of a woman's arms and legs and the size of her shoulders, hands, and feet contribute to a woman's overall beauty score. They are not the most important aspects but do influence beauty ratings to some degree.

Arms appear to be an important body part in women. Research found that women with long arms are highly attractive, even more so than women with long legs. The study involved having volunteers rank women based on their looks. Arm length was found to be an important contributing factor to attractiveness. Hip and waist size were also regarded as important, along with a woman's weight and age.[43] Women with abnormally short arms can consider an arm-lengthening cosmetic procedure. Women with thick upper arms can consider liposuction to slim the upper arms.

Men are attracted to long legs in women[44] since leg length may indicate a woman's biological quality. Wearing high heels, especially nude-colored heels, will make the legs appear relatively longer. Women with large thighs can consider liposuction to slim the thighs.

Although long legs are considered attractive, this is true only for a slight (5 percent) leg length increase; excessively long legs decrease attractiveness. Excessively long legs might indicate maladaptive biological conditions such as genetic diseases, health problems, or weak immune responses.[45] Women with excessively long legs should wear flat shoes and long dresses or skirts.

While broad shoulders are a masculine trait, narrow shoulders are very feminine. The easiest method for hiding broad shoulders is to wear tops with sleeves and avoid wearing sleeveless tops. You can also wear your hair down and long to cover your shoulders.

A study found that men were highly consistent in choosing the most attractive female hands. Therefore, there appears to be a strict consensus among men about what female hands should look like. Hands with long fingers were preferred.[46] Shape averageness and femininity also increase hand attractiveness.[47] Fingers can be made to appear longer by wearing nude-colored nail polish.

Small feet are considered more feminine.[48] For a period of time in China, extremely small feet were considered very beautiful. Women would endure extremely painful footbinding to have small feet and be considered "beautiful" in those times. Wearing dark-colored shoes will help make the feet appear slightly smaller.

Studies show that, just like fashion dolls, the ideal female body is hair-free in all areas, resembling a prepubescent female.[49] The absence of body hair is highly attractive since it indicates low androgen and high estrogen levels, a signal of fertility.[50] A hair-free body also indicates health since excessive body hair (hirsutism) is sometimes associated with medical conditions such as polycystic ovary syndrome (PCOS), Cushing's syndrome, congenital adrenal hyperplasia (CAH), hyperthecosis, and cancer of the adrenal gland or ovaries.

Chapter 5: Breasts

B is for breasts of which ladies have two;
Once prized for the function, now for the view.
- Robert Paul Smith, American author

*B*reasts are composed of fat that serve as energy stores for the body and secrete milk to feed infants. Large breasts indicate that a woman is ready for reproduction.[1] [2] Research shows that women with large breasts and a small waist are about three times more likely to get pregnant than other women.[3] Women with small breasts, usually the result of low levels of female hormones, have reduced fertility.[4] Therefore, men are attracted to large and firmly shaped breasts because they signal fertility.[5]

Although the ideal breast size has fluctuated dramatically over the ages,[6] the majority of studies reveal that men prefer medium or large-sized breasts.[7] [8] [9] [10] The majority of men do not like excessively small or excessively large breasts.

Men rate a C cup as the most attractive breast size in a woman. Research found that men showed little interest in a woman with an A or B cup but gained interest when her breast size was altered to a C cup.[11]

Men rate breasts larger than a D cup as not particularly attractive. Researchers speculate that breasts that are enormous signal reduced fertility since breasts grow larger during pregnancy and lactation.[12] Women with enormous breasts are also negatively perceived as being unintelligent, incompetent, and immodest.[13]

Women with slim bodies, small waists, and moderately large breasts are rated the most attractive and desirable for a relationship.[14] Researchers found that large breasts alone will not increase attractiveness, unless accompanied by a small waist.[15] Research shows that the breasts and waist received more initial male visual fixations than the face or the lower body.[16]

SIZE

A woman's breast size attracts male attention and influences male judgments of attractiveness. Breast size marks an important distinction between men and women. Therefore, breast size is an important visual aspect of femininity.

Breast implants tend to carry the most risks of all cosmetic procedures. Breast implant risks include excessive bleeding, infection, rupturing, deflation, implant displacement, symmastia, Mondor's cord, loss of sensation, scar complications, extrusion, hematoma, seroma, necrosis, and traction rippling.

When a foreign implant is placed into the body, the body naturally forms a capsule or scar tissue around the implant. The scar tissue can contract, which is known as capsular contracture and is the most common complication with breast implants. There are varying grades of capsular contracture, from the implant feeling slightly firm to the implant becoming hard and distorted in shape.

Stem cell breast augmentation is an option for breast enlargement. Fat and stem cells are injected into the breast, which results in a permanent one or two bra cup size increase. The end result is enlarged breasts that are very natural in appearance without the complications associated with implants. The technique does not require general anesthesia and has a short recovery period.

A breast enlargement program consisting of herbs, glandular therapy, or suction devices can be used to enlarge the breasts naturally. However, they may take two to four years of consistent effort to achieve desired results.

Breast growth occurs most efficiently with the balanced presence of estrogen, progesterone, prolactin, human growth hormone (HGH), and growth factor (GF). After puberty, when the body ceases to produce a significant amount of these hormones, breast growth ends. By supplementing these hormones, breasts can grow even during adulthood. Hormone testing should be done to determine the most appropriate natural breast enlargement program to follow.

Reducing androgen levels can also encourage breast growth since excessive androgens in the body can hinder breast growth. Symptoms of excess androgens include acne, excess hair on the arms and face, thinning hair on the scalp, polycystic ovary syndrome (PCOS), and hypoglycemia.

For the majority of women, increasing estrogen levels is the most effective way to increase breast size since estrogen (specifically estradiol) is the hormone that contributes most to the growth of the breasts.[17] Three naturally occurring estrogens in women are estrone (E1), estradiol (E2), and estriol (E3). Estradiol (E2) is the primary form in nonpregnant females, estrone is produced during menopause, and estriol is the primary estrogen of pregnancy.

Synthetic estrogens used for hormone replacement therapy (HRT) list breast enlargement as a side effect. However, synthetic estrogens are not recommended because they come with health risks. Studies show that synthetic HRT increases the incidence of breast cancer,[18] ovarian cancer,[19] and endometrial cancer.[20]

Herbs with estrogenic activity are called phytoestrogens. Many herbalists recommend fenugreek, wild yam, hops, fennel seed,

MACROMASTIA

Macromastia is a condition resulting in the development of extremely large breasts, typically H cup size or bigger. The cause of the rapidly growing breasts, resulting in enormous breasts, is thought to be an abnormal sensitivity of the breast tissue to female hormones.[21] Macromastia may also result from the presence of unusually high amounts of female hormones in the bloodstream.

and shatavari extract for natural breast growth. Ethnobotanist James A. Duke, PhD, author of *The Green Pharmacy*, says that phytoestrogens have a centuries-old reputation as breast enlargers.

The herb *Pueraria mirifica* is the strongest phytoestrogen available. The components that make *Pueraria mirifica* different than other phytoestrogens are miroestrol and deoxymiroestrol, which have a structural similarity to estradiol. Deoxymiroestrol is the most estrogenic plant molecule known. *Pueraria mirifica* has helped women grow an average of two cup sizes per year. Some women confuse Pueraria lobata (kudzu) with Pueraria mirifica, but Pueraria lobata is not effective for breast enlargement.

Unlike other phytoestrogens, *Pueraria mirifica* needs to be taken on a very specific schedule. *Pueraria mirifica* should be taken on the fifth day of the menstrual cycle and then stopped on the twelfth day. *Pueraria mirifica* should be taken two times per day, one dose in the morning and another dose in the evening. *Pueraria mirifica* may result in missing or irregular menstrual periods; therefore, regular breaks from its use are essential. For every three months on Pueraria mirifica, the herb vitex should be used for one month.

Pueraria mirifica appears to work better when combined with the herb goat's rue. Goat's rue does not contain any known phytoestrogens but acts as an estrogen enhancer. Goat's rue is a galactagogue that can increase the production of prolactin.

Some women may have tried natural breast enlargement and achieved minimal results. This is because insulin-like growth factor-1 (IGF-I) levels appear to be the determining factor for successful breast enlargement. A study found that estradiol enhances expression of IGF-1 in some women, which promotes breast enlargement. In the study, 46.7 percent of women experienced breast enlargement of three cup sizes after six months with estradiol. The remaining women did not experience growth because IGF-1 levels were not elevated in their body with the use of estradiol.[22] Another study found that during the follicular phase, breast enlargement was associated with high IGF-1 levels. During the luteal phase, breast enlargement was associated with higher estradiol and progesterone levels and lower testosterone levels.[23] Growth factors along with phytoestrogens may help stimulate breast enlargement.[24] Bovine colostrum can increase IGF-1 levels. Human growth hormone (HGH) can also be taken to help promote breast enlargement.

Mucuna pruriens (velvet bean) may be one of the best natural substances for raising HGH levels. It contains L-dopa, which is a precursor for dopamine. Dopamine increases the production of HGH within the body.

Certain amino acids stimulate the release of HGH. A good blend contains at least 1,200 milligrams of L-arginine, 1,200 milligrams of L-lysine, 1,200 milligrams of L-ornithine, 500 milligrams of L-tyrosine, and 2,000 milligrams of L-glutamine. Take this blend every night before bedtime. Women over thirty years of age can take GABA instead of the amino acid blend. Take 1,500 milligrams every night before bedtime.

For women who have tried phytoestrogenic herbs and not had success, there is another breast enlargement method. Bovine ovary extract is the freeze-dried ovaries from female cows. It works by stimulating the ovaries to produce more estrogen. It can also stimulate the pituitary gland, resulting in an increase in prolactin and growth hormone levels. On average, breasts grow one cup size in three months. Bovine ovary must be certified organic to avoid unnecessary contaminants.

Many women have enlarged breasts using a breast suction device. Like any tissue in the body, when the breasts are exercised and blood flow encouraged, they will enlarge. A suction device can be used instead of supplements, or along with supplements, to maximize breast growth. However, suction devices should not be used excessively or they could leave permanent indentations.

A massage method called "chi breast massage" appears to be the most effective type of breast enlargement massage. To do the chi breast massage, apply oil or cream then place your hands over your breasts and massage your breasts in an upward and inward circular motion, three-hundred-sixty times. Move your breasts toward the middle, not outward. The massage takes about five minutes and can be done two to three times per day.

Massaging phytoestrogens into the breasts is an effective method for enlarging the breasts. Commercially prepared breast enlargement creams are available. To make homemade breast enlargement oil, combine alcohol-free liquid extracts of fenugreek with organic borage oil.

BREAST ENLARGEMENT OIL RECIPE

INGREDIENTS

1/2 cup of organic borage oil
20 drops alcohol-free liquid fenugreek extract

DIRECTIONS

Fill a dark glass bottle with organic borage oil then add 20 drops alcohol-free liquid fenugreek extract. Shake well before each usage. Massage in for about five or ten minutes. Cover with saran wrap. Apply heat for thirty minutes from a heated pad set to low. Leave the concoction on all night if possible.

For women who have high levels of estrogen, herbs that increase progesterone should be taken instead of estrogenic supplements. Chasteberry, also known as vitex, has the ability to increase progesterone.[25] Chasteberry has been shown to increase fertility in women.[26] It is also useful for reducing high prolactin levels. Topical natural progesterone cream is also very helpful for estrogen dominance. Progesterone causes lobular-alveolar development, which rounds out the breasts. It determines how much milk the breasts can produce and store.[27]

To prevent estrogen dominance, increased intake of B vitamins and magnesium is absolutely essential during a natural breast enlargement program. Kelp should be also taken for proper thyroid function. The goal is to keep the body temperature in the range of 98.2 to 98.6 degrees Fahrenheit during the day.

Certain supplements can help maximize the growth of breasts. Women who have high levels of testosterone can include antiandrogens such as saw palmetto berries, spearmint herbal tea, stinging nettle root, or pygeum bark in their breast enlargement program. Women have reported good results from adding MSM, vitamin C, collagen, gelatin, and essential fatty acids to their natural breast enlargement program. Some women feel convinced that chicken feet soup has helped them grow tremendously, although supplemental gelatin may have similar effects.

To make a week's worth of chicken feet soup use 28 chicken feet. Add distilled water, a few slices of ginger root, rice wine, and some shiitake dried mushrooms. Rice wine and the shiitake mushrooms are optional and just for flavor. Combine everything in a large cooking pot, bring to a boil, and then simmer for two hours. When the soup is milky white, it's ready. Put the soup in seven containers for seven days. Either discard the feet or eat them together with the soup. You can add the soup to other soup recipes such as chicken soup. You can also pour the soup into ice cube trays and freeze it. You can then

CHICKEN FEET SOUP RECIPE

INGREDIENTS

28 chicken feet
2 tablespoons rice wine
14 cup of distilled water
Shiitake dried mushrooms
Ginger root

DIRECTIONS

To make a week's worth of chicken feet soup use 28 chicken feet. Add distilled water, a few slices of ginger root, rice wine, and some shiitake dried mushrooms. Rice wine and the shiitake mushrooms are optional and just for flavor. Combine everything in a large cooking pot, bring to a boil, and then simmer for two hours. When the soup is milky white, it's ready. Put the soup in seven containers for seven days. Either discard the feet or eat them together with the soup. You can add the soup to other soup recipes such as chicken soup. You can also pour the soup into ice cube trays and freeze it. You can then add an ice cube into a bowl of your chosen soup. Chicken feet soup works best to enlarge breasts if consumed every day.

add an ice cube into a bowl of your chosen soup. Chicken feet soup works best to enlarge breasts if consumed every day.

Try each breast enlargement program for a minimum of one full year. When little improvement is seen after one year, move on to the next program. Choose only one program to follow, but don't mix and combine supplements from other programs because this will confuse the body and cause problems with hormonal balance.

Take phytoestrogens on an empty stomach or wait two to three hours after eating to take them. Bovine ovary is best taken with food. Spread out supplement doses throughout the day.

Alcohol, sugar, and simple carbohydrates increase insulin levels and should be eliminated during a natural breast enlargement program. Increased insulin is directly linked to increased levels of testosterone, which converts into DHT and inhibits estrogen activity.

Caffeine and carbonated drinks like soda can interfere with the proper absorption of herbs. If you must have caffeine then try consuming it at least a couple of hours before or after taking herbal supplements.

Most women have the most success following a breast enlargement program during the spring and summer. During the summer, serotonin levels are higher in the body, which encourages breast enlargement. During the darker days of the year, the serotonin/melatonin ratio is tilted toward melatonin. Melatonin is antigonadotropic, which hinders breast enlargement. To get maximum growth of breasts make sure to get at least fifteen minutes of sunlight per day.

During any natural breast enlargement program, regular cleansing breaks are necessary in order to regulate hormonal levels. Follow each breast enlargement program for three months followed by a one-month cleansing break. A cleansing break should consist of taking only milk thistle, S-Adenosyl methionine (SAM), and 200 milligrams of diindolylmethane (DIM). Women who are on an estrogen program can also take the herb vitex as directed on the label.

Certain tests must be taken while following a breast enlargement program in order to monitor hormonal balance. Estrogen Metabolism Assessment is a test that evaluates how estrogen is being processed in the body and should be taken every four to five months. A Female Comprehensive Hormone Panel Blood Test should be taken every six to eight months to identify hormone imbalances.

Many women get permanent results in the enlargement of their breasts, but some have needed to use a maintenance dosage of 100 milligrams of bovine ovary or 100 milligrams of each phytoestrogen once per day after following a breast enlargement program.

PUERARIA MIRIFICA ESTROGEN PROGRAM

PHYTOESTROGEN

Pueraria Mirifica

Suggested Dose: 500 milligrams morning and 500 milligrams evening (1,000 milligrams per day) on days five to twelve

GALACTAGOGUE

Goat's Rue

Suggested Dose: 1,000 milligrams, three times per day (3,000 milligrams per day) on days five to twelve

PROGESTERONE

Mexican Wild Yam

Suggested Dose: 1,000 milligrams, three times per day (3,000 milligrams per day) on days eighteen to twenty-four

ANTIANDROGEN

Saw Palmetto Berry

Suggested Dose: 500 milligrams morning and 500 milligrams evening (1,000 milligrams per day)

GROWTH SUPPORT

Bovine Colostrum

Suggested Dose: 400 milligrams per day on days five to twelve

MSM and Vitamin C

Suggested Dose: 3,000 milligrams twice per day (6,000 milligrams per day) of MSM along with 1,000 milligrams of vitamin C, twice per day

Gelatin Capsules
Suggested Dose: 3,000 milligrams per day

Flaxseed Oil Softgel
Suggested Dose: 1,000 milligrams, three times per day (3,000 milligrams per day)

Borage Seed Oil
Suggested dose: 1,000 milligrams per day

Multivitamin
Suggested Dose: 400 milligrams of magnesium, 50 micrograms of B12

Kelp Iodine Capsule
Suggested Dose: 225 micrograms per day

CLEANSING BREAK
Every three months, use only DIM, SAM, milk thistle, and vitex for one month

HERBAL ESTROGEN PROGRAM

PHYTOESTROGEN
Hops
Suggested Dose: 1,000 milligrams, three times per day (3,000 milligrams per day)

Fennel Seed
Suggested Dose: 1,000 milligrams, three times per day (3,000 milligrams per day)

Fenugreek
Suggested Dose: 1,000 milligrams, three times per day (3,000 milligrams per day)

PROGESTERONE
Mexican Wild Yam
Suggested Dose: 1,000 milligrams, three times per day (3,000 milligrams per day)

ANTIANDROGEN
Saw Palmetto Berry
Suggested Dose: 500 milligrams morning and 500 milligrams evening (1,000 milligrams per day)

GROWTH SUPPORT
Bovine Colostrum
Suggested Dose: 400 milligrams per day

MSM and Vitamin C
Suggested Dose: 3,000 milligrams twice per day (6,000 milligrams per day) of MSM along with 1,000 milligrams of vitamin C, twice per day

Gelatin Capsules
Suggested Dose: 3,000 milligrams per day

Flaxseed Oil Softgel
Suggested Dose: 1,000 milligrams, three times per day (3,000 milligrams per day)

Borage Seed Oil
Suggested Dose: 1,000 milligrams per day

Multivitamin
Suggested Dose: 400 milligrams of magnesium, 50 micrograms of B12

Kelp Iodine Capsule
Suggested Dose: 225 micrograms per day

CLEANSING BREAK
Every three months, use only DIM, SAM, milk thistle, and vitex for one month

BOVINE OVARY ESTROGEN PROGRAM

GLANDULAR
Bovine Ovary
Suggested Dose: 500 milligrams, four times per day (2,000 milligrams per day)

ANTIANDROGEN
Saw Palmetto Berry
Suggested Dose: 500 milligrams morning and 500 milligrams evening (1,000 milligrams per day)

Spearmint Tea
Suggested Dose: 3 cups per day

GROWTH SUPPORT
Amino Acid Blend
Suggested Dose: 1,200 milligrams of L-arginine, 1,200 milligrams of L-lysine, 1,200 mg of L-ornithine, 500 milligrams of L-tyrosine, and 2,000 milligrams of L-glutamine, every night before bedtime

Whey Protein Powder
Suggested Dose: 25 grams, twice per day (50 grams per day)

MSM and Vitamin C
Suggested Dose: 3,000 milligrams twice per day (6,000 milligrams per day) of MSM along with 1,000 milligrams of vitamin C, twice per day

Gelatin Capsules
Suggested Dose: 3,000 milligrams per day

Flaxseed Oil Softgel
Suggested Dose: 1,000 milligrams, three times per day (3,000 milligrams per day)

Borage Seed Oil
Suggested Dose: 1,000 milligrams per day

Multivitamin
Suggested Dose: 400 milligrams of magnesium, 50 micrograms of B12

Kelp Iodine Capsule
Suggested Dose: 225 micrograms per day

CLEANSING BREAK
Every three months, use only DIM, SAM, milk thistle, and vitex for one month

AYURVEDIC ESTROGEN PROGRAM

PHYTOESTROGEN
Shatavari Extract
Suggested Dose: 1,000 milligrams, three times per day (3,000 milligrams per day)

GALACTAGOGUE
Goat's Rue
Suggested Dose: 1,000 milligrams, three times per day (3,000 milligrams per day)

ANTIANDROGEN
Saw Palmetto Berry
Suggested Dose: 500 milligrams morning and 500 milligrams evening (1,000 milligrams per day)

Spearmint Tea
Suggested Dose: 3 cups per day

GROWTH SUPPORT
Amino Acid Blend
Suggested Dose: 1,200 milligrams of L-arginine, 1,200 milligrams of L-lysine, 1,200 mg of L-ornithine, 500 milligrams of L-tyrosine, and 2,000 milligrams of L-glutamine every night before bedtime

MSM and Vitamin C
Suggested Dose: 3,000 milligrams twice per day (6,000 milligrams per day) of MSM along with 1,000 milligrams of vitamin C, twice per day

Gelatin Capsules
Suggested Dose: 3,000 milligrams per day

Flaxseed Oil Softgel
Suggested Dose: 1,000 milligrams, three times per day (3,000 milligrams per day)

Borage Seed Oil
Suggested Dose: 1,000 milligrams per day

Multivitamin
Suggested Dose: 400 milligrams of magnesium, 50 micrograms of B12

Kelp Iodine Capsule
Suggested Dose: 225 micrograms per day

CLEANSING BREAK
Every three months, use only DIM, SAM, milk thistle, and vitex for one month

HERBAL PROGESTERONE PROGRAM

PROGESTERONES

Chasteberry
Suggested Dose: 1,000 milligrams, three times per day (3,000 milligrams per day)

Mexican Wild Yam
Suggested Dose: 1,000 milligrams, three times per day (3,000 milligrams per day)

ANTIANDROGEN

Saw Palmetto Berry
Suggested Dose: 500 milligrams morning and 500 milligrams evening (1,000 milligrams per day)

GROWTH SUPPORT

Bovine Colostrum
Suggested Dose: 400 milligrams per day

MSM and Vitamin C
Suggested Dose: 3,000 milligrams twice per day (6,000 milligrams per day) of MSM along with 1,000 milligrams of vitamin C, twice per day

Gelatin Capsules
Suggested Dose: 3,000 milligrams per day

Flaxseed Oil Softgel
Suggested Dose: 1,000 milligrams, three times per day (3,000 milligrams per day)

Borage Seed Oil
Suggested Dose: 1,000 milligrams per day

Multivitamin
Suggested Dose: 400 milligrams of magnesium, 50 micro-grams of B12

Kelp Iodine Capsule
Suggested Dose: 225 micrograms per day

CLEANSING BREAK
Every three months, use only DIM, SAM, and milk thistle for one month

FIRMNESS

Firmly shaped breasts are a sign of youth and fertility. After breast-feeding, weight loss, or upon reaching a certain age, breasts begin to sag and lose their shape. In medical terminology, sagging breasts are referred to as breast involution.

Some women avoid breastfeeding believing that it results in sagging breasts. However, a study found that breastfeeding does not result in sagging breasts. In the study, age, BMI, number of pregnancies, and smoking were discovered to be the main factors resulting in sagging breasts. During pregnancy, the Cooper's ligaments, which help maintain the structural integrity of the breasts, may stretch as the breasts get fuller and heavier. The stretching of the Cooper's ligaments contributes to sagging breasts after pregnancy, regardless of whether a woman breast-feeds or not. Being overweight can have a similar effect.[28]

Breasts need proper support during activity to be kept firm. When breasts bounce during active sports, such as tennis or

FIRM BREASTS PROGRAM

MSM and Vitamin C
Suggested Dose: 3,000 milligrams, twice per day (6,000 milligrams per day) of MSM along with 1,000 milligrams of vitamin C, twice per day

Collagen, Types 1 and 3
Suggested Dose: 3,000 milligrams, twice per day (6,000 milligrams per day)

Flaxseed Oil Softgel
Suggested Dose: 1,000 milligrams, three times per day (3,000 milligrams per day)

Borage Seed Oil
Suggested Dose: 1,000 milligrams per day

jogging, the Cooper's ligaments within the breasts can become stretched or even torn. A good sports bra can help prevent this.

Nutritional supplements may be helpful in slowing or preventing the progress of sagging breasts. However, supplements cannot reverse sagging breasts. Vitamin C and MSM are very important for collagen synthesis, which helps the Cooper's ligaments maintain the structural integrity of the breasts. Supplementing with collagen and essential fatty acids (EFAs) may also be helpful.

The most effective method of lifting the breasts is cosmetic surgery. A breast lift, also known as mastopexy, is a surgery performed on the breasts to lift and reshape them. However, keep in mind that a breast lift surgery does not alter the size of the breasts or round out the upper part of the breasts to any significant degree.

Chapter 6: Health

Health is beauty, and the most
perfect health is the most perfect beauty.
- William Shenstone, English poet

*H*ealth is one of the most essential aspects of attractiveness.[1] An improvement in health leads to increased beauty-score ratings. Traditional Chinese medicine (TCM) practitioner and author Dr. Xiaolan Zhao said, "Health is beauty and without health there is no beauty." She preaches, "As long as your health is good, you are beautiful. Your eyes are shining, your hair is shining." Perfect health gives a glow to the skin, a shine in the eyes, a sparkle to the hair, and a lean body shape.

A healthy woman is highly attractive to men because she is more likely to have healthy children and is better able to care for them. Men unconsciously detect health through beauty. Research confirms that a woman with a beautiful face is healthier.[2][3] Symmetry is a sign of genetic quality and health. As a woman gets older, her face deviates from perfect symmetry.[4] Features can also deviate from perfect symmetry due to parasite infection or reduced immunocompetence.[5]

Health can be detected through behavior. A healthy woman has vibrant energy and positive emotions. Illness causes negative emotions and fatigue. Scientists are also discovering that positive emotions can promote health.

Gaining and maintaining health takes commitment and is not always easy. American author Mark Twain said, "The only way to keep your health is to eat what you don't want, drink what you don't like, and do what you'd rather not."

Sages from around the world have taught that nothing is more valuable than health. "Health is the greatest gift," said Indian spiritual leader Gautama Buddha. Chinese philosopher Lao Tzu said, "Health is the greatest possession." American author Harriet Beecher Stowe said, "A woman's health is her capital."

DISEASE RESISTANCE

The foundation of health is being disease resistant since disease renders the body incapable of survival and leads to death. Disease resistance is built through proper diet, supplements, and health treatments. American inventor Thomas Edison said, "The doctor of the future will give no medicine, but will instruct his patients in the care of the human frame, in diet and in the cause and prevention of disease."

The uninformed believe that conventional medicine is the best and most effective system of health care. It is important to examine the motives of powerful health corporations since health care is a very profitable business. John Dalberg-Acton said, "Power tends to corrupt, and absolute power corrupts absolutely."

The pharmaceutical companies (Big Pharma) are an enormously powerful force. They have the power to control which "peer-reviewed" research gets published, which in turn has an influence on which drugs get prescribed. They also have the power to produce advertising campaigns that influence opinions about health care.

Although conventional medicine is useful for severe pain and medical emergencies, it should be used with great caution. According to an extremely comprehensive report entitled "Death by Medicine," the conventional medical system is now the number one cause of death, followed by heart disease and cancer. The number of deaths caused by conventional medicine is an astounding seven hundred thousand per year. Each year, approximately two million American hospital patients experience adverse drug reactions (ADRs) to prescribed medications.[6] American sociologist Ivan Illich said, "Modern medicine is a negation of health. It isn't organized to serve human health, but only itself, as an institution. It makes more people sick than it heals."

The World Health Organization (WHO) issued a fact sheet entitled "Medicines: corruption and pharmaceuticals." It reports that US$4.1 trillion is spent globally on health services each year with US$750 billion spent in the pharmaceuticals market. "Corruption in the pharmaceutical sector occurs throughout all stages of the medicine chain, from research and development to dispensing and promotion," the fact sheet reads. According to WHO data, unethical practices such as bribery, falsification of evidence, and mismanagement of conflicts of interest are "common throughout the medicine chain."

An article entitled "Forbidden Cures—Suppressed 'Alternative' Therapies" by Ken Adachi states: "Orthodox or Allopathic Medicine utilizes poisonous substances (drugs) in non-lethal dosages in order to suppress symptoms in an affected area. This approach neither addresses the cause of the disease condition, nor is it responsible for healing the patient. Rather, the use of drugs often will temporarily mask the outer manifestations of the malady, while at the same time, drive the disease deeper into the body...only to reappear at a later date, as a more serious, and chronic health threat. They want people to keep on coming back for more treatments and more drugs. A cured patient is a lost source of income. A sick patient who is marginally 'improved' is a manageable patient. The profits from the so called 'health-care' industry are staggering!"

A naturopathic doctor (ND), holistic physician (MD), herbalist, and holistic health practitioner addresses the main causes of disease, which are toxicity, oxygen deficiency, nutrient deficiency, electromagnetic radiation, and stress. The common belief among many holistic health experts is that if you eliminate the cause of disease then you can effectively treat and prevent disease.

Dr. Richard Schulze, one of the leading authorities in the world on natural healing and herbal medicine, said, "Your body has a blueprint, a schematic of what perfect health is and is constantly trying to achieve this perfect health for you."

Nature has the cure for every disease and "we only have to find those cures," said ancient Greek physician Hippocrates. He is known as the "father of medicine." His therapeutic approach was based on the healing power of nature.

Herbs and natural remedies are the medicine of the past and the medicine of the future. The Bible foretells, "The leaves were used for medicine to heal the nations" (NLT, Revelation 22:2).

> "Your body has a blueprint, a schematic of what perfect health is and is constantly trying to achieve this perfect health for you."
> - Dr. Richard Schulze

Nature offers natural alternatives to pharmaceutical drugs. The roots and leaves of every herb have very specific medicinal properties. Some of the most effective prescription drugs are derived from plants. Digitalis, a drug used to stimulate the heart, comes from the herb foxglove. The tranquilizer reserpine comes from the herb snakeroot. Snakeroot was used for thousands of years in India for its calming effect. Quinine is derived from Peruvian bark and is used for reducing fever, especially malarial fever. Morphine and codeine are made from the herb opium poppy (Papaver somniferum).

Conventional medicine should only be used when absolutely necessary, such as to relieve severe pain. However, there are natural remedies available for the relief and prevention of mild to moderate pain.

Aspirin contains acetylsalicylic acid, which is a semisynthetic derivative of the herb white willow bark, containing salicin. Aspirin is one of the only drugs promoted by some experts of integrative medicine, such as Dr. Andrew Weil, as fairly safe and even beneficial to use. However, as with all drugs, it still has some side effects such as irritating the stomach lining.

Informed women take the herb white willow bark instead of aspirin because it does not appear to be as irritating to the stomach lining and is more effective than aspirin because of other active compounds that are found in the whole herb but not the drug. Meadowsweet is useful for the relief of joint and muscle pain. Magnesium, 5-HTP, feverfew, and butterbur are useful for headaches and migraines.

Peppermint is one of the world's oldest medicinal herbs and is scientifically proven to be effective for relieving headaches when applied topically to the temples and forehead. In a double-blind, placebo-controlled, randomized crossover study, patients who applied peppermint oil experienced pain relief.[7] In a second double-blind, placebo-controlled crossover study, peppermint oil reduced headache intensity after fifteen minutes. There was no difference in effectiveness between peppermint oil and acetaminophen.[8]

CMO (cerasomal-cis-9-cetylmyristoleate) is a naturally derived substance that may be effective for all forms of arthritis, especially osteoarthritis and rheumatoid arthritis. CMO treats the cause of arthritis by reprogramming the immune system so that it no longer views its own tissues as foreign, and stops attacking them. Sea cucumber has also been used as an effective treatment for arthritis.

Proper diet prevents and even reverses disease. Many ancient civilizations have effectively used food as medicine to treat and prevent disease. "Let thy food be thy medicine and thy medicine be thy food," said Hippocrates.

Phytochemicals are compounds that occur naturally in produce. There are many phytochemicals with the ability to treat a variety of diseases. The anticancer drug paclitaxel is a phytochemical initially extracted and purified from the Pacific yew tree.

The Dean Ornish Program, developed by Dean Ornish, MD, is scientifically proven to reverse heart disease.[9] A study conducted in Greece found that those consuming the lowest amount of vegetables had about ten times the breast cancer risk of those consuming the highest amount of vegetables.[10]

The work of Dr. Weston A. Price clearly shows how the excellent health of many native cultures rapidly declined once they began consuming an unhealthy diet consisting of sugar, alcohol, processed grains, pasteurized cow's milk, and packaged foods.

Dr. Weston Price and his wife traveled around the world in search of the secret to health. He investigated some of the most remote areas in the world. He observed minimal tooth decay and overall excellent health in groups of people who ate their indigenous foods. He found that when these people were introduced to an unhealthy diet, signs of poor health quickly became quite evident. Incomplete development of the face and body, crooked teeth, and disease became common. Dr. Price documented his work in the book, *Nutrition and Physical Degeneration*. The book contains photographs of the physical degeneration caused by an unhealthy diet.

Degeneration caused by an unhealthy diet has also been observed through studies on animals. When fed diets that were lacking in essential nutrients, animals produced offspring that had abnormalities such as missing eyeballs, displaced organs, extra or missing limbs, deformed bones, two faces, and intestines outside of the body.

Seneca, a Roman philosopher said, "Men do not die, they kill themselves." This is true today, since many women consume foods that cause disease. Even some natural foods are best avoided due to their naturally high toxin content.

Canned, boxed, and frozen foods have no enzymes. Even raw foods may be enzyme deficient if they are picked before they are ripe. Enzymes develop only when the plant ripens in the soil. Irradiating food or treating it with preservatives can also destroy enzymes. Food lacking enzymes is not digested properly and putrefies in the colon.

Packaged meals contain monosodium glutamate (MSG). The effect of MSG in the body has been linked to strokes, nervous system infections, and a large number of diseases such as lupus, cancer, chronic hepatitis, and neurodegenerative diseases.[11]

All processed foods contain low potassium and high sodium. Max Gerson, MD, a German physician who cured cancer and other diseases nutritionally, believed that excess sodium is a major cause of cancer. He believed that the entrance of sodium and loss of potassium in cells initiates disease. To prevent cancer, Max Gerson recommends keeping potassium levels high and sodium levels low in the body.

Aflatoxins are toxic metabolites produced by certain fungi on foods. Research has shown that aflatoxin can cause liver cancer.[12] [13] Peanuts contain the fungus *Aspergillus flavus* and its mycotoxin, aflatoxin. Corn and edible mushrooms also have high levels of poisonous and carcinogenic fungi.[14] Research has found that corn consumption is associated with death from cancer of the esophagus and gastric cancer.[15] [16] Studies show that mushroom consumption can induce cancer.[17] Commercially stored grains also develop mycotoxins. Researchers found an association between patients consuming stored grains and esophageal cancer.[18] Brewer's yeast has been shown to cause breast cancer. Products containing brewer's yeast include bread, muffins, cakes, pies, pastries, and cookies. It would be best to avoid all commercially prepared baked goods.[19]

Wine vinegar and white vinegar contains acetic acid, which causes anemia and cirrhosis. These vinegars are found in pickled foods. On the other hand, apple cider vinegar contains malic acid, which has beneficial effects on health.[20]

Alcohol consumption is linked to many illnesses.[21] Research has found that alcohol consumption increases the risk of certain cancers, including breast cancer.[22] A study of over one million middle-aged British women concluded that for every additional drink regularly consumed per day, the incidence of breast cancer increases by eleven per one thousand.[23] Binge drinking of four to five drinks increased the risk of breast cancer by up to 55 percent.[24]

Some types of fats are healthy while other types of fats cause disease. Heating unsaturated fats causes them to become toxic and harmful. All hydrogenated and partially hydrogenated oils have been overheated. To prevent disease, avoid all margarine, shortening, foods containing partially hydrogenated vegetable oil, pastry, and fried and deep-fried foods.[25] Saturated fats such as coconut oil, palm oil, and butter are acceptable to use for cooking at higher temperatures. Monounsaturated fats such as olive oil can also stand up to medium heat. Polyunsaturated fats such as vegetable, seed, and nut oils are best left out of cooking.

Oily fish are a good source of vitamins A and D, and are rich in omega-3 fatty acids. For this reason the consumption of oily fish can be beneficial. However, women must be careful about the type of fish they consume, especially when pregnant.

Fish and shellfish have been shown to contain varying amounts of heavy metals, particularly mercury and fat-soluble pollutants from water pollution. They often concentrate mercury in their bodies in the form of methylmercury, a highly toxic organic compound of mercury. Methylmercury is not soluble and thus is not excreted from the body.[26] Methylmercury readily crosses the placenta and can harm an unborn baby.[27] Species of fish that are long-lived and high on the food chain, such as marlin, tuna, shark, swordfish, king mackerel, tilefish, northern pike, and lake trout, contain high concentrations of mercury. Swordfish and bluefin tuna have been found to have the highest concentrations of mercury of all fish species.[28] Fish and shellfish have also been found to possess lead and cadmium.[29]

Women who would like to reap the health benefits of fish can consume wild-caught Alaskan salmon instead of Atlantic or Norwegian salmon. A study found that wild Alaskan salmon had the lowest level of contaminants compared to Atlantic salmon and organically farmed Norwegian salmon.[30] Studies show that farmed salmon has consistently higher levels of contaminants than wild salmon.[31][32][33]

Women should consume fish in moderation (once a week). A study that analyzed mercury levels in humans from thirty-two locations in thirteen countries found that mercury levels were highest in the group that ate fish once or more a day.[34]

A study concluded that the benefits of fish intake exceed the potential risks. Moderate consumption of fish, especially species higher in omega-3, reduces risk of coronary death by 36 percent and total mortality by 17 percent.[35]

Frequent consumption of sugar is very unhealthy. For many women, the main concern is that the consumption of sugar causes premature aging.[36] Sugar causes the skin to age by changing the structure of collagen.[37][38] High sugar intake increases advanced glycation end products (AGEs), which are sugar molecules that attach to and damage proteins in the body. AGEs speed up the aging of cells, which may contribute to a variety of chronic and fatal diseases.[39]

Sugar produces a rise in triglycerides, a leading cause of heart disease.[40] Sugar feeds cancer cells and has been connected with the development of cancer of the breast, ovaries, prostate, rectum, pancreas, biliary tract, lung, gallbladder, and stomach.[41][42][43][44][45][46] Sugar can also cause arthritis, multiple sclerosis,[47][48] diabetes,[49][50] osteoporosis,[51] Alzheimer's disease,[52] cataracts,[53] kidney damage,[54] and adrenal glands dysfunction.[55]

Natural and artificial sugar substitutes are available. However, artificial sweeteners have been linked to increased cancer risk.[56][57] Long-term, high-dose use of artificial sweeteners have been linked to headaches, seizures, blindness, and cognitive and behavioral changes.[58]

Natural sugar substitutes are highly recommended by naturopathic doctors. Coconut palm sugar, stevia, and raw organic manuka honey are the best natural sweeteners to use and even have some health benefits.

Coconut palm sugar is a very good sugar substitute. It is low on the glycemic index (GI of thirty-five), and is rich in potassium, magnesium, zinc, iron, and B vitamins.

Stevia has been widely used for centuries in South America as well as in Japan. It has zero calories and has a glycemic index of zero, which means it does not raise blood sugar levels at all. Unlike sugar, which has a negative effect on those with diabetes, stevia has been shown to have a positive effect on those with diabetes.[59] Studies have found that stevia improves insulin sensitivity,[60] promotes additional insulin production,[61] and helps to reverse diabetes and metabolic syndrome.[62]

Ancient scriptures promote the use of honey. According to the Bible, "eat honey, for it is good" (NLT, Proverbs 24:13). The Quran calls honey a healing food (Saheeh International English Translation, Surah an-Nahl 16:68–69). In many ancient cultures, raw organic honey was used for medical purposes.[63] The medicinal use of products made by honeybees is called apitherapy. The use of honey and propolis in the treatment and prevention of numerous diseases has been documented.[64][65][66] Honey has demonstrated bactericidal activity against salmonella, shigella, *Escherichia coli*, and *H. pylori*.[67]

Research demonstrates that propolis has the highest antioxidant power followed by royal jelly and honey.[68] Propolis has antibacterial, antifungal, antiviral, antioxidative, antiparasitic, immunomodulating, anti-inflammatory, analgesic, hepatoprotective, and anticarcinogenic effects.[69] Royal jelly has antitumor effects.[70][71][72]

The antibacterial activity in manuka honey is much stronger than in other types of honey.[73] "UMF" stands for "Unique Manuka

Factor" and is a property that gives manuka honey its special healing quality. UMF manuka honey with a rating of 16+ has the highest level of antibacterial activity. Manuka honey is best consumed raw since heat destroys the nutrients in honey.[74]

Cooking foods destroys their nutrients.[75] A German study found that high consumption of raw vegetables appears to decrease the risk of breast cancer. However, the increased intake of cooked vegetables did not contribute to the reduced risk of breast cancer, probably due to the loss of nutrients.[76] If one still chooses to cook vegetables, then steaming appears to be the best cooking method for the retention of nutrients in vegetables.[77]

The International Agency for Research on Cancer (IARC) has concluded that toxic compounds present in cooked meats may cause cancer.[78] Researchers found that high consumption of well-done, fried, or barbecued meats was associated with increased risks of colorectal[78] and pancreatic[79 80] cancers.

A healthy diet consists of at least 80 percent raw foods. It should include a variety of fruits, vegetables (especially dark greens such as kale, broccoli, and collards), whole grains (especially amaranth and quinoa), seaweeds, super foods, nuts, seeds, dark chocolate, and tea. A comprehensive study found that berries, fruits, vegetables, nuts, and dark chocolate have the highest antioxidant levels of all common foods.[81]

The soil on the earth has been depleted, but the sea is rich in minerals. Seaweeds are the richest source of minerals on the planet. They contain higher amounts of both macrominerals and trace elements than do land plants.[82]

The consumption of seaweed is an important factor contributing to the relatively low breast cancer rates reported in Japan.[83] Research suggests that edible seaweeds prevent cancer.[84] Dulse (*Palmaria palmata*) is especially useful for preventing cancer.[85] Kelp has been shown to prevent breast tumors.[86] Wakame and kombu inhibited growth of cancer cells significantly.[87] Mekabu (wakame root) may prevent breast cancer.[88]

The Mediterranean diet is one of the healthiest ways of eating and leads to a longer life.[89] Healthy fats, staples of the Mediterranean diet, keep you feeling fuller longer than diets that restrict or forbid fat altogether. Monounsaturated fats are found in olive oil, nuts, and avocados. Polyunsaturated omega-3 fatty acids are found in fatty fish (salmon, mackerel, and halibut).

Organic produce is nutritionally superior to conventional produce. Organic food is produced without antibiotics, artificial ingredients, chemical preservatives, genetic engineering, irradiation, synthetic fertilizers, synthetic hormones, and pesticides. According to the Environmental Protection Agency, fungicides, herbicides, and insecticides can be carcinogenic. Pesticides can be neurotoxins, endocrine disruptors, and immune system suppressors. When you are not eating food that is 100 percent organic, you are consuming food that contains poisonous chemicals.[90]

Researchers found that antioxidant levels were higher in those consuming a Mediterranean diet consisting of organic food versus one consisting of conventional food.[91] Organic foods contain higher concentrations of antioxidants.[92] Organic foods contain significantly more nutrients with lower amounts of some heavy metals compared to conventional foods.[93 94]

The best possible thing to do is to grow your own fruits and vegetables. Watering the soil with ozonated water and treating it with volcanic or humic shale and seawater will ensure produce that is rich in nutrients.

Many people do not digest and assimilate pasteurized cow's milk properly. Many people do much better on goat's milk.[95] Goat's milk has a higher nutritional value and is better digested than cow's milk.[96]

One of the healthiest foods is organic, raw milk from grass-fed goats. Raw milk was actually used as a medicine in the past to treat, and frequently cure, some serious chronic diseases.[97] Raw milk is superior to pasteurized milk since heating milk destroys some of the nutrients found in milk.[98]

Women who would rather not consume milk can get their calcium from arame, kombu, or sesame seeds. Arame and kombu are extremely high in calcium. Arame contains 1,170 mg/100 g, kombu contains 800 mg/100 g, and sesame seeds contain 630 mg/100 g. Milk (2 percent) only has 297 mg/1 cup.

Drinking tea daily increases disease resistance.[99][100] Drinking between one and six cups per day provides the most health benefits.[101] Tea contains catechins, a type of antioxidant, which provides protection against disease. Green and black teas are especially high in catechins.

The consumption of green tea may be effective in preventing cancer.[102] It may prevent cancer of the breast, esophagus, stomach, pancreas, and colon.[103] It may also be effective in preventing and fighting heart disease, liver disease, Parkinson's disease, diabetes, and inflammatory bowel disease (IBD).[104]

Pu-erh (Yunnan Tuocha) tea is high in antioxidants.[105][106] In China, Pu-erh tea is widely believed to counteract the unpleasant effects of heavy alcohol consumption. It is traditionally used to strengthen the spleen and stomach as well as remove toxins from the body, improve eyesight, and promote blood circulation.

Researchers found that white tea had more catechins than many other types of tea.[107] Green and black teas undergo fermentation after harvest, while white tea is unfermented. Therefore, white tea has the highest concentration of antioxidants.

"[The Budwig Diet] is far and away the most successful anti-cancer diet in the world."
- Dan C. Roehm, MD

Drinking fennel tea after meals is very beneficial, as it is one of the most effective natural aids for digestion. It promotes functioning of the kidneys, liver, and spleen.

Nettle tea is rich in nutrients, natural antihistamines, and anti-inflammatory substances. It is a powerful blood purifier. Herbalists use nettle to treat a wide variety of illnesses.

Johanna Budwig, a German pharmacologist, chemist, and physicist, developed a special diet called the "Budwig Diet" to prevent and cure cancer. The Budwig Diet was reexamined by oncologist, Dr. Dan C. Roehm, MD. He concluded, "This diet is far and away the most successful anticancer diet in the world." The basis of Dr. Budwig's program is the use of flaxseed oil blended with cottage cheese. Dr. Budwig says the absence of essential fatty acids in the human body is responsible for the production of oxydase, which induces cancer growth and is the cause of many other chronic diseases.

BUDWIG BLEND

INGREDIENTS
1 cup organic cottage cheese
2-5 tablespoons of unrefined, cold-pressed flaxseed oil
1-3 tablespoons of freshly ground flaxseed

DIRECTIONS
Mix the organic cottage cheese with the flaxseed oil in a blender.

Women who eat too much meat tend to have red blemishes, bloodshot eyes, thinning hair, and dark circles under the eyes, indicating allergies and a weakened immune system. Meat contains uric acid, hormones, and chemicals. Women who desire a more healthy appearance can consume less meat and eat more organic, plant-based foods.

The most comprehensive study on nutrition ever conducted, *The China Study*, found that diseases such as cancer, heart disease, diabetes, autoimmune diseases, as well as bone, kidney, eye, and brain diseases could be prevented and reversed by avoiding animal-based foods and eating mainly a whole foods, plant–based diet.[108]

An Indian study found that when all rats had been predisposed to get liver cancer after being given aflatoxin, only the animals fed 20 percent protein got liver cancer while those fed 5 percent got none.[109] Tumor growth in rats was greatly enhanced by diets containing 10 percent animal protein and was completely repressed with either 5 percent animal protein or 20 percent plant protein.[110] [111]

The low-protein diets of the Hunza in Pakistan and the East Indian Todas contribute to the world's highest average life expectancy of about 100 years. A diet high in animal protein, common in the Eskimos, Greenlanders, and Laplanders, results in the lowest life expectancy of thirty to forty years.[112]

The glycemic index (GI) is a numerical system of measuring how much of a rise in circulating blood sugar a carbohydrate triggers—the higher the number, the greater the blood sugar response. A low GI food will cause a small rise, while a high-GI food will trigger a dramatic spike. A GI of seventy or more is high; a GI of fifty-six to sixty-nine is medium; and a GI of fifty-five or less is low. Choosing low-GI carbohydrates—the ones that produce only small fluctuations in blood glucose and insulin levels—is the secret to long-term health.

Food combining is a very important nutritional principle to follow. Proper food combining allows the body to digest and utilize the nutrients in foods to their full extent since different food groups require different digestion times. In chemistry, when acids and alkalines come in contact, they neutralize each other. In the same way, when starches and proteins are combined at the same meal, they neutralize each other and result in poor digestion. Improper food combining often leads to indigestion, bloating, gas, abdominal discomfort, and poor absorption of nutrients.[113]

RULES OF FOOD COMBINING

1. Eat carbohydrates and proteins at separate meals.
2. Eat only one type of protein at each meal.
3. Eat proteins and fats at separate meals.
4. Eat fruit alone.
5. Eat melons alone.

Achlorhydria (no stomach acid) and hypochlohydria (low stomach acid) are very common digestive problems leading to

PERFECT 10 DIET

- Organic vegetables (all except corn, mushrooms)
- Organic fruits
- Organic seaweeds (dulse, kelp, wakame, kombu, mekabu, arame)
- Organic dairy (goat's milk, cottage cheese)
- Wild-caught, omega-3-rich fish (Alaskan salmon, mackerel, halibut)
- Organic beans and lentils
- Organic ancient whole grains (amaranth and quinoa)
- Unsalted, unroasted, organic nuts and seeds (all except peanuts)
- Organic teas (green, white tea, pu-erh, fennel, nettle)
- Budwig blend
- Apple cider vinegar
- Natural sweeteners (coconut palm sugar, stevia, manuka honey)

poor nutrient absorption, food allergies, and parasite infections. A naturopath can perform a gastro-test to determine digestive function. Drinking apple cider vinegar before meals may increase hydrochloric acid (HCL) production.

The "Perfect 10 Diet" combines a variety of the most superior health and nutrition principles to create an ideal diet for maintaining perfect health. The foundation of the diet is consuming at least 80 percent raw foods; combining foods properly; and eating mainly organic produce, whole grains, seeds, nuts, and seaweeds, with lower amounts of fish and dairy. The consumption of tea and the Budwig Blend provide additional health benefits. The avoidance of corn, peanuts, mushrooms, sugar, and high–glycemic index foods is also highly recommended.

Annual health testing is vital for the early detection and prevention of disease. A combination of various health tests will provide an accurate and comprehensive picture of current health status. Select at least five different health tests to perform annually.

An annual physical examination involving a visit to a general practitioner and/or an internist will determine general health status.

A comprehensive metabolic panel (CMP) is a panel of tests, frequently part of an annual physical examination that provides important information about the current health status of the kidneys, liver, as well as blood sugar and blood proteins. Complete blood count (CBC) determines general health status and checks for disorders such as anemia and leukemia.

Women should go to a gynecologist for a pelvic exam and Pap test to check for precancerous and cancerous processes in the cervical canal. All women should have an annual Pap test beginning at age twenty-one. Women twenty-one to twenty-nine should get a Pap test every year, then every other year from ages thirty to sixty-four.

Medical thermal imaging (MTI), also called medical thermography, is a full-body scan used as an aid for diagnosis and prognosis, as well as for monitoring health conditions and injuries.

Heart rate variability (HRV) analysis is a powerful indicator of overall health. HRV analysis determines the probability of sudden, unexplained death by measuring minor variation in heart rate. HRV has become the standard test for measuring stress levels.

Electrodermal screening (EDS), also called bioresonance therapy (BRT), is a fairly quick and effective health-testing method. Electrodermal screening measures the electrical resistance on the skin's surface. The purpose is to detect energy imbalances along invisible lines of the body called meridians. It can detect food sensitivities or allergies, nutritional deficiencies, organ stress, parasites, candida, heavy metals toxicity, hormone imbalance, and more.

Live blood analysis (LBA) is the use of high-resolution dark-field microscopy to observe live blood cells. It provides information on the state of the immune system, nutritional deficiencies, oxygen deficiency, toxicity, pH imbalance, candida, parasites, and organ weakness.

Dry blood analysis (DBA) accurately assesses the level of free radical activity or oxidative stress. Excessive levels of free radical activity are associated with strokes and memory loss, as well as with degenerative diseases such as cancer, heart disease, and arthritis.

The complete digestive stool analysis (CDSA) is a test that provides an overview of digestion, absorption, intestinal function, and microbial flora, as well as identifying pathogenic bacteria, parasites, and yeasts.

Biological terrain assessment (BTA), also called quantitative fluid analysis (QFA), is an analysis of blood, urine, and saliva specimens to help detect fungi, pollutants, viruses, environmental poisons, and nutritional and oxygen deficiency.

Quantum biofeedback provides a comprehensive assessment of potential stressors such as viruses, parasites, nutritional deficiencies, allergies, and mental and emotional stress.

Applied kinesiology (AK) is a technique using the manual muscle test (MMT) as a diagnostic tool and for determining appropriate health treatments for the individual. There are many different branches of applied kinesiology. There is considerable evidence about the reliability and validity of manual muscle testing as a diagnostic tool.[114]

A medical intuition evaluation can provide information on current health status, and also identify any mental and emotional factors that could be causing health issues. Many times, a medical intuitive can identify imbalances within the body long before it manifests as disease. Some conventional medical doctors call on medical intuitives for second opinions.

Iridology analysis is a test conducted by a certified iridologist that examines the iris to determine current health status and future health issues. Iridology reveals constitutional strength, inherited strengths and weaknesses, toxicity levels, levels of inflammation, organ structure, and much more. The iridologist will then make personalized recommendations for the improvement of health and prevention of disease.

Hair analysis is a screening test that identifies vitamin, mineral, and nutritional deficiencies as well as heavy metal toxicity. When new hair cells are forming in the hair follicle, they take in traces of substances going through the blood stream of the individual.

The ELISA (enzyme-linked immunosorbent assay) test can determine food allergies accurately. Testing for food allergies is very important. Many women unknowingly consume foods that are harmful to their body.

The indican scale test will determine intestinal or digestive problems. Peter D'Adamo mentions in his book *Eat Right 4 Your Type* that eating according to your blood type can improve the indican scale test score.

A cavitat scan, performed by a biological dentist, is an ultrasound of the jawbone and shows how healthy the bone is under each tooth. Biological dentistry takes into account the impact that dental toxins and hidden infections can have on overall health. Biological dentists believe that many illnesses and some types of cancer can be linked to silver-mercury fillings, allergy-producing dental materials, root canals, hidden infections, and the misalignment of the teeth and jaw. A digital panoramic X-ray will indicate dental toxicity.

Besides annual health testing, other health tests can be administered based on genetic risk for certain diseases. Determine which tests you must have done and how often you must have them done.

The EndoPAT (peripheral arterial tone) system is a noninvasive test that examines the lining of the arteries. Endothelial cells line the inner walls of the heart and blood vessels. Damage to these cells is the earliest clinically detectable stage of heart disease.

Digital pulsewave analysis (accelerated plethysmography) will give early warning signs of heart disease. The test will also help assess nutraceutical and pharmaceutical needs, as well as show the effectiveness of lifestyle changes.

The carotid intima-media thickness (CIMT) test can provide a direct measurement of vascular disease, even in its earliest stages before it causes symptoms or starts to block blood flow.

An oxidata test will measure the free radicals in the body. Oxidation can contribute to cardiovascular disease.

The AMAS test, an early cancer detection test, is useful for women at high risk for cancer, and for follow-up purposes on women already diagnosed with cancer.

Annual breast health checkups are very important for women over the age of forty-five. However, a study showed that 29 percent more women died of breast cancer in those who had been subjected to routine X-ray mammograms for eleven years than in those never having received X-ray mammograms.[115]

Instead of X-ray mammograms, computed tomography laser mammography (CTLM) can be conducted annually. CTLM is a method of looking at the blood flow to the breast. It does not use ionizing radiation (X-ray) or breast compression. CTLM images through breast implants and dense breast tissue.

The circulating tumor cells (CTCs) test can immediately inform physicians if a patient's cancer treatment is working or needs modification. Research suggests that the CTC test can predict overall survival in those with metastatic breast cancer.[116]

Colonoscopy examinations should start at age fifty and be done every ten years. Regular screenings should start at a younger age for women with a family history of colon cancer or polyps. A simple test called a fecal occult blood test (FOBT) can be done every year to screen for changes that may lead to colon cancer.

All women need to undergo an assessment of bone density at the onset of menopause. A woman could lose a large percentage of bone mass during the first few years of menopause and may reach the state of bone loss called osteoporosis. An NTx urine test will determine the rate at which the bones are undergoing bone resorption.

Toxicity of the body is a major cause of illness. The World Health Organization (WHO) has acknowledged that environmental pollution is the underlying cause in nearly 80 percent of all chronic degenerative diseases. In the environment there are tens of thousands of synthetic chemicals. Every year millions of pounds of chemical pollutants are released into the environment, which gets into our water and food. The body is designed to filter some of the toxins, because if it didn't, it would not survive. Health problems occur when toxins are being absorbed into the body faster than they can be eliminated. Therefore, body detoxification is vital in protecting health and preventing disease.[117]

ANNUAL HEALTH TESTING

- Comprehensive Metabolic Panel (CMP)
- Complete Blood Count (CBC)
- Heart Rate Variability (HRV) analysis
- Medical Thermal Imaging (MTI)
- Live and Dry Blood Analysis (LBA)
- Comprehensive Digestive Stool Analysis (CDSA)
- Electrodermal Screening (EDS)
- Biological Terrain Assessment (BTA)
- Quantum Biofeedback
- Applied Kinesiology (AK)
- Medical Intuition Evaluation
- Iridology Analysis
- Hair Analysis
- Indican Scale Test
- Cavitat Scan

Just like the body needs to be regularly cleansed on the outside, the body needs to be regularly cleansed on the inside as well. American athlete Lee Haney said, "A systemic cleansing and detox is definitely the way to go. It is the key to fighting high blood pressure, heart disease, cancer, and other health-related illnesses."

Many naturopaths highly recommended daily cleansing the body internally with warm water and lemon juice. Half a lemon is squeezed into a full glass of warm water and taken first thing in the morning on an empty stomach. Jethro Kloss, author of *Back to Eden*, said, "The medicinal value of the lemon is as follows: It is an antiseptic. It is also anti-scorbutic, a term meaning a remedy which will prevent disease and assist in cleansing the system of impurities."

A woman should perform complete internal body cleansing every three or four years. However, she must remember that before she feels better she will feel worse as the body is eliminating toxins. "The first couple of days on the detox diet aren't pleasant," said Carol Vorderman, a British media personality. During internal body cleansing avoid pasteurized dairy, meat, fried foods, sugar, artificial sweeteners, and table salt.

INTERNAL BODY CLEANSING

COLON (TWO MONTHS)
- Take a complete digestive enzyme complex with every meal.
- Drink one cup of aloe vera gel mixed with one tablespoon psyllium and one tablespoon chlorophyll every night before going to bed, three hours after meals.
- Do one colonic session every week for two months.

CANDIDA/PARASITES (TWO MONTHS)
- Take a tincture of black walnut, wormwood, wormseed, cloves, male fern, goldenseal, and quassia daily.
- Take oil of oregano daily as directed on label.

- Take grapefruit seed extract daily as directed on label.
- Take Compound X Indian salve (American Indian healing formula) herbal paste internally as directed on label.

KIDNEY/BLADDER (TWO MONTH)

- Drink one cup of hydrangea root, uva ursi, gravel root, and marshmallow root twice daily.
- Take hydrangea root capsules as directed on label.

LYMPHATIC SYSTEM/BLOOD (TWO MONTH)

- Take a tincture of cleavers, redroot, red clover, stillingia root, astragalus root, and mullein leaf daily.
- Do rebounding exercise daily.
- Get lymphatic drainage therapy done by a professional twice per week.
- Get matrix regeneration therapy (MRT) done by a professional once per week.
- Use a far-infrared sauna twice a week for forty-five minutes.

HEAVY METALS/CHEMICALS (TWO MONTHS)

- Take indole-3-carbinol capsules as indicated on the label.
- Drink one to two cups of miso tea daily. Prepare by adding one tablespoon of unpasteurized miso paste to one cup of hot water.
- Eat organic dulse and kelp daily. You can add them to soups and salads.
- Take chlorella, apple pectin, and rutin capsules as directed on label.
- Take oral EDTA chelation daily.

Women who would like a quick and simple full-body cleanse can use quantum magnetization technology. Wu Qing Tong Ti Suite is a Chinese detoxification system. It does the work of one hundred internal cleanses in just twenty-four hours. Within twenty-four hours, a variety of brightly colored, toxic substances are excreted from the body.

Women who would like to treat disease and detoxify the body at the same time can use Compound X Indian salve (American Indian healing formula) herbal paste. It has been used successfully for treating many diseases, including cancer, diabetes, lupus, chronic fatigue syndrome, and viral diseases. For the prevention of illness, it is best used once or twice a year for one to two months.

The liver tends to be the most toxic organ in the body and is best cleansed every month. According to many of the top holistic experts and naturopathic doctors, the liver is considered one of the most important organs in the body.

The "Perfect Liver Cleanse" is based on the Gerson Therapy, a therapy that has helped many patients reverse terminal illnesses.[118] Max Gerson, the German physician who developed the Gerson Therapy, wrote, "Cancer develops in a body that has lost the normal functions of the metabolism as a result of chronic daily poisoning accumulated especially in the liver."[119]

The most profound effect that is seen as a result of doing the "Perfect Liver Cleanse" every month is the amazing glow of the skin, a sure sign of good health.

The "Perfect Liver Cleanse" is a comprehensive liver cleanse consisting of vegetable juicing, lemon water, herbal liver tincture (milk thistle, artichoke, dandelion root, burdock, yellow dock, blue flag, Oregon grape root, celandine, boldo, barberry, fringe tree, *Phyllanthus amarus*, picrorhiza, arjuna bark), triphala churna powder, Liv 52, black radish extract, SAM-e capsules, and coffee enemas.

For women with very high levels of chemical contamination, a thoroughly deep internal cleanse can be conducted with the use of a far-infrared sauna. This is best done under the supervision of a medical professional familiar with this cleansing method. Heat from a far-infrared sauna stimulates the body to release toxins through sweating.

The purification rundown, also known as the Hubbard Method, is a regimen of detoxification aimed at removing chemical contamination. Numerous studies on the Hubbard Method consistently show that it is safe and effective in removing toxic contaminants from the body.[200] [201] [203] [204] [205] During the therapy many individuals report noticing yellowish, tan, or even black stains on their towels deposited from their sweat, which indicates a release of toxins.

PERFECT LIVER CLEANSE

For four days consume nothing but fresh organic vegetable juices prepared with a juicer. Use mostly green vegetables, dandelion greens, carrots, beets, apples, and add two drops of organic herbal liver tincture and one teaspoon of triphala churna powder. Drink as much as you want, the more the better. The recommended amount is thirteen glasses. Take Liv 52, black radish extract, and SAM-e capsules as recommended on the label. Apply a castor oil pack over the liver every night. Undergo a coffee enema daily while on this cleanse.

The Hubbard Method consists of using nonflush niacin dosages starting at 100 milligrams and rising to 5,000 milligrams. Dr. Max Gerson used niacin as part of his therapy to treat cancer. A study found that niacin deficiency was common among cancer patients, occurring in 40 percent of the patients studied.[206] However, high dosages of any one vitamin can be toxic. At dosages of over 2,000 milligrams of niacin there are certain health risks.

Cleansing the liver of gallstones is a powerful cleanse for improving health. It is very common for the biliary tubing to be choked with gallstones. When the gallbladder is scanned or X-rayed, no stones are seen. Most gallstones are too small or not calcified and thus not visible on X-ray. Definitive diagnosis of gallstones can be made with ultrasound imaging.

A gallstone flush may be performed every two weeks for up to one full year until the stones are completely removed. Then, a gallstone flush can be performed annually or as needed.

GALLSTONE FLUSH

PRECLEANSE

A parasite cleanse must be done three weeks before doing the gallstone cleanse. Without removing parasites, cleansing of the gallbladder won't be as effective. For one week before doing the gallstone flush take the Chinese herb Gold Coin Grass or drink four glasses of homemade apple juice to soften the gallstones; otherwise, the cleanse may be painful.

DAY 1

Eat very lightly until 2:00 PM, consuming only apples and apple juice. Do not eat any fat or oils. By not eating any fat you allow the bile in the liver to build up and develop pressure. High pressure pushes out more stones. Do not eat anything at all after 2:00 PM. At 6:00 PM, drink a glass of water with one tablespoon of epsom salt. At 8:00 PM, drink another glass of epsom salt in water. At 10:00 PM, prepare half a cup extra-virgin olive oil and half a cup lemon juice. Shake well and drink it within five minutes. Go to bed immediately and lie down on your right side with your knees up to your chest. Try to keep still for at least twenty minutes. Try not to get up during the rest of the night.

DAY 2

Drink a glass of epsom salt in water first thing in the morning. Two hours later, drink another glass of epsom salt in water. After another two hours food can be consumed.

Stress is a definite culprit of disease and has been linked to almost every illness. Studies have found strong associations between psychological stress and cardiovascular disease.[207]

The death of a family member, job loss, or other high-stress event has been shown to occur before the start of an illness. It isn't possible to avoid stress, but there are ways to counteract it.

The most important method of counteracting stress is having a sense of humor and positive thinking.[208] The Greek philosopher Epictetus once said, "It's not what happens to you, but how you react to it that matters." You have the power to choose how you think and feel about any stressful situation.

"Man is ill because he is never still," said German-Swiss physician Paracelsus. It is important to take the time to relax and sit quietly in prayer, yoga, or meditation.

The use of anti-stress herbs will reduce the chances of developing a stress-related illness during periods of high stress. Adaptogenic herbs support the organs and systems affected by stress, causing the body to become more resistant to stress. Calming herbs have a positive effect on the nervous system; they may reduce feelings of nervousness, anxiety, stress, and insomnia. Choose one anti-stress herb or combine a few.

Providing adequate nourishment to the body will prevent illness. Studies show that inadequate intake of several nutrients is associated with chronic disease.[209]

ANTI-STRESS HERBS

ADAPTOGENIC HERBS
American ginseng
Siberian ginseng
Schisandra
Ashwagandha
Rhodiola

CALMING HERBS
Passionflower
Kava kava
Valerian
Skullcap
Motherwort

Nutrients from whole foods have been shown to be superior to synthetic vitamins or minerals.[210] [211] [212] However, the next best thing to consuming whole foods is to take a whole food supplement. Whole food supplements are made from concentrated whole foods. A whole food supplement is absorbed and assimilated by the body better than synthetic supplements.

In the early 1900s, the average person had a one in fifty chance of getting cancer. Today, one in three people in the United States gets cancer.[213] One of the main reasons is the lack of minerals in the soil. Food is grown in mineral-depleted soils, which result in mineral-depleted food, which then result in mineral-depleted people. Some holistic health experts estimate that you have to eat approximately seventy-five bowls to equal the nutritional value of one bowl of salad sixty years ago.

Juicing organic vegetables is an effective way to nourish the body with minerals. Invest in a high-quality masticating juicer, and juice a variety of different vegetables every day. A masticating juicer eliminates the fiber from vegetables and leaves only the concentrated nutrients. You can juice apple, pear, pomegranate, kiwi, carrot, broccoli, beet, kale, chard, collard greens, spinach, celery, cucumber, cabbage, parsley, arugula, dandelion greens, watercress, wheatgrass, and ginger.

Another effective way to nourish the body with minerals is to take ionic minerals. Ionic minerals are one thousand times smaller than colloidal minerals.

Spirulina and chlorella are highly nutritious and a rich source of minerals.[214] Spirulina is about 51 to 71 percent protein, depending on its source. It is a complete protein containing all essential amino acids.[215] [216] Spirulina has immunomodulation, anticancer, antiviral, and cholesterol-reduction effects.[217]

Essential amino acids are not produced by the body and need to be taken in through diet or supplements. Vegans are especially at risk of developing an amino acid deficiency. The nine essential amino acids are histidine, isoleucine, leucine, lysine, methionine, phenylalanine, threonine, tryptophan, and valine.

Free-form amino acid supplements are the best. Free-form amino acids don't require digestion. The term "free-form" means the amino acids move quickly through the stomach and into the small intestine, where they're rapidly absorbed into the bloodstream.

Essential fatty acids (EFAs) are nutrients that humans need to obtain from food or supplements because the body cannot synthesize them.[218] Holistic health experts says that are many illnesses that are associated with a deficiency of omega-3 fatty acids.

Omega-3 is best obtained through wild salmon oil, cod-liver oil, or krill oil. Flaxseed oil can be included in the diet but is not the best source for essential fatty acids (EFAs). Research found that the omega-3 fatty acids in fish oil "are more biologically potent than alpha-linolenic acid," or ALA, found in flaxseed, primrose, and borage oil. In other words, the body uses EPA and DHA from fish oil much more efficiently than omega-3 ALA from flaxseed, primrose, or borage.[219] In

ESSENTIAL DAILY SUPPLEMENTS

- Whole food supplement
- Homemade vegetable juices
- Nano-ionic full-spectrum minerals
- Spirulina/Chlorella
- Free-form amino acid supplement
- EFAs (wild salmon oil, cod-liver oil, or krill oil)

one study, women were given 15,000 milligrams of flaxseed oil (ALA) daily. At the end of twelve weeks not one of the participants had an increase of EPA or DHA within their blood plasma or the red blood cells.[220]

Besides taking essential nutrients daily, certain supplements can be taken to help prevent illness. Select supplements to take based on your genetic health risk and current health status.

There is much evidence showing that pine bark extract has many health benefits.[221] Pine bark was found to be thirteen times more effective as an antioxidant than vitamin C. It was also found to have higher potency as an antioxidant than catechin, grape seed, and grape skin extracts.[222]

Studies show that red ginseng may be effective in preventing cancer.[223] [224] It also helps reverse liver damage.[225] [226]

Numerous research studies and clinical trials have shown alpha lipoic acid (ALA) to have many health benefits and the ability to treat cataracts and various diseases such as cancer, diabetes, heart diseases, neurodegenerative diseases, liver diseases, and AIDS. It elevates tissue levels of glutathione (GSH), the most powerful antioxidant, often referred to as the master antioxidant.[227] Alpha lipoic acid detoxifies the liver. It decreases susceptibility to the damaging effects of ionizing radiation. It increases the effectiveness and life span of other antioxidants, including vitamins C and E, quercetin, and coenzyme Q10.[228]

Coenzyme Q10 is helpful in maintaining a healthy heart. It has been shown to lower blood pressure without significant side effects.[229] Coenzyme Q10 is well documented as a useful treatment for congestive heart failure.[230] Coenzyme Q10 may also be effective in preventing and treating cancer.[231] Supplementing with coenzyme Q10 has resulted in partial and complete regression of breast cancer.[232] Coenzyme Q10 works better when taken with coenzyme A.

Metabolic therapy, which includes coenzyme Q10, alpha lipoic acid, magnesium orotate, and omega-3, has been shown to protect the heart.[233]

Red yeast rice extract lowers cholesterol. Red yeast rice is a source of naturally occurring statins and is less likely to cause the side effects that can occur with cholesterol-lowering drugs.

Ellagic acid is an antioxidant found in blackberries, raspberries, strawberries, cranberries, walnuts, pecans, pomegranates, and wolfberries. Ellagic acid offers protection against cancer.[234] It has been shown to prevent the growth of breast cancer.[235]

Garlic has hypolipidemic, antiplatelet, and procirculatory effects.[236] Aged garlic extract prevents cancer.[237] Natural killer cells are a part of the immune system and play an important role in eliminating viruses and cancer cells from the body. Aged garlic extract increases the number of natural killer cells and improves natural killer cell activity.[238]

Inositol hexaphosphate (IP6) may be an effective substance for the prevention and treatment of cancer. IP6 enhances the anticancer effect of conventional chemotherapy.[239] IP6 has been shown to inhibit the metastasis of human breast cancer.[240] Minerals will be poorly absorbed when taken with IP6; therefore, minerals should be taken two hours away from taking IP6.

Diindolylmethane (DIM) is a compound derived from indole-3-carbinol, found in cruciferous vegetables. DIM promotes healthy estrogen metabolism. It has been found to prevent breast cancer.[241] It also inhibits the growth of ovarian cancer.[242] The combination of DIM and butyrate may be an effective strategy for the prevention of colon cancer. [243]

Many women are found lacking the element germanium. Germanium has been known to aid in the prevention of cancer. Germanium has been reported to boost the immune system, oxygenate the body, destroy free radicals, and detoxify heavy metals.[244] A hair analysis should be done before supplementation with germanium to confirm that the body is depleted in this nutrient. Long-term intake of germanium is not recommended due to increased risk of kidney failure.[245]

A healthy liver is vital to good health. Numerous diseases and conditions are associated with a weakened, damaged, or diseased liver. All women incur some threat of damage or disease to the liver due to environmental pollution, poor eating habits, alcohol, and pharmaceutical drugs. Women with a poorly functioning liver should support the liver on a daily basis.

Glutathione is a key element of the liver's detoxifying process and protects the liver from damaging toxins.[246] The aged and diseased have the lowest levels of glutathione in their body.[247] Reduced glutathione is the best form to take.

Research has shown that silymarin from milk thistle can increase glutathione levels by more than 35 percent.[248][249] Research suggests that milk thistle extract both prevents and repairs damage to the liver from toxins. It improves liver function in those with chronic toxic chemical exposure.[250] Dandelion root also protects the liver and improves liver function.[251][252]

Punarnava (*Boerhaavia diffusa*) prevents damage to the liver.[253][254] Katuki (*Picrorhiza kurroa*), also called hu huang lian in China, has been found to be helpful in recovery from acute hepatitis. Bhumyamalaki (*Phyllanthus niruri*) improves liver function in acute hepatitis and in some cases eliminates the hepatitis B virus (HBV).[256]

Liv 52 prevents and reverses liver toxicity.[257][258] It reduces the harmful effects of gammaradiation.[259] It has been shown to be effective in the treatment of hepatitis, alcoholic liver disease, and liver cirrhosis.[260]

Turmeric and curcumin were found to have anticancer effects[261] and to reverse liver damage.[262] Daruharidra is often combined with tumeric for a more powerful remedy.

Amla, also called Indian gooseberry, is useful for supporting the health of the liver. It also increases disease resistance and prevents cancer.[263] It has important medicinal values and is useful in the treatment of various diseases.[264]

An overwhelming amount of research has firmly established that the consumption of berry fruits prevents disease and improves health.[265] Exotic superberries such as mangosteen, mulberry, noni, goji, and acai have many health benefits and build disease resistance.

Studies have demonstrated that extracts of mangosteen have antioxidant, antitumoral, antiallergic, anti-inflammatory, antibacterial, and antiviral activities.[266] Mangosteen has potential for cancer reversal and prevention.[267]

Research shows that mulberries may play a role in preventing neurological diseases[268] and reducing the risk of cancer.[269] [270]

Noni is reported to have a broad range of health benefits, including the reduced risk of developing diabetes[280] and protection against brain damage.[281]

Goji berries have been shown to contain high levels of antioxidants.[282] In particular, they are high in carotenoids, specifically beta-carotene and zeaxanthin.

Acai berry has been shown to contain high levels of phytochemicals and nutrients.[283]

One of the main causes of disease is oxygen deficiency. Humans were designed to live in perhaps 38 to 50 percent oxygen. Bruce Fife, ND, says, "The earth's atmosphere contained 38 percent oxygen as recently as the mid-nineteenth century. By the 1950s the percentage of oxygen in the atmosphere dropped to 21 percent due to the increase in pollution."[284]

Dr. Otto Warburg was awarded two Nobel Prizes for his lifelong research showing that cancer is caused by damaged cell respiration due to lack of oxygen at the cellular level. Dr. Otto Warburg explains: "The growth of cancer cells is initiated by a relative lack of oxygen. Cancer cannot live in an oxygen-rich environment. Cancer has only one prime cause. It is the replacement of normal oxygen respiration of the body's cells by an anaerobic (i.e., oxygen deficient) cell respiration." Going into greater detail in *The Prime Cause and Prevention of Cancer*, he writes: "...the cause of cancer is no longer a mystery, we know it occurs whenever any cell is denied 60 percent of its oxygen requirements."

In *Flood Your Body With Oxygen*, Ed McCabe explains that healthy cells within the body have an antioxidant shield and are safe from the effects of oxidation. Oxygen selectively attacks only diseased cells due to their damaged or missing antioxidant shielding. It appears that the mechanisms for defense against oxygen damage are impaired in human cancer cells.[285] McCabe states that there are a variety of ways to increase oxygenation in the body. He suggests active oxygen (O1) supplements, medical ozone, or high-dose intravenous vitamin C. When given intravenously, high levels of vitamin C in the blood generate the production of hydrogen peroxide.

Medical ozone is bactericidal, fungicidal, and virucidal. Some studies prove that ozone infused into donated blood samples kills viruses 100 percent of the time.[286] Dr. James Boyce turned two hundred and fifty-four people from HIV+ to HIV- using ozone therapy. He used IV ozone and put them in a hyperbaric oxygen chamber right after injections. He had them on oxygen supplements and made them bathe in a bathtub full of water mixed with a gallon of 35 percent food-grade hydrogen peroxide.

Extracorporeal recirculatory hemoperfusion, also known as ozone RHP, is the most powerful oxygen therapy. It is like a dialysis machine except it oxygenates and cleanses the blood. Ozone IV and ozone RHP have been shown to cure even the most serious illnesses such as AIDS and cancer.[287] Combining ozone therapies with ionic cesium rapidly alkalinizes the body. An alkaline pH of eight is deadly to cancer.

Ionized oxygen therapy (IOT) is an inhaled therapy using medical grade oxygen. It is effective for all illnesses related to oxygen deficiency such as heart disease, cancer, and AIDS.

Chinese or Indian herbal elixirs consumed daily can help prevent disease and aging. A traditional Chinese medicine (TCM) doctor or Indian herbalist can devise a personalized formulation.

Chinese foxglove root (*Rehmannia glutinosa*) has been considered an elixir in Chinese medicine for more than two thousand years, primarily in combination with other herbs. It is used to combat the effects of aging.[288]

Cistanche (rou cong rong) is a Chinese herb that also helps prevent aging.[289] Chinese foxglove root combined with cistanche is a powerful elixir for the prevention of aging.

Shilajit reverses the aging process.[290] Ancient holy texts, over three thousand years old, make reference to shilajit as the "destroyer of weakness." Shilajit has been used by the longest-living people in the world in the Hunza Valley in Pakistan.

Chyawanprash is a comprehensive herbal elixir that increases disease resistance. It improves health when taken frequently.[291]

Some women may benefit from vitex. Vitex acts on the pituitary gland, which regulates the levels of progesterone and estrogen in the blood. It increases the production of luteinizing hormone (LH) and also mildly inhibits the release of follicle-stimulating hormone (FSH). The result is a shift in the ratio of estrogen to progesterone, in favor of progesterone.[292 293 294] Studies have shown that using vitex once in the morning over a period of several months helps normalize hormone balance and thus alleviates the symptoms of PMS.[295] The amount in most of these trials was 20 milligrams per day.[296 297 298]

A number of herbs help treat menstrual problems. When taken internally, shepherd's purse and agrimony can reduce heavy menstrual bleeding, as well as treat postpartum hemorrhage. Cramp bark relaxes the uterine muscle and relieves cramping. Dong quai has been used for centuries in China for regulating the menstrual cycle for women with excessive or suppressed menstruation.[299] Lady's mantle is also effective for excessive bleeding and cramps.

North American Indians have used false unicorn root (*Chamaelirium luteum*) for centuries. It is one of the best elixirs for strengthening the female reproductive system. It is recommended for dysmenorrhea (painful menstruation), menstrual irregularities, PMS, fibroids, endometriosis, infertility, and morning sickness. It may also help prevent miscarriages.[300]

Pueraria mirifica is very useful for women in menopause. Dr. Wichai Cherdshewasart, a biomedical researcher, has found that 100 milligrams of *Pueraria mirifica* per day helps with menopausal symptoms.[301]

Ginkgo biloba is useful for mature women. It may improve short-term and long-term memory and enhance concentration. It helps in the prevention of neurodegenerative diseases and has cardioprotective, anticancer, and antioxidant effects.[302] Clinical trials have shown ginkgo to be effective in treating dementia.[303]

Pure water is essential for promoting health. The human body is approximately 57 to 75 percent water, depending on age.[304] Ultrapure water should be used for drinking, cooking, tea/coffee water, and bathing/showering.

Tap water contains a multitude of poisonous chemicals. A report by the Ralph Nader Study Group stated, "U.S. drinking water contains more than two thousand toxic chemicals that can cause cancer."[305] The U.S. Council on Environmental Quality said, "Cancer risk among people drinking chlorinated water is as much as 93 percent higher than among those whose water does not contain chlorine." Scientific evidence shows a link between consumption of toxins in drinking water and elevated cancer risk.[306]

The purest water in the world is triple-distilled water. Distilled water has been put through the process of distillation once while triple-distilled water has been put through the process of distillation three times.

Harvey and Marilyn Diamond, authors of *Fit For Life II: Living Health*, said the following in their book: "Distillation provides us with the purest water obtainable." Peter A. Lodewick, MD, author of *A Diabetic Doctor Looks at Diabetes*, says, "Distillation is the single most effective method of water purification."

Distillation, when combined with carbon filtration, will kill and remove 100 percent of bacteria, viruses, cysts, as well as heavy metals and volatile organic compounds. Reverse osmosis is the next best water filtration system. Reverse osmosis, when combined with carbon filtration, provides drinking water that is 98 to 99 percent free of chemicals.

Ultrapure water can be ozonated to make it even purer and turn it into a healing substance.[307] Ozone destroys viruses, bacteria, parasites, and fungi.

There are many myths about ultrapure water obtained from reverse osmosis and distillation. A common myth about ultrapure water is that it leaches minerals from the body. Dr. Andrew Weil said, "While pure water helps to remove minerals from the body that cells have eliminated or not used, it does not 'leach' out minerals that have become part of your body's cell structure."

Another false belief is that ultrapure water has an acidic pH. "As far as acidity goes, distilled water is close to a neutral pH and has no effect on the body's acid/base balance," says Dr. Andrew Weil. The body regulates pH levels constantly to find balance. A healthy body will restore homeostatic pH quickly and easily.

Swimming in chlorinated pools or sitting in a chlorinated hot tub may induce genotoxicity (DNA damage).[308] Carcinogenic by-products have been detected in the blood of those swimming in chemically disinfected water.[309]

Ozone is a much more powerful and safe oxidant than chlorine. Ozone is made from oxygen, or O2, which is converted through electricity to ozone or O3.

It is extremely important to have a shower filter since toxic chemicals evaporate out of the water and are inhaled.[310] Up to one hundred times more toxic chemicals are taken in by showering than by drinking.[311] Women should also avoid steam rooms. Steam rooms are like toxic gas chambers. Use a dry sauna instead of a steam room.

Laptops, microwaves, HD televisions, cell phones, power cables, and high-voltage power lines are sources of electromagnetic frequencies, a form of environmental pollution. Studies strongly confirm that electromagnetic field (EMF) exposure is genotoxic and carcinogenic.[312] Studies show that EMF exposure promotes the development of certain cancers.[313 314]

Ionizing x-radiation, like that used for chest X-rays and other medical procedures, is on the carcinogen "Group 1" list compiled by the International Agency for Research on Cancer (IARC). High-frequency radiation is a source of serious biological damage and can cause diseases such as leukemia or bone, breast, and lung cancer.[315] Since X-rays are a proven carcinogen, it is best to stay away from them whenever possible. CT scans have even stronger radiation than regular X-rays. Select X-ray alternatives whenever possible such as ultrasound or magnetic resonance imaging (MRI).

Microwave ovens should not used for heating foods or liquids. Microwaving food damages its nutritional value. Broccoli heated in the microwave lost up to 97 percent of its beneficial antioxidants. By comparison, steamed broccoli lost 11 percent or fewer of its antioxidants.[316]

Cell phones emit radiofrequency electromagnetic fields (RFEMF), a form of nonionizing radiation. Tissues nearest to where the phone is held can absorb this energy. Tissue damage from wireless microwave radiation is known to be as cumulative as that from ionizing radiation. A substantial number of published studies have convincingly demonstrated that radiofrequency electromagnetic fields have a genotoxic effect.[317] [318 319] Any agent that has a genotoxic effect is suspected to be cancerogenic.

Studies found a consistent association between the use of mobile or cordless phones and brain tumors (astrocytoma and acoustic neuroma). The risk is highest among those who had used a cellular phone for ten years or more.[320 321 323]

A study found that cellular phone use increases the risk of parotid gland tumors (PGT). Approximately 70 percent of these tumors are of a benign nature, while the remaining cases are malignant and the prognosis is poor with an average survival of four to seven months.[324] The risk of getting a parotid tumor is 58 percent for those that made more than five thousand calls during their lifetime.[325]

Swedish scientists found highly significant evidence for serious neuronal damage in the brains of exposed rats after exposure to microwaves from cellular phones.[326]

Every woman who cares about her health will use an EMF radiation-protection chip on her cell phone. A radiation-protection chip will neutralize harmful effects of EMF. Women can also wear a personal EMF protection shield in the form of a necklace or bracelet. All commonly used electronic devices such as laptops and tablet PCs should also have a protection chip applied onto it.

The body regenerates through rest and relaxation, which tends to be done in the home. Creating a healthy home environment will promote good health.

Mikhail Tombak, PhD, author of *Can We Live 150 Years?* considers the health of the spine to be the foundation of good health. To keep the spine healthy and strong, sleeping on a firm mattress and low pillow is vital. The vertebrae are correctly positioned on a firm mattress and a low pillow. Sleeping on a soft mattress and high pillow bends the thoracic vertebrae and worsens the liver's function.[327]

Conventional mattresses contain flame retardants, carcinogenic chemicals, and pesticides. An organic and chemical-free mattress is grown, processed, and manufactured with no synthetic chemicals.

A magnetic mattress pad uses the power of magnetic therapy to improve sleep. Several clinical trials have found that sleeping on a magnetic mattress pad can greatly improve the quality of sleep. After six weeks of sleeping on a magnetic mattress pad, women with fibromyalgia reported less pain, sleep disturbance, fatigue, and next-day tiredness.[328] The weight of evidence from well-conducted controlled trials suggests that static magnets have the ability to provide pain relief.[329]

Indoor air is often more polluted than outdoor air, which can be a dangerous health threat.[340] A high-quality, high-efficiency, particulate air (HEPA) purifier will filter indoor air. A study found that a HEPA filter and electrostatic precipitator systems removed dust particulates and gaseous contaminants better than other air-filter technologies.[341]

Houseplants are very beneficial for filtering indoor air. Plants can also reduce dust accumulation by as much as 20 percent. Indoor dust can contain microbes, allergens, and numerous other substances that can cause health problems.[342]

Research by NASA showed that certain houseplants are more efficient at filtering the air than others. The best houseplants for filtering indoor air include gerbera daisy (*Gerbera jamesonii*), peace lily (*Spathiphyllum* 'Mauna Loa'), bamboo palm (*Chamaedorea sefritzii*), Janet Craig (*Dracaena deremensis* 'Janet Craig'), mother-in-law's tongue (*Sansevieria laurentii*), Red-edged dracaena (*Dracaena marginata*), florist's chrysanthemum (*Chrysanthemum morifolium*), and English ivy (*Hedera helix*).[343]

According to NASA, one plant should be used for every 100 to 120 square feet of office or living space, and the plants should be in at least six-inch containers with nothing covering the potting soil.[344]

Volatile organic compounds (VOCs) are solvents that get released into the air as paint dries. These compounds vaporize and emit gases, even long after paint has dried. According to the U.S. Environmental Protection Agency, some VOCs are suspected carcinogens. Select nontoxic, zero-VOC paint and finishing products for indoor painting.

There are many effective health treatments and devices that help improve or restore health. French physician Jacques-Arsène d'Arsonval said, "I am convinced that the therapy of the future will employ heat, light, electricity and other physical agents yet unknown."

Electromedicine is the medical field concerning application of electromagnetic energy (electricity or magnetics) to the body to restore health. Dr. Robert C. Beck and Royal Rife have promoted electromedicine as being able to kill or disable pathogen-

> ## THE PERFECT HOME ENVIRONMENT
>
> - EMF radiation home protection
> - Organic, chemical-free, firm mattress
> - Magnetic mattress pad
> - High-efficiency particulate air (HEPA) purifier
> - Air-cleaning houseplants
> - Non-toxic paint

ic microbes (viruses, bacteria, fungi) and parasites in the body. Electrical engineer and inventor Nikola Tesla said, "You see, electricity puts into the tired body just what it most needs— life force, nerve force. It's a great doctor, I can tell you, perhaps the greatest of all doctors." Electrotherapeutic devices come in different forms for different uses.

The clinical use of electrochemical treatment (EChT) in China indicates that it is a safe and effective therapy for treatment of localized malignant as well as benign tumors. The five-year survival rates after having received EChT for thyroid tumor is 99 percent, skin cancer is 80 percent, laryngeal cancer is 67 percent, and breast cancer is 50 percent.[345] EChT treatment of cancers in mice resulted in at least partial regression or disappearance of tumor.[346] Research shows that the combination of electrotherapy with immunotherapy resulted in higher cure rates in mice.[347]

Microcurrent electrical therapy (MET) may be the best treatment for many pain-related disorders, providing fast relief of symptoms and promoting healing.[348]

TENS stands for transcutaneous electrical nerve stimulation. It is a method of pain relief. TENS therapy has been useful for almost every type of pain. The most common reason for prescribing TENS is for chronic low-back pain.

The SCENAR device is medical technology that stimulates the nervous system to teach the body to heal itself. It can be effective for a very broad range of diseases.

Some use the violet ray daily to increase their disease resistance and to treat various diseases. One of the major benefits of the device is stimulating superficial circulation.

Intranasal light therapy (ILT) is a portable personal-use technology that delivers light of a selected wavelength and dosage into the nasal cavity, stimulating the body to heal itself. When used on a daily basis it boosts the immune system. It has been applied for blood stasis syndrome of coronary heart diseases[349] and brain diseases.[350]

Low-level laser therapy (LLLT) is showing promise in the treatment of a wide variety of medical conditions. It is effective in relieving short-term pain for rheumatoid arthritis and osteoarthritis.[351]

Many patients testify to the benefits of therapeutic touch (TT). A study found that patients receiving TT had significantly greater reduction in pain and greater reduction in anxiety than did those who received a placebo TT treatment.[352] Another study found that 90 percent of patients receiving TT experienced a sustained reduction in headache pain.[353] TT was found to decrease pain in elders with degenerative arthritis, compared with progressive muscle relaxation (PMR) or routine treatment.[354]

Chiropractic treatments treat and prevent disorders of the neuromusculoskeletal system. They are effective for the treatment of low-back pain, neck pain, headaches, and a number of extremity joint conditions.[355]

Myotherapy is a form of manual medicine focusing on the diagnosis, treatment, and management of musculoskeletal pain.

Myofascial release is used to improve the health of the muscles and fascia, improve circulation, and restore good posture.

Myofascial release was specifically designed to relax the fascia throughout the whole body. Myofascial release therapy has been used effectively for low-back pain, neck stiffness, shoulder injuries, arthritic conditions, and sports injuries.

Prolotherapy is a nonsurgical and permanent treatment for chronic pain. Prolotherapy uses a dextrose (sugar water) solution, which is injected into the ligament or tendon where it attaches to the bone. This causes localized inflammation in these weak areas, which then increases the blood supply and flow of nutrients, and stimulates the tissue to repair itself. It is successful with many different types of musculoskeletal pain such as arthritis, back pain, neck pain, fibromyalgia, sports injuries, unresolved whiplash injuries, carpal tunnel syndrome, chronic tendonitis, partially torn tendons, ligaments and cartilage, degenerated or herniated discs, TMJ, and sciatica.

Swedish massage has been shown to be helpful in reducing pain, joint stiffness, and improving function in those with osteoarthritis of the knee over a period of eight weeks.[356] It also increases circulation.

Deep tissue massage physically breaks up very tight and tense areas in the muscles using targeted, firm pressure to affected areas. Deep tissue massage can help those with stiff backs, tightness in the shoulders, and low-back pain.

Acupressure involves placing physical pressure, by hand, elbow, or with the aid of various devices, on different pressure points on the body. Acupressure may be beneficial for pain, postoperative nausea and vomiting.[357]

Acupuncture involves the insertion of very thin needles into the skin at specific points on the body to restore proper energy flow. According to the World Health Organization (WHO), acupuncture is effective for treating certain conditions. Clinical evidence suggests that acupuncture is effective for treating some conditions.[358] Acupuncture appears to be most effective for reducing certain types of pain such as migraines,

183

neck disorders, tension-type headaches, and peripheral joint osteoarthritis.[359]

Amma massage therapy is one of the oldest forms of massage therapy. It combines various body massage techniques such as pressures, frictions, vibrations, or tapping. Amma massage removes energy blockages by applying pressure at specific points to restore health.

Shiatsu massage therapy is very similar to amma massage and may be equally effective. There are different types of shiatsu massage. A study found that shiatsu is effective for body structure problems, tension, and stress.[360]

The Bowen Technique is a dynamic system of muscle and connective tissue therapy. It decreases musculoskeletal pain and improves joint mobility. There is a link between limited flexibility and development of neuromusculoskeletal symptoms. A study found that a single treatment of the Bowen Technique was found to increase flexibility, and continuing increases in flexibility levels were observed over one week.[361]

The Jaffe-Mellor Technique (JMT) reduces the pain and in many cases completely removes all the symptoms associated with osteoarthritis, rheumatoid arthritis, fibromyalgia, Crohn's disease, and other autoimmune diseases.

Neural therapy can often instantly resolve chronic pain, in many cases permanently. It is successful in eliminating migraine headaches. It works by eliminating "interference" fields in the body through the injection of anesthetics in specific areas of the body.

Polarity therapy is a natural health care system based on the human energy field. Polarity therapy clears any blockages and restrictions in the human energy field. The undisturbed flow and balance of the electromagnetic energy in and around the body is the basis for health. Gamma radiation decreased in 100 percent of patients during polarity therapy.[362]

NeuroModulation Technique (NMT) is a method of accessing and modulating the autonomic control system. It appears to be effective for allergies, arthritis, multiple sclerosis, Crohn's disease, IBS, and gastric reflux disease.

Mild allergies are very common in women and cause symptoms such as red eyes, itchiness, runny nose, eczema, and hives. The Nambudripad's Allergy Elimination Technique (NAET) is a noninvasive, natural solution to eliminate allergies of all types. A published case study has shown that four weeks of NAET treatment relieved eczema that was caused by food allergies. After three years, foods that had previously caused allergic reactions no longer caused any reactions.[363]

Homeopathic remedies are highly diluted substances. There has been no strong evidence to support homeopathy in many cases.[364] A systematic review concluded that "homeopathy cannot be viewed as an evidence-based form of therapy."[365] However, homeopathy may be effective for treating allergies and influenza.[366]

A clinical trial found that patients diagnosed with moderate to severe seasonal allergies who were treated with homeopathy for four weeks showed significant improvement.[367] One study found a success rate of 87.6 percent in one hundred and forty-seven patients who received homeopathic allergy treatment.[368] Another study found a response rate of 82.6 percent in the homeopathy group compared to 67.3 percent in those receiving conventional medicine for allergies.[367]

Allersodes are homeopathic preparations of highly diluted allergens used to desensitize the body to the allergen gradually. Annual desensitization may be necessary. Allersodes can be used along with methylsulfonylmethane (MSM) to reduce symptoms of allergies.[368] Start taking at least 6,000 milligrams of MSM per day for three weeks and then reduce to 3,000 milligrams per day.

Immunotherapy, consisting of sublingual immunotherapy (SLIT) or allergy injections, is an effective allergy treatment method.[367] It is similar to homeopathic allergy treatment. A small dose of an allergen is given under the tongue or through an injection, which reduces sensitivity to allergens.[368]

Sufficient amounts of sun exposure can help prevent disease. According to William B. Grant, PhD, breast cancer risk could be cut in half by sufficient vitamin D levels from sun exposure.[369] Scientific evidence shows that vitamin D deficiency has been associated with increased risks of deadly cancers, cardiovascular disease, multiple sclerosis, rheumatoid arthritis, and type 1 diabetes mellitus.[370] [371]

Women need 3,000 to 5,000 IU of vitamin D daily. Brief daily exposure to the sun (ten minutes) without sunscreen is the preferred source of vitamin D. For vitamin D supplementation, blood testing of vitamin D levels is recommended to help determine the correct amount of supplemental vitamin D to take daily.

Moderate sun exposure is healthy and necessary, but excessive sun exposure is known to cause skin cancer. Nutritional supplements will help increase resistance against skin cancer.[372] Use a sun protection supplement, also known as a sunscreen pill, when exposed to the sun.

Exercise is extremely important for the maintenance of good health and prevention of disease. "Those who think they have not time for bodily exercise will sooner or later have to find time for illness," said English statesman Edward Stanley. Increasing frequency of exercise was associated with reduced risk of death.[373] Women who exercise more frequently lived longer.[374] Improving fitness can reduce the risk of death by 44 percent.[375]

American cartoonist Randy Glasbergen said, "What fits your busy schedule better, exercising one hour a day or being dead twenty-four hours a day?" Regular exercise decreases risk of cardiovascular disease, type 2 diabetes, osteoporosis, colon, and breast cancer. Exercise has been shown to improve insulin sensitivity, reduce blood pressure, reduce inflammation, and decrease blood coagulation.[376]

Breast cancer risk was reduced among women who engaged in seven or more hours of moderate-to-vigorous exercise per week.[377] Among patients with cancer, physical activity equivalent to walking one or more hours per week was associated with improved survival compared with no physical activity. The greatest benefit was observed among cancer survivors who performed exercise equivalent to three to five hours per week at an average pace.[378]

Regular exercise slows down aging.[379] "We do not stop exercising because we grow old—we grow old because we stop exercising," said Dr. Kenneth H. Cooper, MD. Exercise is a natural anti-aging therapy. A lack of exercise actually speeds up aging.[380] Chronic stress is known to accelerate aging. However, exercise can buffer the impact of stress on aging.[381]

Aerobic exercise is known to strengthen and enlarge the heart muscle, which improves the efficiency with which it pumps, resulting in better circulation. Better circulation results in better health. American athlete Jack LaLanne said, "Yes, exercise is the catalyst. That's what makes everything happen: your digestion, your elimination, your sex life, your skin, hair, everything about you depends on circulation."

Exercise promotes positive change in all aspects of health, whether physically, emotionally, or mentally. "Movement is a medicine for creating change in a person's physical, emotional, and mental states," said Carol Welch, founder of BioSomatics Education, a method that supports the body's capacity to be posturally functional by overcoming neuromuscular conditions.

Exercise should be gentle on the joints and increase lymph flow. Rebounding, which consists of jumping on a mini trampoline, is one of the most effective types of exercise, especially because of the effect it has on the lymph.[382] Research comparing rebounding exercise to treadmill jogging found no significant difference between the benefits of these two exercises.[383] However, the main benefit of rebounding is low trauma to the joints.

Rebounding is a good alternative for those who have joint problems or have been told to avoid high-impact exercise.[384]

Swimming is a low-impact exercise since it places no pressure on the joints. Regular swimming builds endurance, muscle strength, cardiovascular fitness, posture, and flexibility.

Meditative movement (MM) is a type of exercise that has many proven health benefits. MM includes qigong, tai chi, and yoga. What categorizes MM as different from traditional forms of exercise is the coordination of body, breath, and mind to achieve deep relaxation.[385] MM is classified as a mind-body intervention.

Qigong is a relaxing form of exercise with anti-aging benefits.[386] [387] Qigong means "working with the qi." Regular qigong practice is very beneficial for long-term health and longevity.[388]

Qigong and tai chi are close relatives; however, qigong is designed for building health while tai chi places more emphasis on the self-defense aspects of the training.

There are a wide range of health benefits from doing either qigong or tai chi. A comprehensive review of studies on qigong and tai chi found over one hundred different physiological and psychological health outcomes.[389]

Yoga is a combination of breathing exercises, physical postures, and meditation that has been practiced for thousands of years in India. Studies comparing the effects of yoga and exercise seem to indicate that yoga may be as effective as or even slightly more effective than exercise at improving a variety of health-related outcome measures.[390]

A study showed that practicing yoga improves cardiovascular function, reduces stress, improves sleep patterns, as well as enhances muscular strength and body flexibility.[391] An Indian study found that yoga treats and prevents heart disease.[392] Salivary cortisol (a measure of stress) decreased significantly after participation in a yoga class. Women also reported lower stress levels and anxiety after three months of practicing yoga.[393]

Negative emotions are like poison in the body. Hate injures the one who hates far more than the one hated.[394] "Good humor is the health of the soul, sadness is its poison," said British statesman Lord Chesterfield. Every cell in your body is affected by every single thought you have and can make you feel good or bad. Those who have negative thoughts are more likely to get cancer.[395]

German New Medicine (GNM) is a healing protocol based on the idea that disease has its root in negative emotions. Dr. Ryke Geerd Hamer, the founder of GNM, discovered that all diseases, including cancer, originate from unexpected shock experience. This is verifiable and visible on brain scans.

Ancient wisdom has taught that positive emotions promote health. The Bible says, "A cheerful disposition is good for your health" (MSG, Proverbs 17:22). English essayist Joseph Addison said, "Cheerfulness is the best promoter of health." Swiss philosopher Henri Frédéric Amiel said, "Happiness gives us the energy, which is the basis for health." Research has shown that positive emotions and happiness have positive health benefits.[396]

Researcher Barbara Fredrickson suggests relaxation therapies and finding meaning in life to produce positive emotions. Traditional forms of relaxation such as prayer, yoga, qigong, or meditation have proved helpful.[397]

New Thought spiritual leader Emmet Fox said, "If you have no time for prayer and meditation, you will have lots of time for sickness and trouble." There is strong scientific evidence that relaxation strengthens the immune system.[398]

Spiritual or religious beliefs, or otherwise appreciating the meaning of life, can also increase positive emotions. American gospel singer Mahalia Jackson said, "Faith and prayer are the vitamins of the soul; man cannot live in health without them."

Comprehensive research shows that those who are religious or spiritual have better physical health, decreased risk of disease, and longer life span, regardless of other variables such as social support or financial status.[399] [400] [401] [402] There have been very few studies to show any negative effects of having religious beliefs.[403]

A woman must have a belief system for her "own good" (ERV, Isaiah 48:17). Formulate a belief system by selecting a religion or philosophy that resonates well with you. Do a thorough search and study all the major world religions and philosophies. God says, "For I know the plans I have for you...plans to prosper you and not to harm you, plans to give you hope and a future. You will seek me and find me when you seek me with all your heart" (NIV, Jeremiah 29:11, 13).

HIGH ENERGY

High energy levels are a sure sign of good health since illness results in low energy levels and fatigue. High energy levels allow a woman to accomplish tasks effortlessly and engage in social activities. At times, energy levels may be low due to stress, excessive work, or lack of sleep, and quick energy boosts are required.

Nutritionists warn that stimulants such as energy drinks and soft drinks contain high amounts of caffeine and sugar, which are unhealthy and cause multiple health problems when overused. Sugar can be considered a poison. It weakens the immune and endocrine systems, and is the cause of various diseases and chronic conditions.[404]

Daily consumption of 500 to 600 milligrams of caffeine represents a significant health risk.[405] In large doses, caffeine can be profoundly toxic, resulting in hypertension, vomiting, arrhythmia, tachycardia, cardiac arrest, convulsions, coma, and death.[406]

A systematic review found that consumption of soft drinks was associated with an increased risk of several medical problems such as the development of type 2 diabetes, hypocalcemia, and hypertension. In a study of over ninety-one thousand women followed for eight years, those who consumed one or more servings of soft drink per day were twice as likely to develop type 2 diabetes.[407]

Energy drinks have been reported in association with serious adverse effects.[408] A study found that healthy adults who drank two cans per day of a popular energy drink experienced an increase in their blood pressure and heart rate.[409] Another study found that the consumption of energy drinks increases the risk of heart attacks.[410]

Instead of consuming energy drinks, which are filled with sugar and artificial additives, you can get the specific energy-boosting nutrients from supplements. Caffeine, taurine, glucuronolactone, B vitamins (niacin, pantothenic acid, B6, B12) are the functional ingredients in energy drinks that reduce tiredness.[411] These ingredients work particularly well in the first hour of consumption to boost energy and alertness.[412] The mixture of these four ingredients improves mental performance, mood, and social extrovertedness.[413] These four ingredients also increase physical performance, endurance, and alertness.[414] Energy drinks also contain herbs like guarana and ginseng, and nutrients like amino acids and B vitamins.[415]

Taurine is a sulfur-containing semiessential amino acid that has been found to increase energy levels, alertness, and concentration.[416] Taurine has been shown to increase endurance and performance in athletes.[417] Exercise capacity increased in patients with heart failure who received 500 milligrams of taurine three times a day.[418] Taurine has health benefits as well. A study found that taurine supplementation in combination with exercise prevents hypertension.[419] Taurine can also prevent acetaminophen-induced liver damage.[420]

Glucuronolactone is a substance naturally occurring in the body by metabolism of glucose in the liver. Glucuronolactone is a popular ingredient in energy drinks. Glucuronolactone works best when combined with caffeine and taurine. Those supplementing with 500 to 3,000 milligrams of glucuronolactone typically report higher energy levels and alertness. Research suggests it is safe even with long-term use.[421]

D-ribose is a natural sugar that acts as a source of cellular energy for the synthesis of ATP. It is a popular supplement among endurance athletes. A study found that D-ribose increased energy an average of 45 percent in those with fibromyalgia and chronic fatigue syndrome. Two-thirds of the patients reported improvement of their symptoms in the first twelve days of using D-ribose.[422] Take five grams three times daily to increase energy.

Carnitine has been shown to increase exercise performance.[423] It also appears to have many health benefits. It may be of benefit in treating Alzheimer's disease, HIV infection, chronic fatigue syndrome, and cognitive impairment. It has also been shown to prevent and treat various heart problems.[424]

Guarana is widely used throughout South America. It is a plant that contains caffeine, theophylline, and theobromine. Guarana is a stimulant that increases mental alertness, fights fatigue, and increases stamina. A study found that guarana improved memory, mood, and alertness at low dosages (37.5 milligrams, 75 milligrams) even better than higher dosages (150 milligrams, 300 milligrams). This suggests that the effects cannot be attributed to caffeine alone.[425] A study found that 50 milligrams of guarana extract taken twice daily reduced fatigue in breast cancer patients undergoing chemotherapy.[426] Guarana is safe for long-term use.[427]

Yerba maté contains caffeine, theobromine, and theophylline. It is said to increase energy levels and is less likely to result in jitters, stomach discomfort, or headaches than with other caffeinated drinks like coffee. Yerba maté has many health benefits, including anticancer effects, and may be a better source of antioxidants than green tea or red wine.[428]

Ephedra, also called ma huang, contains a chemical called ephedrine that is chemically related to amphetamine, a drug used to treat attention deficit hyperactivity disorder (ADHD). Ephedra increases energy, alertness, and concentration. It is also known to reduce appetite and promote weight loss. Ephedra is not for long-term use because it has many reported side effects such as hypertension, tachycardia, CNS excitation, arrhythmia, myocardial infarction, and stroke.

NADH, also known as coenzyme 1, is synthesized from niacin, nicotinamide, and tryptophan. It is used to increase energy, mental clarity, alertness, concentration, and reduce jet lag. A study found that NADH improved the symptoms of patients with chronic fatigue syndrome.[429] Another study found that NADH improves cognitive functioning in those with Alzheimer's disease.[430] For those women simply looking to increase their energy levels, they can take 2.5 to 5 milligrams of NADH once in a while when needed. NADH should not be used every day since some women have reported that prolonged use causes mood swings, anxiety, and insomnia.

Coenzyme A (CoA) increases energy and motivation. Coenzyme A plays a vital role in the process by which the cells generate energy from glucose.

Octacosanol might help improve the way the body uses oxygen. It is used to increase energy levels as well as improve strength, stamina, and reaction time.

Myers' Cocktail is an intravenous push that consists of a combination of vitamins and minerals. It boosts energy levels and can also be used to treat conditions such as chronic fatigue syndrome and fibromyalgia.

Deficiency in B vitamins, especially vitamin B12 deficiency, results in low energy levels. B vitamins are water-soluble, which means they are not easily stored in the body and need to be taken from food or supplements. Holistic nutritionists and naturopaths highly recommend food-based sources of B vitamins such as bee pollen or a whole food B-complex formula for increasing energy levels. Vitamin B12 injections may also be recommended, especially for vegans.

Lecithin supplementation increases energy levels. Lecithin is a crucially important nutrient found in every cell in the body. It plays an important role in regulating and controlling the flow of nutrients, as well as waste materials, in and out of a cell. Take one tablespoon of lecithin granules three times daily before meals.

Malic acid is known for its ability to boost energy through its involvement in the Krebs cycle. Malic acid, an organic acid, is sometimes referred to as a fruit acid because it is found in apples and other fruits.

Supplementing with branched-chain amino acids (BCAAs) prior to exercise or physically demanding tasks will increase energy levels and endurance.[431] A pre-workout supplement consisting of amino acids, as well as creatine, taurine, caffeine, and glucuronolactone can improve endurance during exercise.[432]

The caffeine in coffee is a stimulant that increases alertness, energy, and concentration, and is beneficial for treating fatigue.[433] [434]

ENERGY SUPPLEMENTS

- Myers' cocktail
- Taurine
- Glucuronolactone
- D-ribose
- Carnitine
- Guarana
- Yerba maté
- Ephedra
- NADH
- Coenzyme A
- Octacosanol
- Bee pollen/Whole food B complex
- Vitamin B12 injections
- Lecithin granules
- Malic acid
- Branched-chain amino acids (BCAAs)

There is little evidence of health risks and some evidence of health benefits for the moderate consumption of coffee (three to four cups per day).[435]

Several studies have found that moderate coffee consumption may help prevent diseases such as certain types of cancer, type 2 diabetes, Parkinson's disease, Alzheimer's disease, and liver disease.[436] Research suggests that there is an ingredient in coffee that protects against liver cirrhosis.[437] Those drinking four cups of coffee per day had an 84 percent lower risk of cirrhosis,[438] 67 percent lower risk of developing diabetes,[439] 42 percent lower risk of liver cancer,[440] and a 57 percent reduced risk of (non-hormone-responsive) breast cancer.[441] A meta-analysis found that regular coffee drinkers had a reduced risk of bladder, breast, buccal, pharyngeal, colorectal, endometrial, esophageal, hepatocellular, leukemic, pancreatic, and prostate cancers.[442] A meta-analysis found that coffee intake is associated with a reduced risk of endometrial cancer.[443] Women who consumed four cups of coffee per day had a 25 percent lower risk of endometrial cancer than those who consumed less than one cup per day. However, the addition of sugar and cream to coffee could counteract any potential benefits.[444]

Drinking coffee can raise blood pressure briefly, right after consumption.[445] However, a fifteen-year study of over forty-one thousand women found that the risk of death from cardiovascular disease was 24 percent lower among those consuming one to three cups of coffee daily.[446]

A study based on a major European investigation into the effects of diet and lifestyle on health found that people who drank four or more cups of coffee a day were at no higher risk for chronic disease, compared with those who drank less than a cup of coffee a day.[447]

Many holistic health experts and naturopathic physicians have no major concerns with moderate coffee consumption but are against heavy coffee consumption. Naturopaths warn that heavy coffee consumption can lead to adrenal gland exhaustion, digestive disorders, nutrient deficiency, acidic body pH, and dehydration. Naturopaths also warn about the chemicals found in coffee. Coffee is also one of the most heavily chemically sprayed crops. There are more carcinogens in a single cup of coffee than carcinogenic pesticide residues in the average American diet in a year.[448] These chemicals burden the liver so it is less able to detoxify toxins. Organic coffee is a much better option for coffee lovers.

For those who would like to limit their coffee intake, there are coffee substitutes. Maca root boosts energy levels, stamina, and alertness. Maca powder can be added to a fruit smoothie or protein shake. Maca is also available in the form of an instant beverage known as maca coffee, which has a coffee-like flavor.

For women who want mental alertness, matcha green tea is the best option. Matcha green tea has higher concentrations of catechins than other types of green tea. Buddhist monks have drunk matcha green tea for centuries since it helps provide focused attention and alertness for meditation.

There's a difference between the caffeine found in coffee and the caffeine found in green tea. Green tea contains tannin, which slows down the absorption of caffeine into the bloodstream. This means that the caffeine from green tea is released gradually over

MATCHA ENERGY TEA

INGREDIENTS
Organic matcha green tea powder
Rice milk
Raw honey

DIRECTIONS
Put one teaspoon of matcha powder in a bowl. Add a splash of water and mix it thoroughly into a creamy paste. Then pour in hot water or rice milk and mix again until it is frothy and creamy. Add a little raw honey.

the course of six to eight hours, unlike the short burst from coffee. Matcha also contains two special amino acids called theophylline and L-theanine. L-theanine helps to create a state of mental alertness while keeping you relaxed at the same time.[449] Not only does green tea boost mental alertness, it helps prevent cancer and heart disease,[450] making it the healthiest beverage to consume daily. An ancient Chinese proverb says that it is "better to be deprived of food for three days, than tea for one."

Women who are constantly fatigued should visit a medical doctor or naturopathic doctor. Constant fatigue could be a symptom of a medical condition such as chronic fatigue syndrome (CFS), fibromyalgia, anemia, hypothyroidism, hypoglycemia, adrenal fatigue, or depression.

STRONG IMMUNE SYSTEM

The immune system is the body's guardian against illness. It is designed to protect against bacteria, microbes, viruses, toxins, and parasites that invade the body. When the immune system is compromised due to stress, the body no longer has full protection against illness. During high-stress periods, it is vital to boost the immune system.

Sugar suppresses the immune system. Research found that the amount of sugar consumed in two sweetened drinks lowers the immune system by 50 percent for up to five hours after consumption.[451] [452] Sugar contributes to the reduction in defense against bacterial infection.[453] Those consuming sugar are bound to get infections more often.

Instead of snacks made with sugar, eat snacks made with stevia. Stevia does not lower immune system function. Healthy snacks are another option. Nori is a type of seaweed that is full of nutrients (carotene, vitamins A, B, C) and makes a good alternative to chips. Organic nori can be found in snack-sized pieces in health food stores. Kale is one of the healthiest vegetables. It contains vitamins A, C, and K. Kale can be made into delicious-tasting chips.

Vaccines for the prevention of influenza offer no protection against influenza caused by new virus strains. Drugs used to combat influenza may be ineffective for treating influenza pandemics, due to drug resistance.[454]

KALE CHIPS

INGREDIENTS
Kale
Coconut or olive oil
Sea salt

DIRECTIONS
Break kale leaves into bit-sized pieces, and then sprinkle with coconut oil and sea salt. Spread the kale pieces on a baking sheet and bake at 250°F (120°C) for two hours.

Research shows that certain herbs, extracts, and nutrients boost the immune system and are effective in preventing and treating colds and flus.[455]

Echinacea (*Echinacea purpurea*) is one of the most popular herbal products worldwide. Echinacea decreases the incidence and duration of the common cold. Research shows that echinacea decreased the odds of developing the common cold by 58 percent.[456] Echinacea contains potent antiviral agents against the influenza virus.[457]

Astragalus (*Astragalus membranaceus*) has been used in traditional Chinese medicine for thousands of years. It was often combined with other herbs to strengthen the immune system. Goldenseal (Hydrastis canadensis) is a Native American medicinal plant used as an immune stimulant. These two herbs act differently on the immune system, but both are useful for fighting colds and flus.[458]

Cat's claw (*Uncaria tomentosa*) has the ability to stimulate the immune system.[459] It has proven immunoregulatory and antiviral effects.[460] Peruvian Indians have used cat's claw for thousands of years to treat a wide variety of health problems associated with the immune system.

Elderberry (*Sambucus nigra*) has been used for centuries to treat flus and colds. It has been shown to activate the immune system in healthy individuals as well as in those with cancer or AIDS.[461] It has antimicrobial and antiviral activity.[462] A study found that elderberry extract was effective in treating the influenza A and B virus infections.[463]

Ginger (*Zingiber officinale*) stimulates the immune system.[464] [465] It has a long history of medicinal use in various cultures for treating colds, fever, diarrhea, and nausea.[466]

Licorice root (*Glycyrrhiza glabra*) has antiviral effects. It is used in China, India, and Greece for symptoms of viral respiratory tract infections. Studies found that licorice root has a protective effect against the influenza virus.[467] [468] Research suggests that it may be a potential drug for the treatment of bird flu (H5N1).[469] It has been shown to inhibit replication of the SARS virus and may be a potential treatment for SARS.[470]

Schizandra (*Schisandra chinensis*) strengthens the immune system.[471] Schizandra has a stress-protective effect against a broad spectrum of harmful factors.[472]

Picrorhiza kurroa is a medicinal plant that has immunomodulatory activity.[473] [474] It may even be a useful adjuvant for vaccines.[475] In traditional Chinese and ayurvedic medicine, it is used to treat upper respiratory conditions.

Suma (*Pfaffia paniculata*), also known as Brazilian ginseng, has been shown to enhance the immune system and inhibit the development of leukemia.[476] It contains a wide range of essential vitamins, minerals, amino acids, and trace elements, as well as high levels of the element germanium, a powerful natural antioxidant.

Pau d'arco (*Tabebuia impetiginosa*), also known as lapacho, is considered a natural antibiotic. The native Indians have used pau d'arco to treat colds, flus, and fungal infections. Research suggests it is effective against the stomach bacterial infection *Helicobacter pylori*.[477]

Baikal skullcap (*Scutellaria baicalensis*) has been shown to inhibit the influenza virus.[478] It has been shown to provide protection against influenza virus infections, especially when combined with ribavirin, an antiviral drug for severe RSV infection.[479]

Andrographis (*Andrographis paniculata*), also called chuan xin lian in Chinese medicine, is considered a natural antibiotic. It has the ability to enhance immune function.[480] It may even be a potential cancer therapy because of its stimulating effect on the immune system.[481] Research suggests it may be a safe and effective treatment for the symptoms of upper respiratory tract infection.[482]

Mistletoe (*Viscum album*) extract injections strengthen the immune system. A study found that individuals who took mistletoe extract in addition to their standard medical treatment for cancer lived 40 percent longer.[483] It has been shown to enhance immune responses.[484] It has antiviral activity on human parainfluenza virus type 2 (HPIV-2).[485]

β-glucans, also known as beta-glucans, are naturally occurring polysaccharides that are produced by bacteria, yeast, fungi, and many plants. Intensive research has shown that β-glucans enhance immune function as well as reduce susceptibility to infection and cancer.[486] Studies indicate that β-glucans improve the body's immune system defense against foreign invaders such as bacteria, viruses, fungi, and parasites.[487] The role of glucans in cancer treatment, infection immunity, stress reduction, and restoration of damaged bone marrow has already been established.[488] It is well established that mercury suppresses the immune system. β-glucans were able to lower the immunotoxic effects of mercury significantly.[489]

Olive leaf (*Olea europaea*) extract has antioxidant and antimicrobial properties.[490] Research shows that olive leaf extract is effective against *Campylobacter jejuni*, one of the most common causes of stomach flu; *Helicobacter pylori*, which is linked to the development of duodenal ulcers and stomach cancer; and *Staphylococcus aureus*, which can cause a range of illnesses.[491]

Oregano (*Origanum vulgare*) is used for fighting fungal infections, as well as some bacterial infections. It has shown antimicrobial activity against strains of the food-borne pathogen Listeria monocytogenes.[492] It has antibacterial activity against *Staphylococcus saprophyticus*, often the cause of urinary tract infections, and *Bacillus circulans*, which can cause life-threatening blood poisoning.[493] Enteric-coated oil of wild oregano is the best quality available.

Research shows that grape seed extract has antibacterial activity against respiratory diseases.[494] It also has antiviral activity.[495]

Garlic has many beneficial health effects. It prevents colds and flu by boosting the immune system.[496] Aged garlic extract is considered better than raw garlic in boosting the immune system.[497] Research shows that aged garlic extract reduces the severity of colds and flu.[498] Those who take garlic capsules are less likely to get a cold and recover faster if infected.[499]

Oscillococcinum (*Anas barbariae hepatis et cordis extractum*), an extract of duck liver and heart, is a homeopathic medicine that is known to work well if taken at the very first signs of influenza. Research suggests it reduces the duration of influenza.[500]

Influenzinum is an option for those who want to prevent the flu but do not want to be vaccinated. It is a homeopathic remedy used to prevent and treat the flu. It is updated each year based on the flu strains predicted by the World Health Organization. It contains a dilution of the same viral strains as the flu vaccine. The French Society of Homeopathy conducted a survey for the use of Influenzinum over a ten-year period. About 90 percent of those that took Influenzinum preventively did not get the flu and 97 percent had no side effects.[501]

The difference between Influenzinum and Oscilococcinum is that Influenzinum is prescribed for flu prevention and treatment, while Oscilococcinum reduces the symptoms of those who already have the flu.

Scientists have found that acidic ozone water (AOW) can deactivate the influenza A (H1N1) virus very effectively. Acidic ozone water is made from water mixed with a small amount of acid and an ozonized gas.[502]

Research has shown that beta-carotene may be useful for the prevention and treatment of influenza.[503] Beta-carotene improves immune function and helps prevent infections caused by bacteria, viruses, or parasites.[504]

Carotenoids such as lutein, canthaxanthin, lycopene, and astaxanthin have been shown to be as effective, or more effective, than beta-carotene in stimulating the immune system.[505]

Chyawanprash is an ayurvedic formula containing natural herbs, including amla. It enhances the immune system and reduces the chances of infection.[506]

Dimethylglycine (DMG), an amino acid, stimulates the immune system.[507] Scientists found that it increased immune function fourfold.[508]

Vitamin C and zinc are both important for proper immune function and resistance to infections. These two nutrients reduce the risk, severity, and duration of infectious diseases.[509]

A meta-analysis revealed that vitamin C appears to reduce the duration and severity of colds.[510] Research also shows that for those under significant physical stress, vitamin C reduces the incidence of the common cold by 45 to 91 percent and reduces the incidence of pneumonia by 80 to 100 percent.[511] In one study, those reporting cold and flu symptoms were treated with hourly doses of 1,000 milligrams of vitamin C for the first six hours and then three times daily. Cold and flu symptoms decreased by 85 percent.[512]

The best way to take vitamin C is through a whole food supplement vitamin C complex containing amla, camu camu, acerola, and rose hip. Camu camu contains more natural vitamin C than any other edible botanical on the planet.

Zinc plays an important role in maintaining a healthy immune system.[513] When taken within twenty-four hours of the onset of cold symptoms, it reduces the duration and severity of the cold.[514] One placebo-controlled study found that 86 percent of those who took 23 milligrams of zinc gluconate lozenges were symptom-free after seven days.[515]

Zinc acetate, in daily doses of over 75 milligrams, reduced the duration of colds by 42 percent. Zinc salts other than acetate, in daily doses of over 75 milligrams, reduced the duration of colds by 20 percent. A total daily zinc dose of less than 75 milligrams had no effect.[516] It needs to be supplemented for at least five months to reduce the incidence of colds.[517]

Zinc lozenges slowly dissolving in the mouth over a twenty minute period, releasing adequate iZn (18 milligrams), used every two hours, could shorten common colds by six to seven days, but brands of zinc lozenges that do not release adequate iZn have no effect on the common cold.[518] It is important to measure copper levels while taking zinc long-term.

N-acetylcysteine (NAC), a precursor of reduced glutathione, has been in clinical use as a mucolytic drug. The use of N-acetylcysteine during the winter appears to reduce influenza symptoms.[519]

B vitamin deficiency impairs immunity, specifically vitamin B5 (pantothenic acid) and vitamin B6 (pyridoxine).[520] The most absorbable form of B vitamins is a whole food vitamin B complex.

Probiotics enhance the body's immune system[521] and may be useful for disease prevention and treatment, and the prevention of viral infections.[522]

Colloidal silver is considered a natural antibiotic and may be useful for the prevention and treatment of multidrug-resistant pathogenic bacteria.[523] Colloidal silver has been proven effective against several types of viruses and has a lower possibility of resistance compared to antiviral drugs.[524]

Medicinal mushrooms have been used in Chinese medicine for thousands of years. Research has shown that medicinal mushrooms stimulate the immune system and also have antitumor, antiviral, antibacterial, antiparasitic, and antifungal effects.[525] Organic, freeze-dried medicinal mushrooms are the best type available.

Thymus extract has been shown to boost the immune system.[526] It may be helpful for preventing respiratory infections.[527] Sublingual administration of thymus extract allows for better absorption.

Colostrum reduces the incidence of respiratory illness.[528] Colostrum has an antibacterial effect and enhances the immune system.[529]

Lentinan is used widely in Japan and China as a cancer treatment. Lentinan is a beta-glucan isolated from shiitake mushroom (Lentinus edodes) that has immunomodulatory effects.[530] It is useful for those with low immune function, fungal infection, frequent flu and colds, and infectious disease. It has antibiotic, antiviral, and anticarcinogenic effects.[531] Research shows that lentinan stimulates the immune system to help fight bacterial infections such as Listeria monocytogenes.[532] Lentinan must be injected because it is poorly absorbed orally.

Laughter is good medicine and a powerful immune-boosting remedy. British poet Lord Byron said, "Always laugh when you can. It is cheap medicine." Research has shown that laughter improves the functioning of the immune system.[533][534] Norman Cousins, an American political journalist, used laughter and high-dose vitamin C to recover from the chronic disease ankylosing spondylitis.[535] Some hospitals are incorporating humor therapy programs into their therapeutic regimens.

The body naturally makes hydrogen peroxide to fight infections. A hydrogen peroxide bath will increase immunity as it slowly absorbs through the skin. Place one cup of 35 percent food-grade hydrogen peroxide in the bathtub.

IMMUNE-BOOSTING REMEDIES

HERBS

Echinacea

Astragalus

Goldenseal

Cat's claw

Ginger

Licorice root

Schisandra

Picrorhiza kurroa

Brazilian ginseng

Pau d'arco

Elderberry

Baikal skullcap

Andrographis

Mistletoe extract

EXTRACTS

β-glucans

Olive leaf extract

Enteric-coated oil of wild oregano

Grape seed extract

Aged garlic extract

Oscillococcinum

Influenzinum

Acidic ozone water

NUTRIENTS

Carotenoid complex

Chyawanprash

Dimethylglycine

Whole food vitamin C

Zinc lozenges

N-acetylcysteine

Whole food vitamin B complex

Probiotics

Colloidal silver

Organic, freeze-dried, medicinal mushrooms

Raw organic thymus extract

Organic colostrum

Lentinan injections

Humor therapy

Medical doctors give immunization for infectious disease prevention. However, some holistic health experts view vaccines as dangerous. Dr. Viera Scheibner, PhD, is one of the most respected scientists and scholars of vaccine medical data. Dr. Viera Scheibner calls vaccinations "an illness industry," causing degenerative diseases and behavioral problems.

For those who want conventional immunization, it is effective to monitor the level of defense gained by immunization. Antibody titer tests assess the level of defense that the body has developed against infectious disease. This test can determine whether a recent vaccine caused a strong enough response from the immune system. It can also determine whether booster immunization is needed.

Women who choose to avoid vaccinations can use homoeopathic immunization, known as homeoprophylaxis.

Research shows that homeoprophylaxis offers 95 percent protection in the first six months and 91 percent protection over the year against meningococcal disease.[536] During a 2007 leptospirosis epidemic in Cuba, large-scale application of homeoprophylaxis was "strongly associated with a drastic reduction of disease incidence resulting in complete control of the epidemic."[537]

Precaution is essential during travel since travel exposes the body to infections unknown to the immune system. Visit a travel medicine clinic before each and every trip. Travel medicine clinics offer vaccinations that are required or recommended for international travel. Review travel health websites for health and safety information before each and every trip.

Proper hygiene is very important during travel. Frequently disinfecting hands with a hydrogen peroxide spray will prevent infections. It inactivates 99 percent of influenza viruses.[538]

Every woman should have a travel health kit that consists of echinacea, charcoal tablets, probiotics, antibiotics, goldenseal, garlic capsules, colloidal silver, and active oxygen (O1).

A study concluded that if echinacea is taken before and during travel, it might help prevent the development of respiratory infections.[539]

Intestinal infections are the most common condition acquired during travel. Taking probiotics during a trip may decrease the chance of developing an intestinal infection.[540][541] Azithromycin is the preferred treatment when an intestinal infection is complicated by dysentery.[542] When the intestinal infection is moderate to severe it can be treated with fluoroquinolone.[543] The preferred drug for prevention and treatment of intestinal infections caused by E. coli is rifaximin.[544]

Activated charcoal tablets are helpful for food poisoning since charcoal absorbs toxins.[545]

Herbalists consider goldenseal to be a natural antibiotic. Research shows that it is helpful for various bacterial infections.[546]

Garlic is also considered a natural antibiotic. It is scientifically proven effective against bacterial, viral, mycotic, and parasitic infections.[547] Garlic has even been shown to be effective against drug-resistant bacteria.[548] Taking garlic capsules before eating out may help prevent bacteria-caused food poisoning.[549]

Bacteria and viruses are anaerobic, which means they can't survive in oxygen. Active oxygen (O1) has been shown to kill bacteria.[550] Colloidal silver combined with active oxygen (O1) may be even more effective.

Scientists discovered that hydrogen peroxide deactivates viruses.[551] Holistic health experts specializing in oxygen therapies recommend 35% food-grade hydrogen peroxide taken internally for short-term treatment of viral infections. They recommend one drop of 35 percent food-grade hydrogen peroxide taken in one full glass of water on an empty stomach. The dosage is increased every day until reaching twenty-five drops in one glass of water.

Chapter 7: Style

Fashion fades, only style remains the same.
- Coco Chanel, French fashion designer

S tyle is a very powerful nonverbal communicator. It tells others about who you are. Canadian actor Shawn Ashmore said, "Style is a reflection of your attitude and your personality." In other words, you are what you wear.

Fashion and style are not the same. As French fashion designer Yves Saint Laurent once said, "Fashions fade, style is eternal." Stylish items can be worn many times, in many different ways, but fashionable items can only be worn for a short period of time. "Fashion is made to become unfashionable," said French fashion designer Coco Chanel.

Style is about wearing what makes you look your best, while fashion is about keeping up with the latest trends that may not make you look your best. Irish writer Oscar Wilde said, "Fashion is a form of ugliness so intolerable that we have to alter it every six months." Once a fashion trend passes, it is unattractive. "Nothing is so hideous as an obsolete fashion," said French writer Stendhal.

Women of style start trends that endure. "Don't follow trends, start trends," said Frank Capra, American film director. Audrey Hepburn is known for her little black dress (LBD) while Marilyn

Monroe is known for her flowing white dress and red lips. Both these women had a signature look and became style icons.

A stylish woman dresses in a feminine manner. She knows that men are attracted to feminine style, consisting of dresses, high heels, lingerie, jewelry, painted fingernails, and perfume.[1]

Looking stylish is simple and fairly affordable. French fashion designer Christian Dior said, "Simplicity, good taste, and grooming are the three fundamentals of good dressing and these do not cost money."

CLOTHING

Attractive clothing gives a good first impression. A study found that women wearing attractive clothing were perceived more positively and received higher ratings for competence and sociability compared to women wearing unattractive clothing.[2] English clergyman Thomas Fuller said, "Good clothes open all doors."

Attractive clothing is not overly trendy or boyish. The "Man Repeller," a blog designed to highlight the latest fashion trends, has found that some fashion trends are repulsive to men. Trends such as baggy and odd-colored clothing should have no place in a woman's wardrobe.

A stylish woman dresses in a fairly conservative manner to convey luxury. "Some people think luxury is the opposite of poverty. It is not. It is the opposite of vulgarity," said Coco Chanel. Women of very high social class and women of royalty dress conservatively. Derek Blasberg, author of the books *Classy* and *Very Classy*, said, "Cultivating some mystery is still one of the greatest weapons of mass seduction there is."[3] Duchess Kate Middleton is a great example of a conservative style that conveys luxury. She is known for wearing long-sleeved dresses, pencil skirts, and skirt suits.

Developing a style of your own is superior to following fashion trends. Scottish novelist Margaret Oliphant said, "Oh, never mind the fashion. When one has a style of one's own, it is always twenty times better." Women who follow fashion trends don't have much of an identity. Quentin Crisp said, "Fashion is what you adopt when you don't know who you are." Queen Marie of Romania said, "Fashion exists for women with no taste."

Italian fashion designer Gianni Versace suggests, "Don't be into trends. Don't make fashion own you, but you decide what you are, what you want to express by the way you dress and the way to live."

A woman without style dresses in an effort to attract attention. "A lady who dresses in such a manner as to attract attention to her dress is always badly dressed," said Lola Montez, an Irish entertainer and author of *The Arts of Beauty.*

To develop a sense of style you can start by learning from a role model. You may choose a celebrity or model from the past or present. Do not copy her outfits, but simply study and examine every outfit she wears and try to understand how and why her sense of style defines her. Then begin wearing items of clothing that define who you are as a person. Take photographs of yourself in different outfits. Study and examine which outfits suit you and get the opinion of others.

Match your personality to your sense of style. Greek philosopher Epictetus said, "Know, first, who you are, and then adorn yourself accordingly." For example, if you are very feminine then dress in pastel colors and girly designs. If you are an extrovert then dress in bright, eye-catching colors.

Style is developed over many years of careful observation and experimentation. Most women develop a good sense of style from their mid-twenties to early thirties when they know themselves better. Personal style is based on lifestyle factors such as age, career, hobbies, social scene, and personality. You can always hire a personal stylist if you have trouble developing a sense of style.

Simplicity is the art of style. American poet Henry Wadsworth Longfellow said, "In style...the supreme excellence is simplicity." You will look more elegant in simple styles and clas-

"In style...the supreme excellence is simplicity."
- Henry W. Longfellow

sic colors than in overly unique clothing. "Simplicity, carried to an extreme, becomes elegance," said American author Jon Franklin. French writer Stendhal said, "Only great minds can afford a simple style."

A simple style allows for people's attention and focus to go directly to a woman's beauty. British statesman Edward F. Halifax said, "The plainer the dress, the greater luster does beauty appear."

Clothing staples are very stylish and attractive. Clothing staples constructed with high-quality natural fabrics should be in every woman's wardrobe. Cloth-

"The plainer the dress, the greater luster does beauty appear."
- Edward F. Halifax

ing staples should be chosen in classic colors so they never go out of style. Classic colors include white, beige, black, very dark gray, very dark blue, and red.

A well-known brand name and high price does not ensure high quality. Some designer clothing items are constructed with cheap synthetic fabrics such as polyester, rayon, viscose, and nylon, which tend to lose their shape quickly. High-quality natural fabrics like cashmere, silk, wool, cotton, linen, mohair, bamboo, and hemp hold their shape and are long-lasting. Some clothing items combine natural fabric with synthetic fabric. Accept no more than 5 percent synthetic fabric content in each clothing item. The best clothing designers use 100 percent natural fabric in each clothing item, including the lining of coats, dresses, and purses. Many British fashion designers take the lead in using high-quality natural fabrics and stylish designs.

Many fabrics (including natural fibers) are treated with toxic chemicals that may involve detergents, petrochemical dyes, formaldehyde, volatile organic compounds (VOCs), dioxin-producing bleach, and chemical fabric softeners. Many of these additives are known to cause illnesses such as cancer. Why pay a high price for designer brand name clothing that may be harmful to your health? To protect your health, select clothing made with organic and natural fabrics that have not been treated with chemicals.

The right shoes are an important finishing touch to an outfit. French fashion designer Christian Dior said, "You can never take too much care over the choice of your shoes. Too many women think that they are unimportant, but the real proof of an elegant woman is what is on her feet." High heels do more than most women realize. "You put high heels on and you change," said Spanish shoe designer Manolo Blahnik. French shoe designer Christian Louboutin said, "Shoes transform

TOP SIX TOXIC FABRICS

1. Polyester is the worst fabric you can buy. It is made from synthetic polymers that are made from esters of dihydric alcohol and terpthalic acid.

2. Acrylic fabrics are polycrylonitriles and may cause cancer, according to the Environmental Protection Agency (EPA).

3. Rayon is recycled wood pulp that must be treated with chemicals like caustic soda, ammonia, acetone, and sulphuric acid.

4. Acetate and triacetate are made from wood fibers called cellulose and undergo extensive chemical processing to produce the finished product.

5. Nylon is made from petroleum and is often given a permanent chemical finish.

6. Many of the stain-resistant and wrinkle-free fabrics are treated with perfluorinated chemicals (PFCs).

your body language and attitude. They lift you physically and emotionally."

The best shoes are constructed with suede or leather upper, lining, insole, and outsole. They tend to be a little more comfortable and longer lasting than shoes made with cheap synthetic materials. You can get shoes resoled once they wear down to make them last as long as possible. For women who are conscious of animal rights and refuse to wear anything animal, vegan shoes are an option.

STYLISH CLOTHING STAPLES

COATS
Trench coat
Dress coat
Double-collar jacket
Double-breasted jacket
Peacoat jacket

TOPS
Blazer
V-neck sweater
Cardigan sweater
Turtleneck sweater
Sleeveless turtleneck top
Long-sleeved scoop-neck top
Shell top
V-neck halter-top

BOTTOMS
Slim-leg pants
Roll-up shorts
Pencil skirt

DRESSES
Skirt suit
Mini dress
Sleeveless, knee-length dress
Sheath dress
Maxi dress
Long evening dress

SHOES
4½–inch high-heel classic pumps
4½-inch peep-toe slingback
4½-inch stiletto-heel ankle-band sandal
4½-inch stiletto-heel knee boot

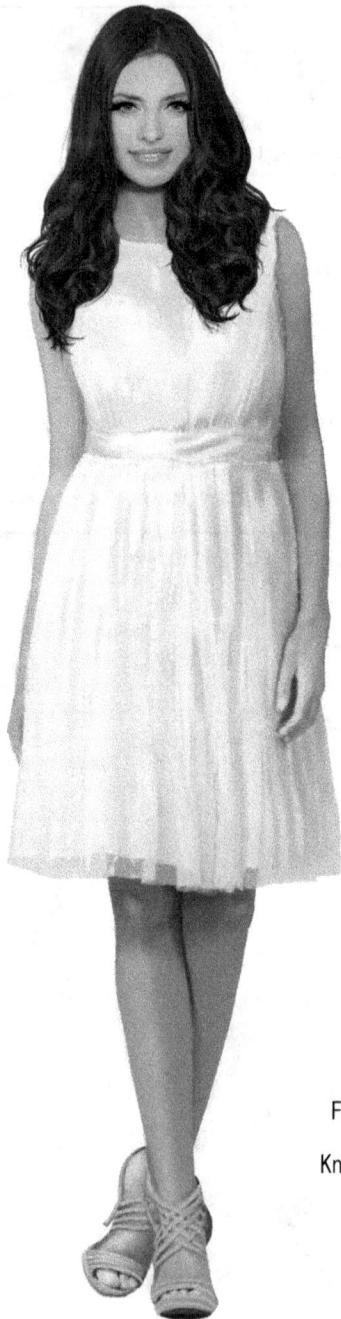

Fashion Figure 1
Sleeveless,
Knee-Length Dress

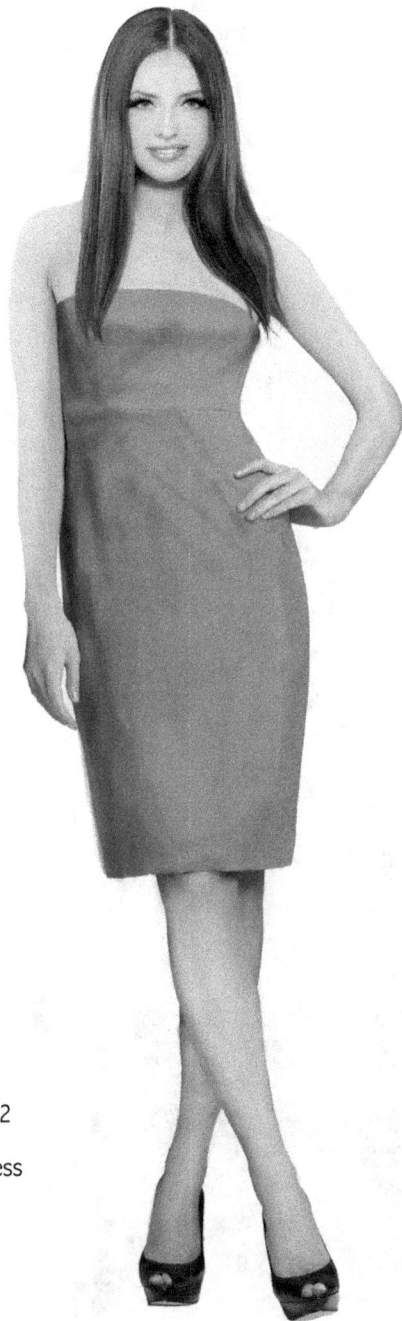

Fashion Figure 2
Strapless,
Knee-Length Dress

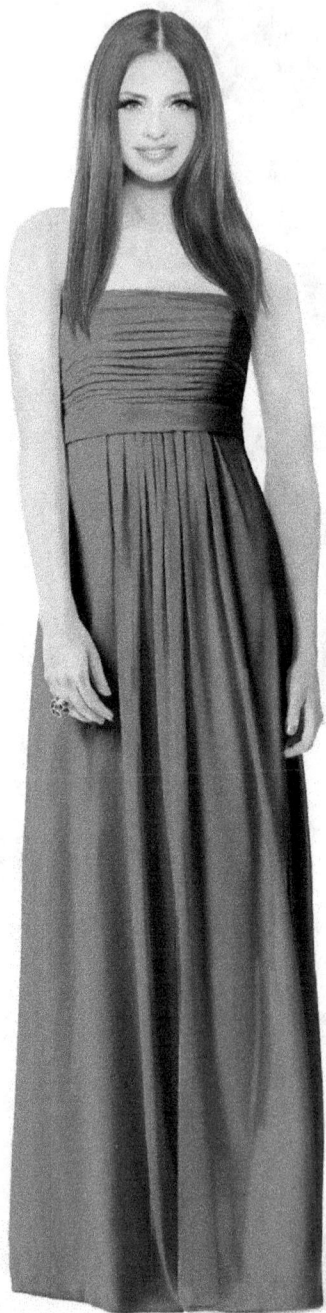

Fashion Figure 3
Strapless, Long Dress

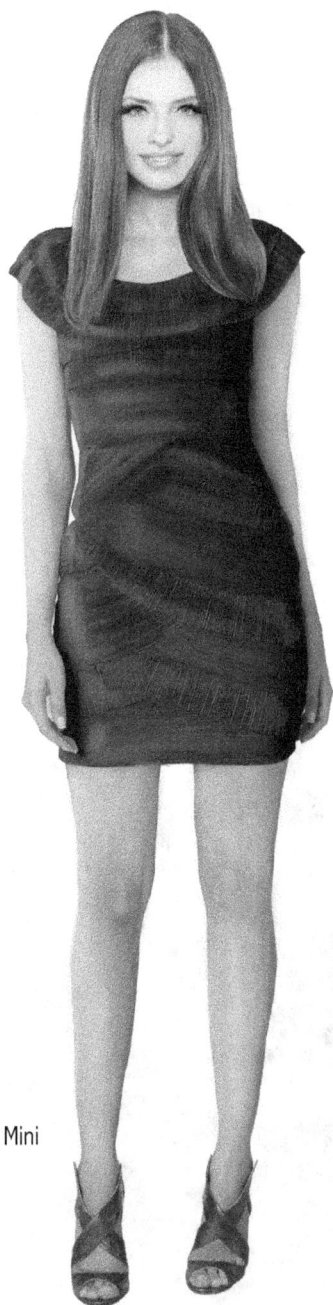

Fashion Figure 4
Cap-Sleeve, Scoop-Neck, Mini

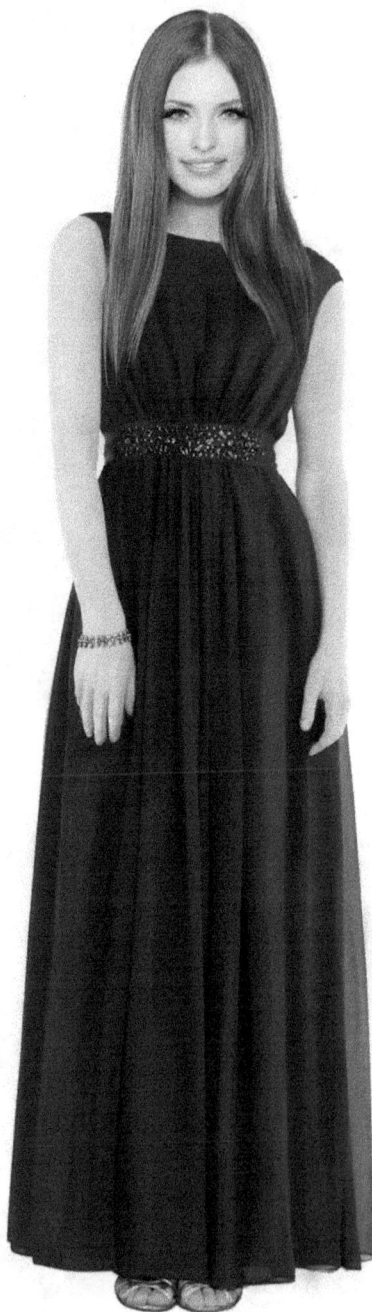

Fashion Figure 5
Maxi Dress

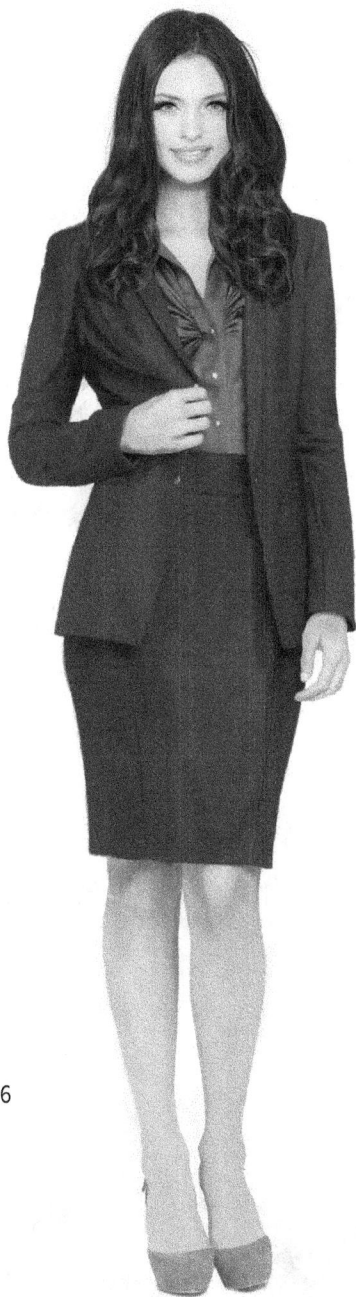

Fashion Figure 6
Skirt Suit

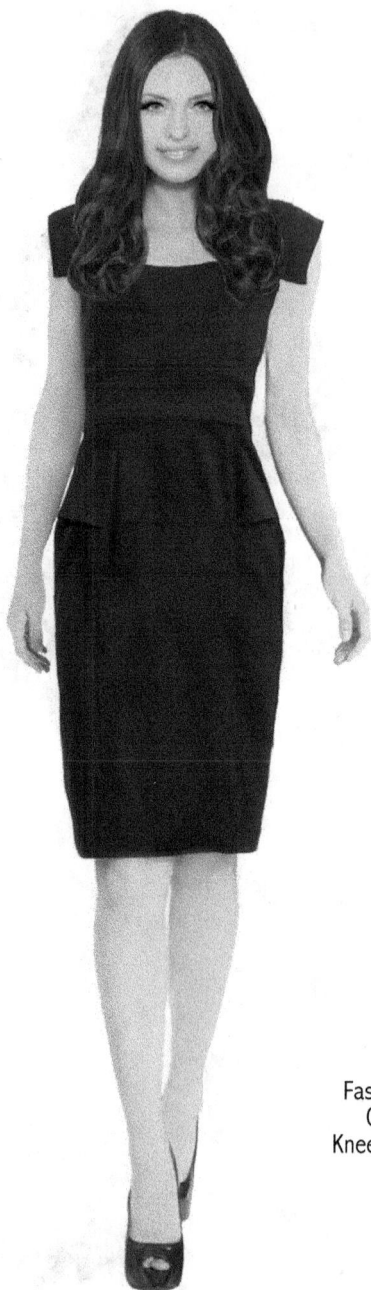

Fashion Figure 7
Cap-Sleeve,
Knee-Length Dress

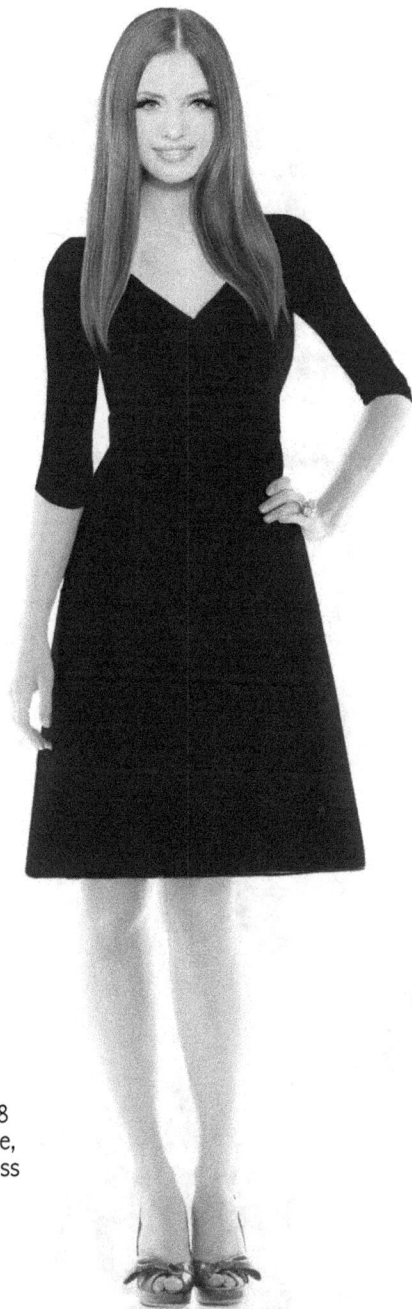

Fashion Figure 8
V-Neck, ¾-sleeve,
Knee-Length Dress

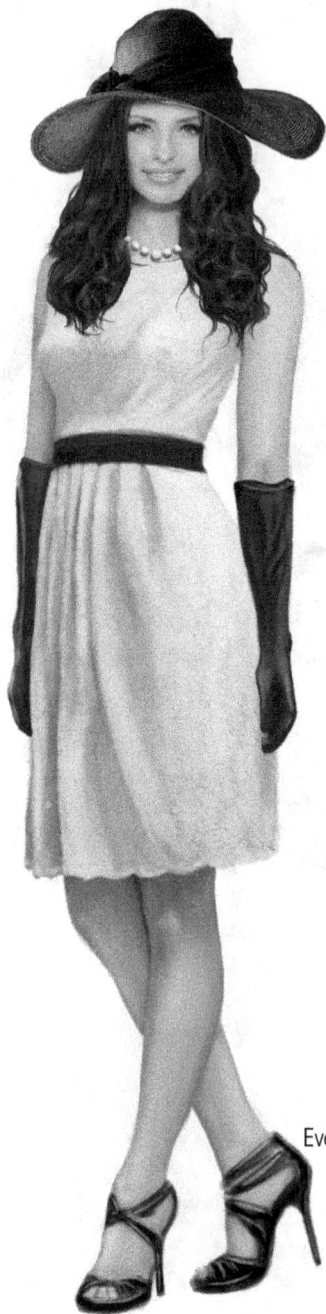

Fashion Figure 9
Evening Gloves, Wide Brim Hat,
Pearl Necklace,
Sheath Dress

Style expert Jill Martin suggests evaluating every single item of clothing you own on a scale of one to ten. Everything in your wardrobe must be a ten. Otherwise, it should be given away to the less fortunate or discarded. Clothing with a score of ten is stylish, fits well, and is in good condition.[4]

A wonderful trick for looking stylish is to wear clothing staples with expensive designer accessories. For example, you can wear a simple black or white halter dress with designer sunglasses, diamond earrings, and a designer handbag. Expensive designer accessories are defining features that can make an outfit look glamorous.

The key to dressing well is to pick one item to be the center of attention in your outfit. For example, if you choose a brightly colored skirt, the rest of your outfit should be subtle and neutral in color.

Italian fashion designer Giorgio Armani said, "The difference between style and fashion is quality." Spend more on stylish clothing staples, which will last a long time. Spend less on fashionable clothing items since they last only a season and may likely be discarded after the trend passes. This suggestion does not apply to accessories such as sunglasses, handbags, and jewelry, as low-quality accessories are a dead giveaway of poor style. It's much better not to purchase accessories at all if you can't afford quality.

You can keep up-to-date with the most fashionable colors, cuts, fabrics, and hemlines by flipping through top fashion magazines such as *Vogue* or *ELLE*. You can also watch the latest fashion shows to pick up on upcoming trends.

Many women can't afford to wear a new outfit every day. However, they can make their outfit look different every time they wear it with belts, scarves, blazers, and accessories. It takes some creativity but it can be done.

Haute couture is a French term that refers to the creation of the most exclusive designs and custom-fitted clothing. Many top celebrities wear haute couture for red carpet events.

Prêt-à-porter is a French term for ready-to-wear that refers to clothing made in standard sizes that fit most women. Fashion houses that produce haute couture also produce ready-to-wear. Sample sales are the best times to buy ready-to-wear designer clothing.

Every social event, location, career, and time of day has a dress code. The most common office dress code consists of business casual and business conservative. The most common social dress codes are cocktail attire, black tie, and white tie. Cocktail attire would include knee-length dresses or cocktail dresses. Black-tie events have a strict dress code that entail wearing a long dress, as do white-tie events, which entail wearing a floor-length evening gown. Many women also wear opera gloves.

A fashion *faux pas* is a French term that means dressing inappropriately. The most common fashion faux pas is excess, such as wearing excessively revealing clothing, excessively tight clothing, excessively high heels, and an excessive amount of accessories.

Another common faux pas is dressing in clothes that don't fit your individual body shape. Go to a tailor to get accurate measurements of your chest, waist, hips, inseam, thigh, upper arm, and sleeve length. Custom-fitted clothing is stylish and luxurious.

Another fashion faux pas is wearing inappropriate undergarments. Visible bra and panty lines look very unstylish. Seamless, invisible undergarments are created to lay flat against the body. They are available in skin-tone-matching colors so they remain undetectable underneath clothing.

Strapless bras tend to slip down. Instead of wearing a strapless bra, wear a seamless, strapless bustier or overbust corset. Be sure to decide if you need a bustier or a corset as their functions are different. A corset reduces the waist size, typically by two to four inches. An overbust bustier lifts up the breasts to create cleavage.

Women looking to attract men should be aware about the color of their clothing. Men are particularly attracted to bright colors.[5] A study found that the color of clothing worn affects attractiveness ratings. Men rated women wearing red, black, and blue shirts as more attractive than several other colors.[6]

According to color consultant Leatrice Eiseman, men are attracted to women wearing the color pinkish peach. It is a color that makes a woman more approachable. The color is "very flattering to most skin tones, it gives you healthy glow," says Leatrice Eiseman. She strongly suggests staying away from yellowish green, which is a color that repels men.

American fashion designer Bill Blass said, "When in doubt, wear red." Red is one of the most attractive colors for a woman to wear. Studies have found that a woman wearing red is more likely to be asked out on a date and have more money spent on her during the date. A study found

"When in doubt, wear red."
- Bill Blass

that men rate women wearing red clothing as more attractive and desirable.[7] Women in red clothing attract more attention from men than those wearing other colors of clothing.[8][9]

An interesting study found that attractive clothing actually increases a woman's facial beauty because of the positive emotions felt when wearing them. The researchers photographed faces of women wearing clothes in which they felt attractive, comfortable, or unattractive while expressing an emotionally neutral face. Men rated the faces of women wearing attractive clothing as the most beautiful, but the faces of women in comfortable and unattractive clothing were ranked as least desirable, even though the clothes were not visible in the photographs.[10] This study may suggest that wearing attractive clothing isn't so much about the clothing itself but the positive emotions it inspires in a woman. American writer Dale Carnegie said, "The expression a woman wears on her face is far more important than the clothes she wears on her back."

Lady Duff-Gordon, an English dressmaker, once said, "Put even the plainest woman into a beautiful dress and unconsciously she will try to live up to it." It's not so much about the dress, but about the confidence displayed, which the dress may help bring out.

ACCESSORIES

Accessories are the secret to great style. They are the finishing touch that enhance a woman's beauty. Accessories even have the power to increase the appearance of status and luxury.

Face-framing accessories such as dangling earrings or a flower in the hair are the most attractive accessories since they draw attention to the face, which is the most important physical feature. The Bible says, "Earrings add to your beauty" (CEV, Song of Solomon 1:10). Flowers are associated with femininity. A study found that the amount of tip increased when a waitress wore a flower in her hair.[11]

"Earrings add to your beauty."
- The Bible (CEV, Song of Solomon 1:10)

Steve Harvey, author of *Act Like A Lady Think Like A Man*, says that men are very simple. Men like shiny things and are attracted to a woman who sparkles. However, never wear more than three pieces of jewelry. If you are wearing a bracelet, a necklace, earrings, and rings, then you are wearing too much jewelry.

A big, floppy designer hat worn with designer opera gloves looks very

MUST-HAVE ACCESSORIES

Diamond stud earrings
Diamond dangling earrings
Diamond watch
Diamond necklace
White pearl necklace
Designer sunglasses
Designer leather handbag
Wide-brim floppy hat
Opera gloves
Silk neck scarf
Faux flower for hair

stylish. Regardless of how simple your outfit, these two vintage accessories will give you an upper-class appearance.

Expressing individual style is a creative process best done through customizing accessories. The most stylish women are inclined to customize their accessories to make each piece completely unique.

Women who are still developing a sense of style can purchase handbags, hats, gloves, and scarves in classic colors—white, beige, black, very dark gray, or very dark blue.

Pearl and diamond jewelry pieces are one of the best style investments a woman will make. However, before purchasing pearl and diamond jewelry, every woman must get educated about quality standards.

Natural pearls are formed randomly and are accidents of nature. When a certain type of irritant, such as a parasite, becomes lodged in the tissue of a mollusk, the animal responds by secreting a calcium carbonate substance called nacre to coat the intruder and protect itself. Over a period of several years, this buildup of nacre forms a natural pearl. It is the nacre that gives pearls their beautiful luster and color. Natural pearls are so rare to find in nature that most pearls sold today are cultured. To create a cultured pearl, a tiny bead is implanted into the oyster, and gradually the oyster coats the bead.

Diamond shape refers to a diamond's form, primarily as viewed from above. All diamond shapes have different attributes. Women can select a shape according to their personal taste and style. They can select a round, princess, emerald, Asscher, marquise, oval, radiant, pear, heart, or cushion-shaped diamond.

The cut is a diamond's most important characteristic since it has the greatest overall influence on a diamond's beauty. The better a diamond is cut, the more sparkle it will have. When a diamond is cut with the proper proportions, light is returned out of the top of the diamond. If it is cut too shallow, light leaks out of the bottom.

DIAMOND CUT

IDEAL CUT
Represents roughly the top 3 percent of diamond quality based on cut. Reflects nearly all light that enters the diamond.

VERY GOOD CUT
Represents roughly the top 15 percent of diamond quality based on cut. Reflects nearly as much light as the ideal cut, but for a lower price.

GOOD CUT
Represents roughly the top 25 percent of diamond quality based on cut. Reflects most light that enters.

FAIR CUT
Represents roughly the top 35 percent of diamond quality based on cut. Still a quality diamond, but a fair cut will not be as brilliant as a good cut.

POOR CUT
Diamonds that are generally so deep and narrow or shallow and wide that they lose most of the light out of the sides and bottom.

Color refers to a diamond's lack of color, grading the whiteness of a diamond. Diamonds that are white, containing little or no color, receive higher-quality grades than those with visible color. Colorless diamonds are the rarest and most valuable of all. Diamonds are graded according to the GIA (Gemological Institute of America) color chart. A color grade of D is the highest possible, while Z is the lowest.

DIAMOND COLOR

Z-N
Noticeable color.

M-K
Noticeable color.

J-I
Near-colorless.

H-G
Near-colorless. Color difficult to detect unless compared side-by-side against diamonds of better grades.

F-E
Colorless. Minute traces of color can be detected by an expert gemologist. A rare diamond.

D
Absolutely colorless. The highest color grade. Extremely rare.

Clarity is a measure of the number and size of the tiny imperfections that occur in almost all diamonds. Gemologists refer to these imperfections by a variety of technical names, including blemishes and inclusions, among others. Diamonds with few or no imperfections receive the highest clarity grades. Less than 1 percent of all diamonds ever found have had no inclusions and can be called flawless (FL) or internally flawless (IF). VVS diamonds are also extremely rare. VS diamonds are of superior quality and are used in extremely fine jewelry. A large percentage of jewelry is made with SI-quality diamonds. According to many experts, clarity generally has the least impact on a diamond's beauty since these imperfections tend to be microscopic.

DIAMOND CLARITY

FL
Flawless

IF
Internally Flawless

VVS1, VVS2
Very Very Slight Inclusion

VS1, VS2
Very Slight Inclusion

SI1, SI2
Slight Inclusion

I1, I2, I3
Included

Carat is a specific measure of a diamond's weight. The weight of a diamond less than one carat in size may also be described in terms of points. There are one hundred points in one carat.

Conflict diamonds, also called blood diamonds, are diamonds that are sold to finance the operations of rebel, military, and terrorist groups. Murder and mutilation are typical of these groups. Conflict diamonds are a symbol of pain, suffering, injustice, terror, fear, war, slavery, and death.

For women who want a 100 percent guarantee that their diamond is conflict-free, synthetic diamonds such as cubic zirconia or moissanite are an option. Natural, white gemstones such as sapphire, zircon, topaz, danburite, and petalite are also an option.

Nail polish is an essential accessory. Polished nails give the appearance of health. Poor health will result in unhealthy-looking nails. Virtually every nutritional deficiency can affect the growth of the nail in some manner.[12]

The most attractive and natural-looking nail polish color is a sheer, pale, peachy pink shade similar to a healthy nail bed. Sheer nail polish will enhance, not hide, your natural nails since your lunula and free edge will still be visible. Nail polish that hides your lunula and distal edge will always look unnatural.

Nearly all men reported that they do not like extremely long nails resembling animal claws. The ideal nail tip is about a sixteenth of an inch in length.

French manicures with very long tips, longer than a quarter inch, are not stylish. Style expert Camilla Morton, author of *How to Walk in High Heels: The Girl's Guide to Everything*, says that French manicures are tacky. Style expert Lucia van der Post, author of *Things I Wish My Mother Had Told Me: A Guide to Living with Impeccable Grace and Style*, also comments that French manicures are considered tacky. However, short French manicures with tips that are a sixteenth of an inch long are acceptable because they enhance the look of the free edge.

Women who want strong nails can select nail products that are composed of half nail polish and half gel. These products are ideal since they don't chip, scratch, or lose shine and are non-damaging to the nails. The procedure may require placing your hands under a UV light to cure the color. Therefore, apply a sunscreen before the procedure to protect your hands from UV skin damage.

Some women use tattoos in an effort to enhance their beauty. Studies show that having a tattoo does not increase attractiveness ratings, even though some women think it does.[13] A study found that a woman without a tattoo was rated significantly more attractive, intelligent, artistic, athletic, motivated, generous, mysterious, and honest compared to the same female with a tattoo.[14] Another study found that women with tattoos received lower ratings on competence, character, and sociability than those without one.[15]

Women with tattoos are perceived to be less credible than those without them. A survey done on employers in occupations of retail and business revealed they were less likely to hire people with tattoos than those without them.[16] These results are also consistent with empirical research suggesting that a conservative appearance enhances the ratings of credibility.[17]

SCENT

Scents trigger memories. When you first smell a new scent, you link it to an event, a person, a thing, or even a moment. When you encounter the smell again, the link is already there, ready to elicit a memory or a mood. A "perfect 10" woman wears a signature scent so that she can be memorable to everyone she encounters. A signature scent is the fragrance that is worn the most often and that your partner and friends associate with you.

Scent has the power to increase a woman's attractiveness. Women's magazine *Cosmopolitan* found that 81 percent of men think fragrance boost a woman's overall attractiveness. "Pleasant aromas can actually stimulate parts of the brain directly connected to sexual desire," says Dr. Alan Hirsch, MD, founder and director of Chicago's Smell and Taste Treatment and Research Foundation.

Various polls by *Cosmopolitan* found that sweet and tasty scents are most favored by men. Fruity notes are the second-most favored and floral scents come in last. "It appears food odors elicit the greatest sexual response," says Dr. Alan Hirsch. He conducted a study and found that the combined odor of lavender and pumpkin pie had the greatest effect, increasing male sexual arousal by 40 percent. The combination of black licorice and doughnut increased male sexual arousal by 30 percent. The combined scent of pumpkin pie and doughnut was third, with a 20 percent increase. Orange, lily of the valley, vanilla, lavender, and musk also elicited male sexual arousal to some degree.[18]

Aromatherapy experts have long believed cinnamon to be an aphrodisiac. According to Laura Davimes, an aromatherapy expert, "certain aromatic plants exude oils similar to our own sexual secretions or pheromones. Wearing cinnamon/vanilla blends increases the presence of pheromone-like substances and dramatically increases attraction."

The key to wearing perfume is to never to wear too much. Wearing perfume every day can make you insensitive to that particular scent, resulting in over-application. Stick to misting your pulse points (inner wrists, elbows, neck, backs of the knees). "The warmth of the skin will slowly release the fragrance into the air as you move," says perfumer Frédéric Malle.

Perfumes should be organic and free of chemicals. Many perfumes are made with a variety of synthetic chemicals that are harmful to a woman's health. Chemicals in fragrances can enter the body through skin absorption and inhalation. Once inside the body, the chemicals can impact any organ or system.[19] Synthetic musk chemicals are known to accumulate in human tissue and are present in breast milk.[20]

ORGANIC PERFUME

INGREDIENTS
5 drops organic essential oil
5 drops organic essential oil
3 drops organic essential oil
1 cup distilled water
5 teaspoons organic vodka

DIRECTIONS
Stir the essential oils slowly into the alcohol, one drop at a time. Stir long enough for the oils to be completely dispersed. Then, let the blend of oil and alcohol stand undisturbed for forty-eight hours. Then, add the distilled water and stir. Leave your perfume to stand for at least three weeks in a cool, dark place. Perfume is like fine wine, it needs to stand and mature before it reaches perfection. After the perfume has matured, bottle it in a glass bottle with a stopper. The strength of the perfume is dependent on the ratio of essential oils, alcohol, and water in the blend. A single drop too much, or too little, will change the scent of the perfume.

You can make your own perfume by combining essential oils of your choice with alcohol and water. The water for making perfume must be distilled.

According to research, an ovulating woman can go without fragrance and still smell attractive. Anthropologist Helen Fisher, PhD, author of *Why We Love*, says, "Men are most attracted to your own special fragrance—they find that combination of sweet and musky incredibly sexy."

In two studies, women wore shirts for three nights during various phases of their menstrual cycles. Men smelled the shirts that had been worn by the female participants. Saliva samples for testosterone analysis were collected before and after the men smelled the shirts. Results revealed that the men who smelled the shirts of the ovulating women had higher levels of testosterone than the men who had smelled shirts worn by non-ovulating women. In addition, after smelling the shirts, the men rated the shirts worn by the ovulating women as having the most pleasant scent.[21]

Chapter 8: Elegance

We must never confuse elegance with snobbery.
- Yves Saint Laurent, French fashion designer

*E*legance is the fine art of social mannerism. It's all about the image a woman projects to others. It defines a woman to a large degree. Elegance expert Lucia Van Der Post describes elegance as "a way of being and behaving." An elegant woman expresses herself in a feminine, soft, polite, dignified, and graceful manner. English critic William Hazlitt said, "Grace in women has more effect than beauty."

Elegance is timeless. For centuries, women of elegance have portrayed a very specific image. Actresses Audrey Hepburn and Grace Kelly are considered by many to be the essence of elegance. Both women had *je ne sais quoi*, a French term meaning an elusive quality that makes a woman very attractive, admirable, and unique. Many believe that elusive quality was elegance.

Women can learn how to be elegant through deportment lessons or finishing school. Learning the art of elegance requires repeated practice until it becomes a habit. Greek philosopher Aristotle said, "We are what we repeatedly do. Excellence, then, is not an act, but a habit."

The sages of the world past and present have taught that what a woman thinks of herself determines who she is and what she becomes. Indian spiritual leader Gautama Buddha said, "The mind is everything. What you think you become." When a woman is mentally elegant it will manifest on the outside. "The only real elegance is in the mind; if you've got that, the rest really comes from it," said American fashion expert Diana Vreeland. An elegant woman must believe that she is beautiful. "Nothing makes a woman more beautiful than the belief that she is beautiful," said Italian actress Sophia Loren.

MOVEMENT

According to Gordon Wainright, author of *Teach Yourself Body Language*, by simply changing the way you carry yourself you can increase your attractiveness. An elegant woman carries herself with the dignity and grace of a queen. However, she never exaggerates her movements.

To walk in an elegant manner, make sure to stand up tall, pull your shoulders back, and lift your chest up. Keep your chin parallel to the floor, and your weight centered in your pelvis. Pick up and put down your feet slowly and softly. Your steps should be light and gentle. Walk in small steps. You can place one foot in front of the other as models do, but this is optional. Let your arms gently move along with your body.

If walking in an elegant manner is a challenge for you, then you should definitely consider ballet lessons. Ballet has many benefits, including sculpting and toning the body, promoting flexibility, and improving bad posture. Ballet is the ultimate method of teaching elegant movement.

If you have a naturally slouched back, you can improve your posture by the exercise of balancing a book on your head and walking around your home like this for half an hour each day. Rolfing is one of the best ways to improve posture since it lengthens the tissues in the body. Hellerwork Structural Integration,

Zentherapy, Alexander technique, and Feldenkrais Method are also helpful for correcting posture.

The raindrop technique (RT) is a method of using essential oils, mixed with a variety of massage techniques, to bring the body back into structural and electrical alignment. It has resolved numerous cases of scoliosis and kyphosis, and eliminated the need for back surgery in some cases. The rainbow therapy is an advanced version of the raindrop technique and may be even more effective.

VOICE

The voice of a woman makes a strong first impression just like physical appearance.[1] Dr. Lillian Glass, body language and communication expert, has found that the way a person speaks significantly affects physical attractiveness. A person with a facial abnormality but a good speaking voice was perceived as being more physically attractive than someone who had a speech problem. Those previously seen as attractive were perceived as unattractive when they were associated with a distortion in their speaking voice. Dr. Lillian Glass says that the most attractive voice is enthusiastic, lively, and has a varied pitch and loudness.

A feminine voice is the defining quality of a woman. "Voice is a profound difference between men and women, and it colors every human interaction we have," says anthropologist David Puts. A woman must learn the difference between a masculine voice and a feminine voice and apply this information to feminize her voice.

The most obvious difference between male and female voices is pitch. The pitch of a male voice ranges from 100 to 150 hertz, while it ranges from 175 to 250 hertz in a woman. Using a chromatic frequency tuner, you can learn to identify your own pitch.

Resonance has to do with the ring of your vocal tone. Males have a larger throat space than do females. This creates a larger resonating chamber, which results in the voice having a fuller, deeper quality to it even when the pitch is the same.

Pacing refers to the speed of speech, while phrasing refers to the number of words per breath. Men tend to speak in shorter bursts followed by pauses, whereas women speak in long and flowing sentences.

Men tend to speak more monotonously while women use more melodic intonation and vary the pitch of their voices within a phrase or sentence. Women talk from their head while men talk from their chest.

Singing is a good way to feminize your voice. Sing along to songs with female voices every day. You can record yourself speaking, and practice refining your voice. Make your voice smaller and higher as you speak. If you have a naturally deep voice, then consciously contract your throat to create a smaller space in the throat. You can also have surgery to make your voice box smaller if you have a serious issue with your voice.

Smoking is the worst thing you can do for your voice, so don't smoke or hang around in smoky places. Smoking and secondhand smoke will damage your voice.

If you are serious about making your voice sound more attractive, then steer clear of dairy products. Cheese, milk, ice cream, and butter all thicken the mucus in your throat. Gargle your throat with saltwater to clear away mucus.

Higher estrogen levels change the pitch of a woman's voice. In one experiment, researcher Dr. Gordon Gallup asked men to rate the attractiveness of female voices. Audio clips were recorded from the same woman at different times during her menstrual cycles. All the men said they preferred the higher-pitched voices. During ovulation when women are the most fertile, they produce more estrogen, which raises the pitch of their voice. Therefore, men are instinctively more attracted to a higher-pitched voice because it indicates a woman will conceive. Consider taking natural estrogen supplements such as *Pueraria mirifica* to increase the femininity of your voice.

SPEECH

An elegant woman speaks in a very polite, sweet, and dignified manner. She is the pure essence of femininity through her speech and diction.

People experience pure pleasure speaking with a woman of elegance. Her speech is filled with sweetness. She speaks in a kind and warm tone of voice. She uses sweet and affectionate nicknames for her girlfriends or her partner such as "honey," "darling," or "sweetheart." Affectionate speech denotes some degree of intimacy or closeness, so a woman would not use such nicknames with strangers or men she is not in a relationship with.

A woman of elegance speaks quietly and softly, especially when around men. Her speech is not too fast-paced and not too loud. She never interrupts when someone is speaking but waits patiently until they finish before she speaks.

An elegant woman does not use dirty, vulgar language. The main purpose of bad language is to give the impression of toughness, defensiveness, and to add humor, emphasis, or shock value. A woman would never want to give such an impression. She does not need to shock people or try to fit in since her physical beauty alone is enough to shock people and claim respect. When she is very frustrated she may respond with feminine words. Acceptable words include "oopsy," "yuck," or "ick". The *Urban Dictionary* defines "ick" as "something gross, a feminine way of saying 'ew'."

A woman should know which subjects to avoid during conversation. Fashion writer and editor Derek Blasberg said, "I'm shocked by how many supposedly sophisticated girls…believe menstrual cycles are appropriate cocktail conversation."

A woman of elegance discusses positive, upbuilding, and interesting issues. She reads a lot and thus has many topics to discuss. She enjoys speaking positively about her passions in life such as her family, friends, pets, or hobbies. However, she is even more interested in learning about the person she is talking to. She asks open-ended questions that get a person talking. Open-ended questions typically begin with words such as "why," "how," or phrases such as "tell me about..." Often they are not technically a question but a statement that implicitly asks for a response. Closed-ended questions get a "yes" or "no" response and stop the flow of the conversation.

MANNERS

Elegance expert Lucia Van Der Post says elegance is "about good manners." Good manners means respecting others. It makes a large impact in the way people perceive a woman.

In the chapter The Art Of Beauty found in *The Love Books of Ovid*, Roman poet Publius Ovidius wrote: "Your first preoccupation, my dears, should be your manners. When a woman's manners are good, she never fails to attract. Manners indeed are more than half the battle."

> "When a woman's manners are good, she never fails to attract."
> - Ovid

Smiling is a sign of kindness and friendliness. People feel good when they receive a smile from a physically attractive woman and their defenses come down. "Beauty is power; a smile is its sword," said Charles Reade, a famous author.

> "Beauty is power; a smile is its sword."
> - Charles Reade

The essence of good manners is being polite and non-demanding. Always say "please" and "thank you," as they are such small but powerful words. Don't expect or demand too much from others; rather, be willing to give of yourself. Learn to forget about yourself temporarily to cater to others.

An elegant woman believes in the law of cause and effect. She acknowledges that what goes around comes around. She is polite and kind, even to those she doesn't like. If she doesn't like someone, she simply tolerates their presence.

An elegant woman knows how to handle negative situations with grace. The Bible says, "Sensible people control their temper; they earn respect by overlooking wrongs" (NLT, Proverbs 19:11). An elegant woman never shows her negative emotions, but simply stops talking and gives "a look." She may simply look at the offending person as if she is high above them and then ignore them completely as if they no longer exist.

Elegance is defined in the dictionary as "restraint and grace of style." A woman of elegance never shows her negative emotions to anyone. When she is upset, she responds with sadness or disappointment but never with anger or aggression. She does not yell, scream, or throw a fit. If she is upset, she simply withdraws from anyone around her and goes somewhere private where no one can hear or see her so that she can express her anger or frustration if she chooses to do so. Controlling negative emotions in front of people can be challenging, but an elegant woman always accomplishes this with perfection.

An elegant woman does not gossip. She acts as if she knows everything but tells no one anything. Occasional gossip on positive subjects is acceptable. Negative gossip is not elegant. Indian spiritual guru Sri Sathya Sai Baba said, "Before you speak, think—Is it necessary? Is it true? Is it kind? Will it hurt anyone? Will it improve on the silence?"

An elegant woman refrains from harsh facial expressions and tries to maintain a peaceful expression at all times. Her smile is neither tight nor causes her to squint. She laughs gently and quietly. If she frowns she expresses it only slightly.

Do not do anything too loudly, too rudely, or too aggressively. A man is allowed to be aggressive at times if needed, especially if he is defending the ones he loves. A woman who takes on a man's role is defeminizing herself. Being the opposite sex means being the opposite of a man.

An elegant woman knows good table manners and etiquette. She places her napkin on her lap. She eats without putting her elbows on the table. She holds and uses flatware properly.

In formal table settings, flatware is used in order from outside to inside, with the exception of oyster forks, which are placed on the right-hand side of the bowl in a spoon. The European style, also called the continental style, is to hold the fork in the left hand and the knife in the right throughout the meal. Once a bite-sized piece of food has been cut, it is brought straight to the mouth by the left hand. There is no need to put down the knife. The knife and fork are both held with the handle running along the palm and extending out to be held by thumb and forefinger. The palm conceals the handle. Once the meal is finished, knife and folk should be placed parallel to each other on the plate.

CLASS

A classy woman is of high rank within society. She is highly respected and valued by others. She is dignified and holds onto certain values. She has great interest in personal development, education, and charity work.

To be a classy woman does not necessarily mean climbing the social ladder or being very wealthy. A woman who simply acts like she is of high value will give the impression of being classy. Admirable behavior and achievements will also give a woman class.

A classy woman dresses conservatively because she knows physical beauty is based mainly on her face and not on revealing outfits. She behaves in a reserved manner but is confident and outgoing in her speech.

In the book *What Turns Men On*, Brigitte Nioche surveyed over five thousand men to find out what qualities they find the most attractive and least attractive. Vulgarity was the least attractive quality, being even less attractive than shyness. It's better to act shy and quiet than loud and vulgar. A vulgar woman shows off her sexuality, dresses provocatively, speaks loudly, and uses dirty language or rude remarks. Women who act vulgar are in desperate need of attention and have not been taught the value of acting classy.

Men place women into two categories: women they sleep with and women they marry. A "perfect 10" woman will attract a man for who she is, not what she offers sexually. Don't offer anything! Just be classy, and quality men will be attracted to you.

Classy women hold strongly to the value of commitment or marriage. Classy women reserve their sexuality for their partner and treat it like a valuable commodity to be given only after a strong commitment. Classy women believe in the concept that rarity increases value. Whatever is very rare is considered very valuable. Diamonds are valuable only because they are rare. One of the reasons some men in today's society do not value women as they should is because some women give themselves away for little or no commitment.

A step above being classy is being part of the elite class, also known as high society. Being a "society girl" or "it girl" requires the gift of being born or marrying into a wealthy family. High society women and their husbands have immense financial power to make things happen.

Within high society there are certain acceptable careers, sports, and hobbies. Acceptable careers for a high society woman include being a model, actress, business owner, fashion designer, artist, writer, or mother/housewife. Some high society women have chosen charity as their "career". Acceptable high society sports typically include tennis, skiing, golf, scuba diving, and horseback riding. Acceptable hobbies include fine art, luxury travel, education, and charity.

245

Some high society women who are very socially active become socialites. A socialite is someone who attends many upscale parties and events, which are reported in magazines and newspapers.

High society women tend to be highly educated and attend prestigious schools. They typically study business, law, languages, literature, history, economics, art, culture, religion, and philosophy. They don't always use their degree in any career path but consider it an important contribution to their social status.

All high society women know how to be good hostesses. The hostess assumes the responsibility for every aspect of a party or event. Hostesses usually get the help of a planner, event coordinator, florist, caterer, musician, and wait staff.

For charity balls, dances, and galas, social secretaries and event planners help with the list, invitations, and plans. Invitations are sent about four to six weeks before the event.

High society women are members of private, elite social clubs and associate with other women of high social status. They know that the type of company they keep influences people's opinion of them.

High society women like to have the best of everything but never brag about it. Showing off is never classy because it gives the impression that you are trying to impress. Volunteering information is bragging. Only when asked is it appropriate to tell someone the details. When a classy woman rides in a limo, she uses the word "car" instead of "limo." She never uses the words "expensive," "exclusive," or "rich." She never talks about brands or labels.

SOPHISTICATION

Sophistication refers to being informed about fashion, culture, literature, and travel. A sophisticated woman is intricate and exceptionally well-developed. She is admired by nearly every-one she encounters.

A sophisticated woman knows what she likes and doesn't like and is very clear about it. She has refined taste and selects things based on her knowledge and experience. "Knowledge is the only elegance," said American writer Ralph Waldo Emerson.

Being sophisticated requires having tried and experienced many different things. It's an attitude of "been there and done that." Sophisticated women are not easily shocked or impressed because they have seen and experienced so much already.

"The World is a book, and those who do not travel read only a page."
- Saint Augustine

Sophistication starts with an interest in life. American author Henry Miller said, "Develop an interest in life as you see it; the people, things, literature, music—the world is so rich, simply throbbing with rich treasures, beautiful souls and interesting people. Forget yourself."

You can become sophisticated by being adventurous and developing a passion for trying new things. Try new restaurants, new wines, and new foods. Try new activities. Visit new museums or art galleries. Explore new countries and cities. Acquire a taste for sophisticated music such as jazz and classical. Go to jazz concerts or lounges where you can meet other sophisticated people.

To be sophisticated you must love learning. Thoroughly educate yourself about wine, food, music, opera, art, fashion, history, philosophy, and travel. Keep up-to-date with the latest topics that are being discussed in social settings. Read the news daily. A sophisticated woman can never be bored because there is so much to learn about.

Knowing more than one language is sophisticated. A woman who speaks several languages gives the impression that she has the time and resources required for learning languages. Not everyone has the opportunity to learn multiple languages. That makes it such an exclusive skill to possess.

Sophistication requires being well-read and well-traveled. Read the latest and greatest books that everyone is talking about. Focus on traveling and seeing the major countries and cities in the world. Traveling expands your mind. Saint Augustine said, "The world is a book, and those who do not travel read only a page." Travel inspires and educates. American businesswoman Ivanka Trump said, "In both business and personal life, I've always found that travel inspires me more than anything else I do." The most sophisticated women have traveled to, or lived in, some of the major cities of the world.

Chapter 9: Personality

*P*ersonality is made up of behavioral patterns and social attitudes. The dictionary defines personality as a pattern of thoughts, feelings, and behaviors that make a person unique. A woman's personality can be measured quite accurately with psychometric tests.

Studies show that an attractive personality is as important as physical beauty.[1] American actress Halle Berry said, "Beauty is not just physical." While outer appearance has an influence on short-term perceived attractiveness, personality has an influence on long-term perceived attractiveness.

An attractive personality has the power to increase beauty-score ratings.[2] "People may see physical beauty differently when they know that person's other qualities, usually invisible to strangers," says anthropologist Kevin Kniffin.

Physical beauty is highly valued for a short-term romantic relationship.[3][4][5] However, men looking for a long-term romantic relationship are interested in an attractive personality because it indicates that a woman will be a high-quality partner.[6][7] When researchers asked couples who had been married for over fifteen years why their marriage lasted, couples said that their partner was their best friend and that they liked their partner as a person.[8]

Physical beauty along with an attractive personality will result in popularity. Popularity tends to refer to having high social status that brings with it admiration and respect from others.

French writer Voltaire said, "It is not sufficient to see and to know the beauty of a work. We must feel and be affected by it." A woman is a masterpiece when she can touch others' feelings and affect them through her personality.

CHARM

You must be charming to be considered beautiful. "A plain woman is one who, however beautiful, neglects to charm," said American writer Edgar Saltus. The dictionary defines charm as "an action thought to have magical power." Being charming has a powerful, almost magical, effect on people. British physician and psychologist Havelock Ellis said, "Charm—which means the power to effect work without employing brute force—is indispensable to women. Charm is a woman's strength just as strength is a man's charm."

Being charming isn't about being the center of attention as some believe. "Charm is a glow within a woman that casts a most becoming light on others," said John Mason Brown, an American critic. Charming women put the spotlight on someone else and make them feel important.[9] Brian Tracy, a personal and professional development expert, said, "Charm is the ability to create extraordinary rapport that makes others feel exceptional." American writer Maya Angelou said, "I've learned that people will forget what you said, people will forget what you did, but people will never forget how you made them feel."

Abraham Lincoln, the sixteenth president of the United States, said, "Everybody likes a compliment." Women who compliment others are more charming, even when the recipient of the compliment is aware of ulterior motives behind the compliment. Compliments make a person feel noticed, appreciated, and important. Humanitarian Mother Teresa said, "Kind words can be short and easy to speak, but their echoes are truly endless."

Listening is the best way to make someone feel important. Charming women listen exceptionally well. Listening means much more than just being able to recall everything a person says. It means indicating your genuine, undivided attention.[10] Making eye contact shows you are genuinely interested.

Conversation should be enjoyable. Constant serious talk is boring, and being boring is a huge turnoff for people. As beauty icon Marilyn Monroe once said, "It's better to be absolutely ridiculous than absolutely boring."

The best way to make conversation interesting and enjoyable is to be witty. Being witty means throwing clever, funny, and short comments into conversation. American author Judith Krantz said, "I'm convinced that it's energy and humor. The two of them combined equal charm."

Being witty requires speed of thought. It's also about voicing your honest opinion about things in a clever way, without seriously putting someone down. It's not like telling a joke. You can learn to be witty by memorizing funny one-liners. You can even use the witty one-liners famous people of the past have uttered.

Most communication is nonverbal. According to prominent psychologist Albert Mehrabian, PhD, the impact our message has consists of the following: words account for 7 percent, tone of voice accounts for 38 percent, and body language accounts for 55 percent.[11] [12]

A smile is a universally attractive, nonverbal gesture. It gives the impression that a woman is kind and friendly. Patti Wood, a respected body language expert, said, "The smile is the international signal of friendliness." Research has found that smiling

WITTY QUOTES

"Never take life seriously. Nobody gets out alive anyway."
- Author Unknown

"There cannot be a crisis next week. My schedule is already full."
- Henry Kissinger, American diplomat

"She got her good looks from her father. He's a plastic surgeon."
- Groucho Marx

"A successful man is one who makes more money than his wife can spend. A successful woman is one who can find such a man."
- Lana Turner, American actress

increases a woman's beauty ratings, while sad facial expressions decrease beauty ratings.[13] [14] [15]

Physical beauty may attract stares, but smiling invites approaches. A study found that women who made thirty-five flirtatious signals per hour were approached by an average of four men. Women who were very physically attractive, but didn't make flirtatious signals, often didn't get approached at all. Smiling was the most effective technique for capturing a man's attention and getting him to approach.[16]

Smiling with the eyes appears the most sincere. According to Dr. Martin Seligman, author of *Authentic Happiness*, there are two kinds of smiles: the "Duchenne smile" and the "Pan American." The most attractive smile is the Duchenne smile, a smile that causes the skin around the corners of the eyes to crinkle.[17]

Relationship expert Dr. Tracy Cabot suggests mirroring to create an instant bond with someone and come across as charming. People tend to trust and like others who are like them. Trust is the most important foundation for a friendship or romantic relationship. A person who is being mirrored will instinctively feel that they can trust the person mirroring them.

Mirroring involves very subtly copying another person's body movements. For example, if you're having coffee with someone and they're sitting forward, talking excitedly about something, you can mirror them by also sitting forward to listen and talking excitedly back to them. The key is to try to share the person's thoughts, feelings, speech rhythm, and behavior as best you can. Once you've created a bond with someone, you don't need to continue to make as much of an effort to mirror them since you will most likely already be doing it naturally without even thinking about it.

Couples in love who've been together for a long time tend to dress and even act the same. They mirror each other without even thinking about it because they're bonded.

The world is full of hardships and stress, so a woman who expresses warmth is very magnetic. Expressing warmth involves drawing people closer in the much the same way a fireplace does on a cold night. Hospitality, sincere care, enthusiastic interest, and physical affection are expressions of warmth. Invite a person over for a meal. Give a gift of homemade cookies. Greet a person with a hug. It promotes bonding and trust between people.[18] "That's why oxytocin is sometimes called 'the love hormone,'" says psychiatrist and psychotherapist Kai MacDonald. "Previously, studies of healthy individuals have shown that intranasal doses of oxytocin reduce activation of brain circuits involved in fear, increase levels of eye contact, and increase both trust and generosity," says Kai MacDonald.

CONFIDENCE

Confidence is one of the most important personality traits for a woman to possess. American singer Beyoncé Knowles said, "The most attractive quality a woman can have is self-confidence. You can be pretty, but if you're not confident you don't come across as sexy." In one study, men rated photographs of women who looked confident as more attractive.[19] "Men and women both prefer a confident date," says psychologist Craig Malkin, PhD.

The way you carry yourself can make a huge difference. Anthropologist Helen Fisher, PhD, says, "The way you carry yourself helps a man determine how attractive you are." Stand up straight, push your shoulders back, hold your head high, and walk at a quicker speed than normal. Look like you have places to go and people to meet.

Confidence is about having good communication skills. Confident communication consists of clearly expressing your thoughts and opinions in a radiant and vibrant way.

Learning a new skill or finding a talent that you become passionate about will help build confidence. Discover what you are good at and spend time doing it. To find out what you are good at you need to try various hobbies such as sports, art, collecting, designing, creating, learning languages, playing musical instruments, or volunteering. When you are passionate about something in life, you will feel more confident. A woman without any interests or skills tends to be insecure and needy.

One of the most important ways to increase confidence is to feel good about yourself. Get into the habit of using positive affirmations. Every day, tell yourself that you deserve the best and that you are an amazing person. Value the qualities you have and be yourself in every way possible. You need to love yourself before others can truly love you. We show people how to treat us by the way we treat ourselves.

Sometimes you don't need to really feel confident to be confident. American Actress Vanessa Hudgens said, "Sometimes, you need to look like you're confident even when you're not." American psychologist William James recommends, "If you want a quality, act as if you already had it. Try the 'as if' technique."

Those with confidence appear to have higher energy levels than those that are insecure. Energy supplements have the potential to increase a woman's confidence. Research shows that the combination of caffeine, taurine, and glucuronolactone, found in energy drinks, increases social extrovertedness.[20] Therefore, caffeine or energy supplements can be taken before socializing.

Practice makes perfect. Therefore, if you want more social confidence, socialize frequently. Associate with those who display confidence and are kind enough to encourage you to develop confidence. You can also hire a "social coach" to help you develop social skills and confidence with people.

Some women may experience social anxiety, also known as social phobia, to varying degrees. This causes them to avoid socializing. The main causes of social anxiety are lack of confidence and fear of being judged.

The most effective treatment for social anxiety is cognitive behavioral therapy (CBT). CBT will improve symptoms up to 75 percent, according to the Mayo Clinic. Cognitive behavioral therapy may include systematic desensitization.

Creative visualization, or imagined interactions, may be effective for treating social anxiety. Creative visualization is the technique of imagining social interactions happening. For example, a woman can visualize acting and communicating with confidence around people.

Research has actually proven that visualization works. In a study on creative visualization, Russian scientists compared four groups of Olympic athletes in terms of their training. Group 1 received 100 percent physical training; Group 2 received 75 percent physical training with 25 percent mental training; Group 3 received 50 percent physical training with 50 percent mental training; and Group 4 received 25 percent physical training with 75 percent mental training. Mental training refers to athletes simply imagining that they were performing. The scientists discovered that Group 4, with 75 percent of their time devoted to mental training, performed the best.[21]

For women who don't respond to behavioral therapy or visualization, a psychiatrist can prescribe medication for women who suffer from severe social anxiety.

Stage fright (public speaking anxiety) is placed even before death as the greatest fear for many people. Some celebrities take propranolol or other beta-blockers before performances, public appearances, or interviews.

SASSINESS

Sassiness is all about feeling worthwhile and being assertive to those who may try to put you down. It's about knowing that you deserve respect. It is an attitude of not caring what others think of you. American actor Bill Cosby said, "I don't know the key to success, but the key to failure is trying to please everybody."

Just as zest adds flavor to something, sassiness makes a woman more interesting and exciting to be around. French fashion designer Christian Dior said, "Zest is the secret of all beauty. There is no beauty that is attractive without zest."

Sassiness is one of the most male-attracting personality traits. In the book *What Turns Men On*, Brigitte Nioche surveyed over five thousand men to find out what qualities they find most attractive in a woman. Men rank assertiveness as the most attractive quality. Helplessness is ranked second. The key then is to strike a balance between being assertive and needing a man. Men want a woman who can be assertive. However, they also want to feel like a "hero" when a woman needs help with something. The classic relationship book *Men Are from Mars, Women Are from Venus* says, "Men are motivated and empowered when they feel needed."[22]

Sherry Argov wrote two of the greatest relationship books, *Why Men Love Bitches* and *Why Men Marry Bitches*. The books use the term bitch not in a derogatory way, but as a catchy word that defines a strong woman who expects respect from men. Sherry Argov writes: "I'm not recommending that a woman have an abrasive disposition. The woman I'm describing is kind yet strong. She doesn't give up her life, and she won't chase a man."[23]

Sherry Argov states, "What women need to understand is that when a man considers a woman to be a prize, looks have very little to do with it." Spanish artist Pablo Picasso said, "There are only two types of women—goddesses and doormats."

In order to be treated like a prize, it is important to act like a prize. It's a simple mind trick. American writer Kurt Vonnegut Jr. wrote, "We are what we pretend to be, so we must be careful about what we pretend to be."

All women must understand how men think. Men are hunters and love the thrill of the chase. A man wants to chase a woman in the beginning stages of dating. If there is no chase, there is no excitement in the relationship. A woman must allow a man to chase her until she captures his heart.

Andrew Trees reveals in his book *Decoding Love* that women who take the initiative with men are perceived negatively. When a man has to make an effort to win a woman over, he will place a higher value on her and treat her with respect and love.

Men love challenge. Therefore, a nonchalant attitude increases a man's attraction to a woman. A nonchalant attitude can be adopted by following specific dating rules. *The Rules* are time-tested dating rules that make a woman appear more attractive to a man. They consist of not calling often, rarely returning calls, ending phone calls or dates first, and not seeing a man more than once or twice a week.[24]

As a romantic relationship progresses, a woman must still maintain her sassiness to prevent or solve relationship problems. Men don't respond to words. They respond to no contact. If a man is acting with disrespect or disinterest, a sassy woman simply starts acting emotionally or physically distant. Distance tends to get a man's attention, and it will renew his respect.

Sherry Argov says, "A little distance combined with the appearance of self-control makes him nervous that he may be losing you." Excitement and fear are similar feelings and come from the same part of the brain. A man who is somewhat afraid of losing a woman is somewhat excited about that woman. "The one who loves the least, controls the relationship," said American writer Dr. Robert Anthony. A woman should regularly get away from her relationship, which can be a weekend getaway or a few weeks vacation. This keeps her mysterious, interesting, and exciting.

Being too nice can actually push people away. Instead, be polar and hard to figure out. Polarity results in popularity. Polarity is defined as being in opposite extremes. Robert Greene, author of *The Art of Seduction*, says, "A mix of qualities suggests depth, which fascinates even as it confuses."[25] Social "Queen Bees," who are leaders of a woman's clique, have a combination of assertiveness and kindness. They also have well-developed social skills, assertion skills, and leadership skills.

People respond to rarity. When something becomes rare, it becomes more valuable. Diamonds are valuable because they are so rare. By making yourself unavailable sometimes, your time becomes a rare commodity and increases in value. Make yourself available only at certain times of the day or week. People will value your time when it is limited.[26]

POSITIVITY

Positivity is the inclination to be in an optimistic and hopeful state of mind. It's about feeling positive emotions such as love, kindness, joy, and peace. Most people are attracted to positivity and repelled by negativity. American educator Henry Van Dyke said, "There is no personal charm so great as the charm of a cheerful temperament."

Positive emotions do more than simply make one feel good; they are necessary for forming and maintaining relationships. Research shows that positive emotions "cultivate social closeness, forge lasting relationships, and build complex understanding of others."[27]

Short-term negative emotions should be expressed freely in private. It is much better to express negative emotions constructively than to suppress them. Research has shown that trying to suppress a thought can cause an increase in the frequency of the thought.[28] Suppressing negative emotions can also result in lowered immunity. There are even a number of studies showing that expressing emotion is associated with better health.[29] Short-term negativity is a normal reaction to negative life events.

Prolonged negative emotions are disturbing and unpleasant. They repel people, and could suggest a personality disorder. Therefore, it is very important to remove the cause of prolonged negative emotions.

A woman must first determine the root cause of her negativity. It could be psychological, physical, or spiritual. A medical intuitive scan, quantum biofeedback, or aura imagery will help determine the cause of negative emotions. Once a cause is found, an appropriate therapy can be selected.

Psychotherapy deals with psychological issues that cause negative thoughts, emotions, and behaviors. Meta-analytic studies have demonstrated that psychotherapy is quite effective.[30] There are many different types of psychotherapy for treating negative emotions. A woman should try the type of psychotherapy she feels will work for her and then assess if it is really working, with the use of a heart rate variability (HRV) test. Research has demonstrated that those with psychological issues consistently show lower HRV scores.[31 32]

Cognitive behavioral therapy (CBT) is a type of psychotherapy that changes thinking patterns. Changing thinking patterns will change emotions and behavior. Research has found cognitive behavioral therapy effective for treating depression, anxiety, panic disorder, social phobia, and post-traumatic stress disorder (PTSD). Cognitive behavioral therapy was found to be superior to antidepressant drugs.[33]

Psychoanalysis and psychodynamic therapy are both similar forms of a type of psychotherapy that discovers the unconscious mind and how it influences negative emotions and behavior. These types of psychotherapy have been proven effective in treating various psychological issues.[34] Patients maintain therapeutic gains and appear to continue to improve even after the treatment ends.[35]

Hypnotherapy is the use of hypnosis in psychotherapy. Hypnosis is a deeply relaxed mental state, with increased suggestibility. Hypnotherapy bypasses the conscious mind to enable communication with the subconscious mind. Hypnotherapy is highly effective in the treatment of psychosomatic disorders.[36]

Research has shown that feeling angry increases the risk of developing illnesses such as heart disease and type 2 diabetes.[37] Indian spiritual leader Gautama Buddha said, "Holding on to anger is like grasping a hot coal with the intent of throwing it at someone else; you are the one who gets burned." Forgiveness therapy (FT) has been shown to be effective in treating emotionally abused women and helps overcome depression, anxiety, and post-traumatic stress disorder symptoms.[38] Forgiveness of self and others may even be effective in preventing suicide.[39]

Trauma results from energy that is trapped in the body that has not been resolved and discharged. Trauma that has not been resolved can cause psychological issues.[40]

Traumatic incident reduction (TIR) is an effective method for the rapid resolution of trauma-related conditions.[41] It helps reduce negative emotions such as panic attacks, depression, and anxiety resulting from unresolved past traumas.

Eye movement desensitization and reprocessing (EMDR) is a form of psychotherapy that can treat traumatic disorders.

EMDR has been found to be effective in the treatment of post-traumatic stress disorder (PTSD).[42]

Somatic experiencing (SE) is a body-awareness approach to trauma. It has been applied to veterans, rape survivors, Holocaust survivors, and car accident survivors. It has been shown to decrease post-traumatic stress disorder symptoms.[43]

Bioenergetic analysis and therapy is a form of psychotherapy that combines work with the body and the mind to help resolve psychological issues. Research shows that it is a highly effective therapy.[44][45][46] It has been shown to reduce symptoms of social insecurity, depression, anxiety, anger, and hostility.[47]

Mindfulness-based therapies are effective in treating a variety of psychological issues such as anxiety, depression, eating disorders, and addiction.[48][49] Mindfulness also enhances relationships. A study found that couples that practiced mindfulness enhanced their relationships with each other. The couples reported improved closeness, acceptance of one another, and relationship satisfaction.[50] Another study also found that mindfulness improved the quality of communication between couples.[51]

Some effective mindfulness-based therapies are mindfulness-based stress reduction (MBSR), mindfulness-based cognitive therapy (MBCT), dialectical behavior therapy (DBT), Gestalt therapy, and Morita therapy. Mindfulness-based stress reduction has been shown to be effective for many psychological issues and for reducing stress levels.[52][53]

Mindfulness-based cognitive therapy (MBCT) incorporates elements of cognitive behavioral therapy with mindfulness-based stress reduction. Research suggests that mindfulness-based cognitive therapy is useful for treating depression and preventing relapse of depression. It may also be effective in bipolar and anxiety disorders.[54][55]

Dialectical behavior therapy (DBT) has been used to effectively treat borderline personality disorder (BPD).[56][57] It may reduce hopelessness, depression, and anger expression in women with BPD.[58] It also appears to be effective in reducing suicide attempts.[59] It has been shown to maintain therapeutic gains after a one-year follow-up.[60]

Gestalt therapy is based on self-exploration and focuses on gaining an awareness of emotions and behaviors in the present rather than in the past. It has been proven effective in treating various psychological issues.[61]

Morita therapy involves accepting our feelings and thoughts without trying to change or "work through" them. It has been shown to be effective for those with hypochondriasis and anxiety neurosis.[62]

Mettā meditation, also known as loving-kindness meditation (LKM), is a popular form of meditation in Buddhism. It increases positive emotions, which has the potential to increase one's personal resources and overall life satisfaction. It may also reduce depressive symptoms.[63] Loving-kindness meditation has been shown to increase positive social behavior and decrease antisocial behavior.[64]

Emotional freedom techniques (EFT) and several other varieties of "emotional acupressure" are rooted in ancient Chinese medicine and applied kinesiology. According to EFT theory, the cause of all negative emotions is a disruption in the body's energy system. EFT can treat any psychological issue. It has been shown to work immediately to reduce phobia-related anxiety.[65] It has also been shown to treat post-traumatic stress disorder effectively, although eye movement desensitization and reprocessing (EMDR) was slightly more effective.[66]

Thought field therapy (TFT) is a type of "emotional acupressure" developed by psychologist Roger Callahan. He treated 97 percent of sixty-eight phobic patients successfully in an average treatment time of four minutes.[67] TFT has been used clinically in the treatment of negative emotions such as phobias, traumas, anxiety, depression, anger, stress, obsessions, and addictions. Heart rate variability (HRV) data obtained before and after TFT treatment in the same session has proven the effectiveness of TFT.[68][69] TFT is reported to be the most rapid treatment, with comparable success to other therapies: traumatic incident reduction (TIR)—254 minutes, eye movement desensitization and reprocessing (EMDR)—172 minutes, visual-kinesthetic dissociation (VKD)—113 minutes, and thought field therapy (TFT)—63 minutes.[70]

Wholistic hybrid of EMDR and EFT (WHEE) is effective for treating psychological issues, reducing negative emotions, and increasing positive emotions.[71] A study found that WHEE reduced anxiety in only two sessions, and cognitive behavioral therapy achieved the same benefits as WHEE did in five sessions.[72]

Neuro emotional technique (NET) is a type of psychotherapy that combines a number of techniques and principles from traditional Chinese medicine, chiropractic, and applied kinesiology. It releases unresolved negative emotional blocks. Research shows than it can reduce traumatic stress symptoms.[73] NET can also reduce anxiety symptoms[74][75] and phobias.[76]

Healing touch is a therapy where the practitioner uses his or her hands, either on or above the patient's body, to rebalance the body's energy field. Studies show that those who received healing touch had an increase in positive emotions and a decrease in anxiety and depression.[77]

Advanced integrative therapy (AIT) is a type of energy psychotherapy. Energy psychotherapy is a quick and effective treatment for a range of psychological issues.[78]

Neuro-linguistic programming (NLP) is capable of addressing problems such as phobias, depression, habit disorders, psychosomatic illnesses, and learning disorders. It has been found to be similar in effectiveness to other well-established practices such as cognitive behavior therapy.[79]

The Silva Method is a personal development program. It may increase positive emotions by increasing alpha brain waves.[80]

DNA Theta Healing is a form of prayer, done in a theta brain wave state that brings about psychological healing. It is believed that emotional and behavioral patterns are also inherited through DNA. As DNA is activated, any negative personality traits can be recoded to clear the negative genetic patterning. It appears that different intentions produce different effects on the DNA molecule.[81]

PSYCH-K stands for psychological kinesiology. It is an effective way to change negative beliefs and dissolve resistance to change in the subconscious mind. It helps reprogram the mind with positive beliefs. Beliefs create your reality, and your reality creates your beliefs.[82]

Music therapy is the therapeutic use of music. A qualified music therapist selects the right treatment program for each individual. Research has shown that music therapy is effective in treating various psychological issues. Music therapy appears to have a positive impact on mood.[83] It has been shown to reduce depressive symptoms[84] and anxiety.[85]

Art therapy is a combination of visual art and psychotherapy. Creating art is a form of self-expression and self-discovery. A study found that art therapy decreased levels of hopelessness, anxiety, and depressed mood in women dealing with fertility problems.[86]

Dance therapy is a form of expressive therapy since movement and emotion are directly related. Dance therapy appears to have positive effects on self-esteem.[87] It has been shown to reduce depression.[88]

Animal therapy can improve positivity by increasing socialization, behavior, and motivation. Animal therapy can help treat depression and anxiety.[89] It can also promote feelings of self-worth.[90]

Negativity and personality disorders could have physical causes such as neurotransmitter deficiencies, nutritional deficiencies, blood sugar imbalances, food allergies, heavy metal toxicity, microbial infection, hormonal imbalances, or physical inactivity.[91] Electrodermal screening (EDS), a form of computerized information gathering, is the simplest method of determining physical causes of negative emotions.

Orthomolecular psychiatry is an effective method for treating negative emotions. Orthomolecular medical researchers say the future of psychiatry is in nutrition because nutrition has such a long, safe, and effective history of correcting many issues.

The brain dramatically influences behavior, thoughts, and feelings. SPECT scans, performed by certain physiatrists, can determine the improper functioning of different parts of the brain and neurotransmitter deficiencies or excesses.

Neurotransmitter deficiencies cause various negative emotions. Symptoms of dopamine deficiency are depression, slow thinking, no motivation, fatigue, excessive sleep, and difficulty getting out of bed. Symptoms of serotonin deficiency are mood swings, depression, feelings of worthlessness, anger, obsessive-compulsive disorder, insomnia, and suicidal thoughts. Serotonin and dopamine levels tend to counterbalance each other, so when serotonin is raised, dopamine tends to get lowered, and vice versa.

Different amino acids make different neurotransmitters. A free-form amino acid supplement will correct neurotransmitter deficiencies. Herbs also work well to correct neurotransmitter deficiencies.

Saint John's wort is a natural herbal supplement that has been used by some psychiatrists with success. It raises serotonin levels in the brain. Studies show Saint John's wort is just as effective as several other anti-depressants. The dose is 300 milligrams three times per day.[92] Mucuna pruriens also acts as an antidepressant since it contains L-dopa, a precursor to the neurotransmitter dopamine.

Vitamins, minerals, and omega-3 fatty acids are often deficient in those with negative emotions. Studies have shown that nutritional therapies can reduce the symptoms of depression, bipolar disorder, schizophrenia, and obsessive-compulsive disorder

(OCD).[93] Depression is a common symptom of vitamin B deficiencies.[94] B vitamins have been shown to reduce mood and psychological strain associated with long-term stress.[95]

Blood sugar imbalances have been shown to be associated with criminal, antisocial, and delinquent behavior in offenders. In an outstanding study, offenders were required to undergo various health tests, and the most common problems were glucose intolerance and zinc deficiency. Every single offender had blood sugar imbalances.[96] Another investigation found that every single offender tested had reactive hypoglycemia.[97]

Studies have found that by correcting blood sugar imbalances, a criminal's behavior improves dramatically. Juvenile offenders were placed on a diet low in sugar and food additives. Behavioral records of over three thousand incarcerated juveniles for the twelve months revealed a 21 percent decline in the incidence of serious antisocial behaviors, and fights declined by 25 percent.[98] Another study found a 44 percent reduction in the incidence of antisocial behavior in over one thousand juveniles during three months on a low-sugar diet.[99]

In many cases, food or chemical allergies and intolerances can cause mental and emotional changes. Symptoms of food allergies can include depression, delusions, hallucinations, mood swings, hyperactivity, irritability, nervousness, or violent behavior. Any type of food consumed daily can become a food allergen.

Nutritional enzyme therapy is an essential part of an effective allergy treatment program since when food is very well digested it is nonallergenic to the body. Allergy desensitization with homeopathic remedies is also helpful in treating allergies.[100]

Heavy metal toxicity can be a physical cause of negative emotions. Mercury, lead, cadmium, and arsenic are the most commonly found heavy metals in the body. Lead toxicity can lead to anxiety, delusions, and mental confusion. Arsenic can cause dementia, apathy, and anorexia. Mercury toxicity may cause depression, anorexia, irritability, and psychosis. Hair analysis will rule out heavy metal toxicity.

Parasite infections can cause insomnia, anxiety, irritability, and depression. Parasite infections can be treated with herbal parasite cleanses.

Candida infection is an overlooked but common cause of depression, mood swings, anxiety, irritability, and hyperactivity, with the most definitive symptom being craving for sweets. The best treatment for candida is a combination of a low dose of nystatin along with oil of wild oregano (*Origanum vulgare*).[101]

Hormonal imbalance can be a cause of negative emotions. Adrenal imbalance can cause temper, anxiety, panic attacks, or mild depression. Hypothyroidism results from insufficient production of the thyroid hormone and can cause insomnia, hallucinations, depression, nightmares, paranoia, mood swings, suspiciousness, and fear. Hyperthyroidism results from an overproduction of the

REMEDIES FOR NEGATIVE EMOTIONS

5-HTP - Antidepressant
Tyrosine - Stress-related negative mood
Lithium - Bipolar disorder
GABA - Anti-anxiety
Calcium/Magnesium - Insomnia, anti-anxiety
SAM-e - Antidepressant
Gamma-linolenic acid - PMS, depression
Kava - Social anxiety
Hops - Insomnia, anxiety, depression
Passionflower - Insomnia, anxiety, hyperactivity
Valerian - Insomnia, depression, anxiety
Skullcap - Anti-anxiety
California poppy - Anti-anxiety
Saint Ignatius bean - Hysteria, grief, shock

thyroid hormone and can cause nervousness, insomnia, mood swings, impatience, hyperactivity, anxiety, and depression.

Bach flower remedies and homeopathic remedies are prescribed by a homeopathic doctor are helpful in treating various negative emotions. Rescue Remedy is the most commonly known Bach flower remedy. It is helpful during times of stress or during a panic attack.

Aromatherapy is the practice of using highly concentrated plant extracts, which are called essential oils. They are said to be approximately one hundred times more concentrated than the original herb. Essential oils can be inhaled into the lungs or applied to the skin during massage to be absorbed into the bloodstream. Aromatherapy has been shown to be effective in reducing anxiety[102] and depression.[103]

Physical inactivity may be a risk factor for depressive symptoms.[104] Exercise is an effective method of increasing positivity. Paul Dudley White said, "A vigorous five-mile walk will do more good for an unhappy but otherwise healthy adult than all the medicine and psychology in the world." Research found that those who exercised have lower levels of anxiety, depression, and were more positive.[105] [106] In a large Japanese study, those who exercised scored higher on extraversion and lower on neuroticism.[107] Award-winning American pop singer Cher said, "Nothing lifts me out of a bad mood better than a hard workout on my treadmill. It never fails. To us, exercise is nothing short of a miracle."

A study found that sixteen weeks of exercise was comparable in effect to antidepressants drugs.[108] Each fifty-minute increase in exercise per week was associated with a 50 percent decrease in depression.[109] Exercise was shown to produce better antidepressant effects when the exercise program was longer than nine weeks and involved more sessions. The strongest antidepressant effect occurred with the combination of exercise and psychotherapy.[110]

The root cause of negativity could be spiritual and not psychological or physical. Spiritual leaders believe that lack of spirituality is a major problem worldwide. The Dalai Lama said, "Lack of spirituality and culture is the main cause behind the rampant corruption in the world."

Spirituality is about being focused on the human spirit and God, and may or may not include religion. Spirituality is an experience that must be deeply felt rather than simply known.

Although invisible and not always proven scientifically, the spirit is more powerful than anything else and does have an impact on emotions. "We do not need more of the things that are seen, we need more of the things that are unseen," said Calvin Coolidge, thirtieth President of the United States.

In the book *Mental Wellness: A Spiritual Journey*, Dr. Hamdy El-Rayes explains that a lack of spirituality can be a cause of depression, and that spirituality can help in recovery from depression. He also goes on to state that one of the main things people struggle with is the lack of love in their life. Many individuals don't know how to love either themselves or other people. Dr. Hamdy El-Rayes also believes that one of the main reasons for depression is a fast-paced lifestyle that brings about distance from our essential self. Dr. Hamdy El-Rayes suggests meditation and living mindfully.

There is strong evidence that practicing a religion increases positive emotions and improves mental health.[111][112] Religious involvement is linked with lower levels of depression, suicide, anxiety, and substance abuse.[113] A study found that religious individuals appear to express more positive social attitudes.[114] However, the type of religion practiced determines the emotional outcomes. Emotional distress is greater in those who practice dogmatic religion.[115] In contrast, those who are spiritually growth oriented or transitional have lower rates of negative emotions.[116]

Research shows that those who are involved in religion by intrinsic motivation have reduced risk of depression. However, those who attend church out of obligation have increased risk for depression.[117]

Studies show that religion and spirituality are usually, although not always, beneficial in healing from trauma.[118]

Prayer is a spiritual and religious practice that is considered a form of communication with God. Studies show that frequent prayer is associated with better psychological health.[119][120] Prayer is also associated with relief of distress.[121]

One spiritual pathway that has been shown to reduce stress and related symptoms in war survivors is meditation on a word or phrase with spiritual significance, which is sometimes called a mantra. Researchers concluded that mantra repetition significantly reduced symptoms of stress, anxiety, and anger.[122]

The study of New Thought literature helps cultivate a strong sense of positivity since it teaches that we are what we are as a result of past thoughts and feelings. New Thought author Henry Thomas Hamblin said, "Concentrate your mind on good and positive thoughts and nothing can go wrong in the future."[123] "Human beings, by changing the inner attitudes of their minds, can change the outer aspects of their lives," said William James, an American psychologist and philosopher. Roman emperor Marcus Aurelius said, "The happiness of your life depends upon the quality of your thoughts." American author Earl Nightingale said, "Our attitude towards life determines life's attitude to us."

Criticizing others puts you into a negative state of mind and may bring about negative future events. Indian spiritual leader Gautama Buddha said, "All that we are is the result of what we have thought. If a man speaks or acts with an evil thought, pain follows him. If a man speaks or acts with a pure thought, happiness follows him, like a shadow that never leaves him."

Instead of focusing on others, focus on improving yourself, knowing that there are always improvements to be made. "Give so much time to the improvement of yourself that you have no time to criticize others," said New Thought leader Christian D. Larson.

In addition to New Thought, the study of religious literature or philosophy helps cultivate positivity because it helps you understand that everything works out for your own good and has a purpose (Romans 8:28). Even negative life events have a purpose. Greek philosopher Democritus said, "Nothing occurs at random, but everything happens for a reason and by necessity." American actress Marilyn Monroe said, "I believe that everything happens for a reason...sometimes good things fall apart so better things can fall together."

The death of a loved one is one of the hardest things to deal with, and yet religious wisdom teaches that even death has a purpose. The Bible says, "Good people pass away; the godly often die before their time. But no one seems to care or wonder why. No one seems to understand that God is protecting them from the evil to come" (NLT, Isaiah 57:1–2).

Associating with positive people has the power to lift you up into a positive mood, but negative people can have a very foul effect on you over time. The Bible says, "Associating with bad people will ruin decent people" (GWT, 1 Corinthians 15:33). American businessman William Clement Stone said, "Be careful the friends you choose for you will become like them."

Positivity is directly related to happiness. Those that are happier are naturally more positive. Short-term happiness can be found through achievement or pleasure. However, these things can easily be lost. "Don't let your happiness depend on something you may lose," said British author C. S. Lewis.

Finding and fulfilling your life purpose brings about long-term happiness since it gives one the feeling that life is worth living. The life mission theory states that everybody has a unique talent to contribute to the world.[124][125] Those who have a near-death experience (NDE) come to realize that everyone

HAPPINESS QUOTES

"There is no cosmetic for beauty like happiness."
- Marguerite Gardiner, Irish writer

"To be happy, make other people happy."
- W. Clement Stone, American businessman

"Happiness...consists in giving, and in serving others."
- Henry Drummond, Scottish evangelist

"There is more happiness in giving than receiving."
– The Jerusalem Bible, Acts 20:35

has a mission in life that no one else can fulfill. They alone are the ones who must fulfill it before they die.[126]

The best route to long-term happiness is making others happy. Albert Einstein wisely said, "A person starts to live when he can live outside himself." All spiritual leaders who have mastered the art of happiness will tell you that giving, not getting, is the secret to happiness. A woman can find happiness through giving to people.

INTELLIGENCE

Intelligence is generally defined as the ability to acquire and apply knowledge. Intelligence is an important personality trait for a woman to possess. "Beauty is only temporary, but your mind lasts you a lifetime," said Alicia Machado, an actress and Miss Universe winner. Research shows that people expect physically attractive women to be more intelligent than unattractive or average women.[127]

American author Dennis Franck said, "There's great value in taking months or years or the rest of your lifetime to develop yourself. Discover your goals and talents. Educate yourself. Improve your body, mind and spirit for God so you can more effectively help and bless others, or do it so you will be more attractive to the opposite sex."

There are different types of intelligence. Every woman has strengths in some areas of intelligence but not necessarily in other areas. The most commonly measured type of intelligence is IQ (intelligence quotient), which can be determined by a standard IQ test.

Fluid and crystallized intelligence are two components of general intelligence. Fluid intelligence is the ability to think logically and solve problems. Crystallized intelligence is the ability to use skills, knowledge, and experience.

Every single woman has a very specific way of learning. The VARK model is one of the most frequently used methods to describe and categorize different learning styles. Visual women learn best by seeing. The Visual Teaching Alliance estimates that approximately 65 percent of the population learns best visually. Auditory women learn best through listening. Kinesthetic women prefer to learn by experiencing and are said to make up around 5 percent of the population.

Reading is one of the best methods of increasing intelligence for visual learners. "Even the worst book can give us something to think about," said the Polish poet Wislawa Szymborska. Women who don't enjoy reading can watch documentaries or informative television shows.

Women who are auditory learners can listen to audiobooks or attend lectures. They can voice their knowledge and listen to other people's knowledge.

Women who are kinesthetic learners can increase their intelligence by doing, experiencing, touching, moving, or being active in some way.

Ancient wisdom teaches that socializing can actually increase intelligence. The Bible says, "Just as iron sharpens iron,

273

friends sharpen the minds of each other" (CEV, Proverbs 27:17). Research confirms the mental benefits of socializing. A study concluded that social interaction "helps exercise people's brains and minds."[128]

Intelligence is displayed to others mostly through speech. Therefore, choose words and subjects of conversation carefully. The most intelligent individuals make a social impact with very few words. This is often why wise quotes become very popular. The Bible wisely says, "The more words you speak, the less they mean" (NLT, Ecclesiastes 6:11).

A woman can appear highly intelligent if she has knowledge on many different subjects. She does not need to know everything about everything, but a little about everything. A daily or weekly overview of the latest news will help a woman know a little about everything. Reading women's magazines and research journals are other means of keeping up-to-date on interesting topics to bring up during conversations.

Conscientiousness is an important part of acquiring intelligence. "To create something exceptional, your mindset must be relentlessly focused on the smallest detail," said Italian fashion designer Giorgio Armani. A woman must be conscious of her decisions every single day, however big or small. Good decisions are based on actions that achieve worthwhile goals.

Determination and patience are necessary personality traits that have the ability to increase intelligence. British statesman Benjamin Disraeli said, "Patience is a necessary ingredient of genius." The main reason some women lack intelligence is that they lack the determination and patience that is required to learn.

Mindfulness meditation has been shown to improve mental processes[129] and memory.[130] It has also been shown to reduce distracting thoughts and mind wandering, which is beneficial during reading and learning.[131] Mindfulness meditation is a research-based form of meditation derived from a twenty-five-hundred-year-old Buddhist practice called insight meditation.

Educational kinesiology (Edu-K) is a simple system for improving learning performance. It appears to speed up response times.[132] It may be able to correct certain learning difficulties. The techniques are known as Brain Gym and brain integration therapy (BIT).

Evidence shows that nutrients can increase fluid intelligence and academic performance.[133] Omega-3 is important for brain health. Higher levels of omega-3 improve intelligence and mental performance.[134 135] Omega-3 also prevents age-related mental decline.[136] A woman can take a whole food supplement as well as an omega-3 supplement daily to ensure optimal brain functioning.

Nootropics, also referred to as smart drugs or memory enhancers, are substances that improve intelligence, memory, attention, and concentration.

Acetylcholine is a neurotransmitter that is important for memory and learning.[137] Acetylcholine deficiency can result in learning difficulties, memory problems, poor attention, and difficulty concentrating. Specific supplements such as alpha-GPC and phosphatidylcholine can increase acetylcholine. Huperzine A helps preserve acetylcholine in the brain. Alpha-GPC or phosphatidylcholine taken with huperzine A may improve mental functioning.

Ashwagandha (*Withania somnifera*) is a commonly used herb in Ayurvedic medicine with many health benefits.[138] It may help to preserve brain function and memory by protecting acetylcholine from breakdown.[139]

Brahmi (*Bacopa monnieri*) was used in ayurvedic medicine for centuries. A study found that brahmi decreases the rate of forgetting newly acquired information.[140] It has also been shown to improve mental functions such as learning and memory.[141]

Gotu kola (*Centella asiatica*) has been used in ayurvedic medicine to improve mental function and memory. Research indicates that it possesses neuroprotective properties and nootropic activity.[142] It enhances learning ability and memory retention power.[143]

Herbalists recommend Panax ginseng, also known as Asian ginseng, to improve mental performance. Evidence shows that ginseng improves cognitive performance, specifically alertness, attention, and memory.[144] A study found Panax ginseng is effective for reducing chronic stress.[145] Therefore, Panax ginseng would be beneficial to women requiring improved mental function during stressful times such as during school tests or work projects.

Ginkgo biloba has been used therapeutically in China for centuries. It has been shown to reduce age-related mental decline.[146] A study found that a ginkgo biloba/Panax ginseng combination improved both working and long-term memory.[147]

Chapter 10: Character

> Character contributes to beauty.
> It fortifies a woman as her youth fades.
> - Jacqueline Bisset, English actress

A woman can be physically beautiful and have a great personality, but it is her moral character that truly defines her. "Beauty has a lot to do with character," said American makeup artist Kevyn Aucoin. Mother Teresa and Princess Diana, both humanitarians, were admired and loved mainly for their beautiful characters. Besides beauty, Miss Universe judges are analyzing the character of each contestant.

Character and personality are two different things. Personality is defined by personal and social attitudes, while character is defined by mental and moral qualities. Personality is what you notice first, and character is what you notice later. Personality is primarily inborn traits, while character consists of learned behavior.

Character development is an ongoing and lifelong process. Marvin W. Berkowitz, PhD., a professor of research-based character education, teaches that being of good character requires knowing what's right, caring about what's right, and doing what's right.

In *The Love Books of Ovid* it is written: "Time will lay waste your beauty, and your pretty face will be lined with wrinkles.

The day will come when you will be sorry you looked at yourself in the mirror, and regret for your vanished beauty will bring you still more wrinkles. But a good disposition is a virtue in itself, and it is lasting; the burden of the years cannot depress it."

English writer Thomas Nash said, "Beauty is but a flower, which wrinkles will devour," but beauty of character lasts. Author Martin Buxbaum said, "Some people, no matter how old they get, never lose their beauty—they merely move it from their faces into their hearts."

WISDOM

The dictionary defines wisdom as the ability to think and act using knowledge, experience, understanding, good judgment, and insight. It is also the ability to discern what is true and right. Researchers in the field of positive psychology have defined wisdom as the coordination of "knowledge and experience" and "its deliberate use to improve well being."[1] Chinese philosopher Confucius said, "I hear and I forget. I see and I remember. I do and I understand."

Every woman has the capacity to be as wise as sages like Albert Einstein, Leonardo Da Vinci, and Helen Keller. A strong desire for wisdom is a good start. You gain wisdom when you ask questions, explore, want to know how things work, and learn valuable lessons from experiences.[2]

The first step toward wisdom is the acquisition of knowledge. Read nonfiction books on a variety of subjects. Stimulate your mind constantly and at every possible time of the day. Don't waste any time doing absolutely nothing. Listen to audio books when doing activities such as driving, exercising, or waiting.

Humility is a key factor in acquiring wisdom. The Bible says, "When pride comes, then comes shame, but with humility comes wisdom" (WEB, Proverbs 11:2). When you are humble, you believe that there is still more for you to learn. You never feel like an "expert" in any one subject. Humble women are teachable, open to change, and never stop learning.

John Piper, a pastor and author, suggests two main ways of acquiring wisdom. First, pray for wisdom. "If you need wisdom, ask our generous God, and he will give it to you" (NLT, James 1:5). King Solomon was not born a wise man. He prayed for wisdom and became one of the wisest men who ever lived (1 Kings 3:7–9). Secondly, think frequently of the shortness of this life and the infinite length of the next. "A wise person thinks a lot about death, while a fool thinks only about having a good time" (NLT, Ecclesiastes 7:4).

SACRED ANCIENT WISDOM

"Let your beauty be not just the outward adorning of braiding the hair, and of wearing jewels of gold, or of putting on fine clothing; but in the hidden person of the heart, in the incorruptible adornment of a gentle and quiet spirit."
- World English Bible, 1 Peter 3:3–4

"There is no capital more useful than intellect and wisdom, and there is no indigence more injurious than ignorance and unawareness."
- Ibn Shu'ba al-Harrani, Tuhaf al-'Uqul, p.198

"Without an acquaintance with the rules of propriety, it is impossible for the character to be established."
- Analects of Confucius, Book 20, Chapter 3

Sacred ancient religious texts are valuable sources of wisdom because they have stood the test of time. Religious studies scholar Huston Smith said, "Religion has preserved history's greatest wisdom teachings."

King Solomon, one of the wealthiest and wisest men who ever lived, wrote the Book of Wisdom (Job, Psalms, Proverbs, Ecclesiastes, Song of Solomon). Read a chapter from Proverbs every day for a few years and your life is bound to improve.[3] Ecclesiastes is also a very valuable source of wisdom. Choose a simple Bible translation such as the New Living Translation (NLT), God's Word Translation (GWT), The Message (MSG), or Easy-to-Read Version (ERV).

Read biographies of wise individuals. Try to understand how and why wise individuals did things the way they did. Read and memorize inspiring quotes by wise individuals daily.

WISDOM FOR CHARACTER DEVELOPEMENT

"Character contributes to beauty. It fortifies a woman as her youth fades. A mode of conduct, a standard of courage, discipline, fortitude, and integrity can do a great deal to make a woman beautiful."
- Jacqueline Bisset, English actress

"Personality can open doors, but only character can keep them open."
- Elmer G. Letterman, business author

"Character isn't something you were born with and can't change, like your fingerprints. It's something you weren't born with and must take responsibility for forming."
- Jim Rohn, American entrepreneur

"Any fool can criticize, condemn, and complain...but it takes character and self control to be understanding and forgiving."
- Dale Carnegie, American writer

"People grow through experience if they meet life honestly and courageously. This is how character is built."
- Eleanor Roosevelt, American First Lady

"The depth and strength of a human character are defined by its moral reserves."
- Leon Trotsky, Russian revolutionary

"Character is doing the right thing when nobody's looking. There are too many people who think that the only thing that's right is to get by, and the only thing that's wrong is to get caught."
- J. C. Watts, American politician

"The measure of a man's real character is what he would do if he knew he would never be found out."
- Thomas B. Macaulay, English historian

Books and sages give knowledge, but wisdom comes from within. Martial arts instructor Dan Inosanto said, "Knowledge comes from your instructors, wisdom comes from within." World-champion athlete Dan Millman said, "Everything you'll ever need to know is within you; the secrets of the universe are imprinted on the cells of your body."

SELFLESSNESS

Being selfish means being far more interested in what we can get rather than what we can give. It's about being concerned about our own interests without considering others. "Selfishness is the greatest curse of the human race," said British statesman William E. Gladstone. Many people consider selfishness in a woman very unattractive and repelling.

Selflessness is the opposite of being selfish. Selflessness means we act without thought for how we will benefit or be rewarded. Johann Wolfgang von Goethe, a German writer, said, "You can easily judge the character of a man by how he treats those who can do nothing for him." Abigail Van Buren, an American journalist, said, "The best index to a person's character is (a) how he treats people who can't do him any good, and (b) how he treats people who can't fight back." Selflessness means we help others because we identify with their problems and their suffering.

Personal fulfillment is found in service to others. "The best way to find yourself is to lose yourself in the service of others," said Indian spiritual leader Mahatma Gandhi. The fourteenth Dalai Lama said, "Our prime purpose in this life is to help others." As German physicist Albert Einstein once noted, "Only a life lived for others is a life worthwhile."

When we give to others, we receive in return. American political journalist Theodore H. White stated, "You can't get unless you give. And you have to give without wanting to get."

In a poem by Maya Angelou entitled, *The Beauty of a Woman*, true beauty in a woman "is reflected by her soul./ It's the caring that she cares to give,/ the passion that she shows." A woman of beautiful character cares about family, friends, and strangers in need.

A woman who cares for others can achieve perfection in character. Scottish economist Adam Smith said, "To feel much for others and little for ourselves; to restrain our selfishness and exercise our benevolent affections, constitute the perfection of human nature."

To learn selflessness, you must learn compassion. Compassion means "to suffer with." Compassion is the ability to understand the suffering or pain of others and maintain a strong desire to help. Most women learn compassion when they experience hardships themselves. For example, if a woman loses a family member in death, she is more likely to understand how another person feels when someone loses a family member in death. Compassion can also be acquired by listening to others without judging them.

Cultivating a humble attitude will cause you to think about yourself less and about others more. "Humility is not thinking less of yourself, it's thinking of yourself less," said American writer Rick Warren.

Selflessness can be learned through developing spirituality. "The brain functions in a certain way during spiritual experiences," said Brick Johnstone, professor of health psychology at the MU School of Health Professions. "We studied people with brain injury and found that people with injuries to the right parietal lobe of the brain reported higher levels of spiritual experiences, such as transcendence." This link is important, Johnstone said, because it means selflessness can be learned by decreasing activity in that part of the brain. He suggests this can be done through conscious effort, such as meditation or prayer.[4]

Selflessness requires some act of volunteering or donating, which causes you to think of yourself less and concern yourself with other people's needs and wants.

Choosing a role model is helpful in developing selflessness. Actress Angelina Jolie is renowned for adopting and raising many children as well as being a goodwill ambassador for the United Nations High Commissioner for Refugees (UNHCR). Actress Audrey Hepburn

SPONSORING A CHILD

Sponsoring a child is very rewarding, especially when you can write letters to them. Not all charity organizations are completely honest. Thus, thorough research on the charity of your choice is required before supporting it. Search for "charity reviews" online, or ask those who work directly for the charity to find one that is honest about contributions. Charities should spend more on program expenses and less on administrative expenses.

devoted a great amount of her time to working for UNICEF as a goodwill ambassador. Top model Joanna Krupa is known for her charity work and deep concern for animal welfare.

Decide how you will contribute to society, and go about doing it. Life ends for everyone at some point. However, what you contribute to society can leave a lasting memory. "The best use of life is to spend it for something that will outlast it," said William James, an American philosopher. American writer Chuck Palahniuk said, "We all die. The goal isn't to live forever, the goal is to create something that will."

INTEGRITY

Integrity means knowing the difference between right and wrong and conforming to a standard of goodness. Goodness is always beautiful. French beauty Ninon de l'Enclos said, "That which is striking and beautiful is not always good, but that which is good is always beautiful."

Integrity gives beauty to the character. Indian spiritual leader Sri Sathya Sai Baba said, "If there is righteousness in the heart, there will be beauty in the character."

Integrity is developed mainly through spirituality since spirituality teaches the value of integrity. Spirituality is about having faith in the unseen, specifically a higher power or God. When

> "If there is righteousness in the heart, there will be beauty in the character."
> - Sri Sathya Sai Baba

you look up to a higher power and make a connection with that power, it causes you to act with integrity.

Spiritual leaders teach that spirituality is essential to life. "Just as a candle cannot burn without fire, men cannot live without a spiritual life," said Indian spiritual leader Gautama Buddha.

There is no spirituality without belief in the existence of a higher power. Evidence of a higher power is seen through all that exists just as evidence of the wind is seen through the movement of the trees. English poet Christina Rossetti wrote: "Who has seen the wind?/ Neither you nor I./ But when the trees bow down their heads,/ The wind is passing by."

Belief in a higher power who created everything is the most reasonable conclusion. Amino acids will not link together to form proteins. It is like saying that, if bricks formed in nature, they would get together to build houses. Proteins never form except in already-living cells. Never! Evidence that life never comes from nonliving materials is so abundant that it is a basic principle of science, called the Principle of Biogenesis.[5]

Some women may not believe in a higher power due to difficult circumstances. However, everyone is responsible for their own life. The Bible says, "People ruin their lives by their own stupidity, so why does God always get blamed?" (MSG, Proverbs 19:3). "God made men and women true and upright; we're the ones who've made a mess of things" (MSG, Ecclesiastes 7:29).

Spirituality is beyond just religion. Religion has, for many, become negatively associated with obligatory creeds and rituals. Spirituality is positively thought of as deeply individual and subjective.[6] "Religion has a great role to play in the encouragement of character development, and often does so admirably. Sometimes, however, religion may actually undermine that process," says David Truman, a spiritual mentor.

True spirituality is developed from within and not by any man-made religion. "All religions have been made by men," said French military and political leader Napoleon.

Religions teach that you need to follow their rituals or teachings to be spiritual. Writer Duane Alan Hahn noted, "They say that you need to follow their teachings because you cannot be good on your own, but you are never alone. There is never a time when you are separate from God." The 14th Dalai Lama, a Tibetan spiritual leader, said, "If you have a particular faith or religion, that is good. But you can survive without it."

You are made of spirituality since your spirit comes from God and goes back to God (Ecclesiastes 12:7). Pierre Teilhard de Chardin, a French priest and philosopher, said, "We are not human beings having a spiritual experience. We are spiritual beings having a human experience."

True spirituality comes from loving motivations, not religious or spiritual practices dictated by time. True spirituality guides your everyday actions, your speech, and your whole life. It is the "deepest values and meanings by which people live."[7]

How a woman treats others is one of the best measures of spirituality. "True spirituality begins where self-serving ego leaves off and where the consideration of others begins," says David Truman. The Bible says, "Religion that God our Father accepts as pure and faultless is this: to look after orphans and widows" (NIV, James 1:27).

Jesus, the founder of Christianity, taught that the greatest commandment is to love others (Matthew 22:36–39). All the teachings found in the Bible are based simply on loving others (Matthew 22:39–40). Our only requirement in life is to love (Luke 10:25–28). "Where love is, there God is also," said Indian spiritual leader Mahatma Gandhi. The fourteenth Dalai Lama said, "Love and compassion are the true religions to me. But to develop this, we do not need to believe in any religion." Franklin D. Roosevelt, the thirty-second president of the United States said, "Selfishness is the only real atheism...unselfishness, the only real religion."

Mother Teresa was once asked, "Can you sum up what love really is?" She replied: "Love is giving." If we stop giving, we stop loving; if we stop loving, we stop growing; and unless we grow we will never achieve happiness and satisfaction as a result of fully developing our character.[8]

The fourteenth Dalai Lama said, "Love is the absence of judgment." Non-judgment comes from being aware that we are all made of the same spiritual energy (Genesis 1:27, 1 John

4:8). Therefore, we are one with God and all in existence (Mark 12:29). We are all one and the same.[9]

To love is to access the great spiritual power of God (1 John 4:16). "Love is the greatest power on earth. It conquers all things," said American activist Peace Pilgrim.

The Bible is an accurate guidebook to spirituality that has stood the test of time. American clergyman Aiden Wilson Tozer said, "The Word of God well understood and religiously obeyed is the shortest route to spiritual perfection."

Approximately two thousand five hundred prophecies appear in the pages of the Bible. About two thousand of them have already been fulfilled. Since the probability for any one of these prophecies having been fulfilled by chance averages less than one in ten and since the prophecies are, for the most part, independent of one another, the odds for all these prophecies having been fulfilled by chance without error are less than one in 10^{2000} (one with 2,000 zeros written after it).[10]

In the book *The Purpose Driven Life*, Rick Warren explains that being spiritual means more than creeds and convictions; it includes conduct and character. "The Bible is more than a doctrinal guidebook...it produces change...[and] builds character," says Warren.

Prayer is a connecting force to God. It is a vital part of spirituality. "Prayer is man's greatest power!" said William Clement Stone. However, some feel that God doesn't answer their prayers.

Prayers may not be answered because of "evil deeds" (Isaiah 1:13–17). Some refer to this as the law of cause and effect. One of the laws of physics is that "to every action there is always an equal and opposite reaction."

The fact is acceptable behavior leads to accepted prayers. The Bible says, "Share your food with the hungry and open your homes to the homeless poor. Give clothes to those who have nothing to wear, and do not refuse to help your own relatives"

(GNT, Isaiah 58:7). "Then when you pray, God will answer" (MSG, Isaiah 58:9).

FORTITUDE

Fortitude is having courage and endurance in dealing with hardships. Serious illness, violent abuse, death of loved ones, or facing natural disasters can lead only to two things: fortitude or breakdown.

Breakdown occurs when challenges paralyze us. "Life's challenges are not supposed to paralyze you, they're supposed to help you discover who you are," said Bernice Johnson Reagon, an American musician.

American model and actress Rita Mero once said, "I think that everything happens to you for a reason. The hard times that you go through build character, making you a much stronger person."

Hardships are the greatest learning experiences. Indian spiritual leader Swami Vivekananda said, "You will find that misery and happiness are equal factors in the formation of... character...and in some instances misery is a greater teacher than happiness."[11]

At times, hardships are meant to test your character. Rick Warren, in his book *The Purpose Driven Life*, said, "When you understand that life is a test, you realize that nothing is insignificant in your life. Even the smallest incident has significance for your character development. Character is both developed and revealed by tests, and all of life is a test. God constantly watches your response to people, problems, conflict, illness, and disappointment."[12]

Throughout the Bible we see how God tested people. The Israelites were tested for forty years! The Bible says, "Remember how the Lord your God led you through the wilderness for these forty years, humbling you and testing you to prove your character" (NLT, Deuteronomy 8:2). God tested Joseph for more than twenty years! The Bible says, "Until the time came to fulfill his dreams, the Lord tested Joseph's character" (NLT, Psalm 105:19).

Consider how God uses the same process of heat refinement on us as on silver and gold. A silversmith must hold the silver in the middle of the fire where the flames are the hottest to burn away all the impurities. God sits as a refiner and purifier of silver (Malachi 3:3). The silversmith has to sit there in front of the fire the whole time the silver is being refined. He knows the silver is fully refined when he sees his image in it. You will be fully refined when God sees his image in you. Just as silver goes through an extensive and complex process of refinement, the fire of hardship refines character. "It is the fire of suffering that brings forth the gold of godliness," said French writer Madame Guyon.

The way you react to any hardships in life will determine the outcome. Do you get bitter or better? Some women become miserable when faced with challenges. They refuse to interpret the lessons these challenges bring. Women who face challenges with a

FORTITUDE BIBLICAL WISDOM

"Fire tests the purity of silver and gold, but the Lord tests the heart." (NLT, Proverbs 17:3)

"But he knows where I am going. And when he tests me, I will come out as pure as gold." (NLT, Job 23:10)

"I will bring this third through the fire. I will refine them as silver is refined. I will test them as gold is tested." (GWT, Zechariah 13:9)

"Sorrow is better than laughter, for sadness has a refining influence on us." (NLT, Ecclesiastes 7:3)

positive attitude will be able to deal with them. American novelist Ellen Glasgow once said, "Nothing in life is so hard that you can't make it easier by the way you take it."

We learn and we grow through life's challenges if we view them as blessings in disguise. Roman lyric poet Horace said, "Adversity has the effect of eliciting talents which in prosperous circumstances would have lain dormant." American psychiatrist Elisabeth Kübler-Ross said, "There are no mistakes, no coincidences. All events are blessings given to us to learn from."

Building fortitude requires understanding that suffering has a purpose and a meaning. Life is full of meaning since we are not here by accident. We are all part of God's plan in some way.[13]

In the book *Man's Search for Meaning*, Viktor E. Frankl, a psychiatrist who wrote of his experiences in a Nazi concentration camp, stated: "Man is not destroyed by suffering; he is destroyed by suffering without meaning." Frankl founded logotherapy, a therapy based on finding meaning in suffering. He believed that "there is nothing in the world that would so effectively help one survive even the worst conditions as the knowledge that there is a meaning in one's life."[14] Frankl also believed that when we are no longer able to change a situation, we are challenged to change ourselves. When an individual discovers their true talent and begins to use it with dedication, they may overcome great hardship in life.[15]

The best way to deal with difficult circumstances is to keep busy. American businessman Lee Iacocca said, "In times of great stress or adversity, it's always best to keep busy, to plow your anger and your energy into something positive."

The beauty of all hardship comes after the suffering. Austrian neurologist Sigmund Freud said, "One day, in retrospect, the years of struggle will strike you as the most beautiful." Peter Marshall, a Scottish clergyman, said, "When we long for life without difficulties, remind us that oaks grow strong in contrary winds and diamonds are made under pressure."

As with muscles, character is strengthened through resistance. American author Helen Keller said, "Character cannot be developed in ease and quiet. Only through experience of trial and suffering can the soul be strengthened, vision cleared, ambition inspired, and success achieved."

Appendix A

THE UNHEALTHY PURSUIT OF OUTER BEAUTY

Women should keep in mind that there is a fine line between the desire to be attractive and just plain vanity. The desire to look beautiful stems from the desire to attract a romantic partner and the need for love and acceptance. All women aspire to be admired. Just as men want power and respect, women want beauty and love.

Vanity is defined as excessive pride in one's appearance, excessive desire for notice or approval, and excessive focus on one's appearance. Notice the repetition of the word "excessive." Everything requires balance or it can become an unhealthy obsession.

Aiming for perfection helps us accomplish more than does a lazy attitude. British statesman Lord Chesterfield said, "Aim at perfection in everything, though in most things it is unattainable. However, they who aim at it, and persevere, will come much nearer to it than those whose laziness and despondency make them give it up as unattainable." However, improvement, not perfection, should be the goal. "Strive for continuous improvement, instead of perfection," said St. Kittitian athlete Kim Collins.

VANITY QUIZ

1. Do you excessively look at yourself in the mirror?
2. Do you excessively feel proud of your physical appearance?
3. Do you excessively need notice or approval from people?
4. Do you excessively spend time on making yourself look beautiful?
5. Do you excessively concern yourself with your imperfections?

Answering "yes" to more than two questions is a sign of vanity. The more "yes" answers you gave, the higher the level of vanity.

Perfection is something all humans are naturally wired to strive for. The closer we get to perfection, the more satisfied we feel. However, only a healthy pursuit of beauty can give a woman satisfaction.

The pursuit of looking attractive can be assessed to see if it is at a healthy or an unhealthy level. Psychologists categorize perfectionists as adaptive (healthy) perfectionists and maladaptive (unhealthy) perfectionists. Healthy perfectionists are motivated, while unhealthy perfectionists are obsessed.

Healthy perfectionists set high but achievable standards for themselves and use these standards to motivate themselves to do their best. Striving to be the best that you can be is a commendable quality. This form of perfectionism, measured by a subscale of the Almost Perfect Scale-Revised (APS-R), called the High Standards scale, is associated with healthy psychological outcomes such as high self-esteem.

Unhealthy perfectionists set unattainably high standards. No level of achievement is ever enough. This form of perfectionism, measured by another subscale of the APS-R, called the Discrepancy scale, is correlated with unhealthy mental conditions.[1]

A study led by Kenneth Rice found that healthy perfectionism leads to high achievement, while unhealthy perfectionism leads to depression and hopelessness.[2] Another study, by Diane

K. Delegard, PhD, a counselor and psychologist, has shown that there is a correlation between unhealthy perfectionism, and anxiety, depression, low self-esteem, and internal shame.[3] Eating disorders such as anorexia nervosa and bulimia nervosa can also result from unhealthy perfectionism.[4]

A study found that some young women felt that it was a must for them to look pretty in order to be accepted by their peers. The researchers concluded that peer and media influences play a key role in appearance-based rejection sensitivity. The results held true even after accounting for self-esteem, self-perceived attractiveness, and sensitivity to rejection in general. Within younger age groups, peers will cast out individuals who do not fit a certain beauty or behavior standard.[5]

> "Strive for continuous improvement, instead of perfection."
> - Kim Collins

The main cause of vanity is the false belief that the pursuit of physical beauty will make you truly happy. Being beautiful will never bring ultimate happiness and satisfaction. The world's most beautiful and truly happy women are those who are able to balance the pursuit of outer beauty with the pursuit of inner beauty.

Appendix B

WHY DOES IMPERFECTION EXIST?

*A*s stated at the beginning of the book, studies have shown that we all have an innate template of what a woman "should" look like. If there is perfection in female beauty, why, then, is there imperfection in female beauty?

Scientists might argue that imperfection in beauty is a result of genetic disorder or illness. Religion may state that all imperfection is caused by sin. New Thought leaders may teach that imperfection is a state of mind. Any one of these or a combination of these factors may be the cause of imperfection in female beauty.

Everything in life appears to have two polar opposites: Good and bad; healthy and unhealthy; beautiful and ugly. Ancient wisdom teaches that everything has positive and negative aspects (Ecclesiastes 3:1–8). We can form our opinion as to what is the purpose of contrast.

One of the most reasonable explanations for the purpose of contrast is found in the book, *Your Soul's Plan*. Robert Schwartz explains that contrast leads to greater appreciation and understanding of the positive. He says, "The physical plane provides us with this contrast because it is one of duality: up and down, hot and cold, good and bad. The sorrow in duality allows us to better know joy. The chaos of Earth enhances our appreciation of peace. The hatred we may encounter deepens our understanding of love." In chapter two of the *Tao Te Ching* it says, "Under Heaven all can see beauty as beauty only because there is ugliness. All can know good as good only because there is evil." Therefore, we can conclude that without contrast to beauty, we cannot fully understand and appreciate the beauty we see.

Acknowledgments

I wish to thank my mother, Krystyna, who always believed in me, encouraged me, and helped to foster my passion for writing. You are the brightest star in the universe.

I would also like to thank Adam, who provided loving support and positive encouragement during the entire creation process of this book. I may have not written this book if it wasn't for him.

I would like to humbly thank Giovanni, who gave me a very valuable suggestion that motivated me to start writing this book. Without his advice, I might never have undertaken the large and time-consuming task of writing this book.

Thank you to my editor Rob Tilley, who did a spectacular job; I couldn't have asked for a better editor. I would also like to thank my two other editors Gina Melissa Fusco and Gail Lennon.

References

INTRODUCTION

1. Saladin, M. E., Saper, Z. L., & Breen, L. J. (1988). Perceived attractiveness and attributions of criminality: What is beautiful is not criminal. *Canadian Journal of Criminology*, 30(3), 251–59.

2. Stewart, J. E. (1980). Defendant's attractiveness as a factor in the outcome of criminal trials: An observational study. *Journal of Applied Social Psychology*, 10(4), 348–61.

3. Sigall, H., & Ostrove, N. (1975). Beautiful but dangerous: Effects of offender attractiveness and nature of the crime on juridic judgement. *Journal of Personality and Social Psychology*, 31(3), 410—14.

4. Gunnell, J. J., & Ceci, S. J. (2010). When emotionality trumps reason: A study of individual processing style and juror bias. *Behavioral Sciences and the Law*, 28(6), 850–77.

5. Cash, T. F., & Kilcullen, R. N. (1985). The aye of the beholder: susceptibility to sexism and beautyism in the evaluation of managerial applicants. *Journal of Applied Social Psychology*, 15(4), 591–605.

6. Chiu, R. K., & Babcock, R. D. (2002). The relative importance of facial attractiveness and gender in Hong Kong selection decisions. *International Journal of Human Resource Management,* 13(1), 141–55.

7. Marlowe, C. M., Schneider, S. L., & Nelson, C. E. (1996). Gender and attractiveness biases in hiring decisions: Are more experienced managers less biased? *Journal of Applied Psychology*, 81(1), 11–21.

8. Judge, T., & Cable, D. (2011). When it comes to pay, do the thin win? The effect of weight on pay for men and women. *Journal of Applied Psychology*, 96(1), 95–112.

9. Feingold, A. (1992). Good-looking people are not what we think. *Psychological Bulletin*, 111(2), 304–41.

10. Dion, K., Berscheid, E., & Walster, E. (1972). What is beautiful is good. *Journal of Personality and Social Psychology*, 24(3), 285–90.

11. Langlois, J. H., Kalakanis, L., Rubenstein, A. J., Larson, A., Hallamm, M., & Smoot, M. (2000). Maxims or myths of beauty? A meta-analytic and theoretical review. *Psychological Bulletin*, 126(3), 390–423.

12. Ramsey, J. L., Langlois, J. H., Hoss, R. A., Rubenstein, A. J., & Griffin, A. M. (2004). Origins of a stereotype: Categorization of facial attractiveness by 6-month-old infants. *Developmental Science*, 7(2), 201–11.

13. Langlois, J. H., Roggman, L. A., Casey, R. J., Ritter, J. M., Rieser-Danner, L. A., & Jenkins, V. Y. (1987). Infant preferences for attractive faces: Rudiments of a stereotype? *Developmental Psychology*, 23(3), 363—69.

14. Rubenstein, A. R., Kalakanis, L. A., & Langlois, J. H. (1999). Infant Preferences for Attractive Faces: A Cognitive Explanation. *Developmental Psychology*, 35(3), 848–55.

15. Slater, A. M., et al. (1998). Newborn infants prefer attractive faces. *Infant Behavior and Development*, 21(2), 345–54.

16. Buss, D. M. (1989) Sex differences in human mate preferences: Evolutionary hypotheses tested in 37 cultures. *Behavioral and Brain Sciences*, 12(1), 1–49.

17. Buss, D. M., & Barnes, M. (1986). Preferences in human mate selection. *Journal of Personality and Social Psychology*, 50(3), 559–70.

18. Berscheid, E., Dion, K., Walster, E., & Walster, W. G. (1971). Physical attractiveness and dating choice: A test of the matching hypothesis. *Journal of Experimental Social Psychology*, 7(2), 173–89.

19. Andersson, M. (1994). *Sexual selection*. Princeton (NJ): Princeton University Press.

20. Roberts, S. C., et al. (2004). Female facial attractiveness increases during the fertile phase of the menstrual cycle. *Proceedings Biological Sciences*, 271(Suppl 5), S270–S272.

21. Kościński, K. (2008). Facial attractiveness: Variation, adaptiveness and consequences of facial preferences. *Anthropological Review*, 71(1), 77–105.

22. Hönekopp, J., Bartholomé, T., & Jansen, G. (2004). Facial attractiveness, symmetry, and physical fitness in young women. *Human Nature*, 15(2), 147–67.

23. Shackelford, T. K., & Larsen, R. J. (1999). Facial attractiveness and physical health. *Evolution and Human Behavior*, 20, 71–76.

24. Thornhill, R., & Gangestad. S. W. (2006). Facial sexual dimorphism, developmental stability, and susceptibility to disease in men and women. *Evolution and Human Behavior*, 27(2), 131–44.

25. Thornhill, R., & Grammer, K. (1999). The body and face of woman: One ornament that signals quality? *Evolution and Human Behavior*, 20(2), 105–20.

26. Buss, D. (2003). *The Evolution of desire: Strategies of human mating.* New York: Basic Books.

27. Sigall, H., & Landy, D. (1973). Radiating beauty: Effects of having a physically attractive partner on person perception. *Journal of Personality and Social Psychology,* 28(2), 218–24.

28. Peterson, C., & Seligman, M. E. P. (2004). *Character strengths and virtues: A handbook and classification.* Washington: APA Press and Oxford University Press.

CHAPTER 1: FACE

1. Confer J. C., Perilloux, C., & Buss, D. M. (2010). More than just a pretty face: Men's priority shifts toward bodily attractiveness in short-term versus long-term mating contexts. *Evolution and Human Behavior,* 31(5), 348–53.

2. Johnston, V. S., & Franklin, M. (1993). Is beauty in the eye of the beholder? *Ethology and Sociobiology,* 14(3), 183–99.

3. Hill, K. R., & Hurtado, A. M. (1996). *Ache life history: The ecology and demography of a foraging people.* Piscataway (NJ): Aldine Transaction.

4. Pessa, J. E., Slice, D. E., Hanz, K. R., Broadbent, T. H. Jr, & Rohrich, R. J. (2008). Aging and the shape of the mandible. *Plastic and Reconstructive Surgery,* 121(1), 196–200.

5. Pallett, P. M., Link, S., & Lee, K. (2010). New "golden" ratios for facial beauty. *Vision Research,* 50(2), 149–54.

6. Jefferson Y. (2004). Facial beauty:establishing a universal standard. *International Journal Of Orthodontics,* 15(1), 9–22.

7. Jasienska, G., Lipson, S. F., Ellison, P. T., Thune, I., & Ziomkiewicz, A. (2006). Symmetrical women have higher potential fertility. *Evolution and Human Behavior,* 27(5), 390–400.

8. Thornhill, R., & Gangestad, S. W. (1993). Human facial beauty: averageness, symmetry, and parasite resistance. *Human Nature,* 4(3), 237–69.

9. Thornhill, R., Møller, A. P. (1997). Developmental stability, disease and medicine. *Biological Reviews,* 72(4), 497–528.

10. Manning, J. T., Scutt, D., Whitehouse, G. H., Leinster, S. J., & Walton, J. M. (1996). Asymmetry and the menstrual cycle in women. *Ethology and Sociobiology,* 17(2), 129–43.

11. Borelli, C., & Berneburg, M. (2010). "Beauty lies in the eye of the beholder"? Aspects of beauty and attractiveness. *Journal der Deutschen Dermatologischen Gesellschaft,* 8(5), 326–30.

12. Cunningham, M. R. (1986). Measuring the physical in physical attractiveness:

Quasi-experiments on the sociobiology of female facial beauty. *Journal of Personality and Social Psychology*, 50(5), 925–35.

13. Jones, D. (1996). *Physical attractiveness and the theory of sexual selection*. Ann Arbor: Museum of Anthropology University of Michigan.

14. Etcoff, N. (2000). *Survival of The Prettiest: The Science of Beauty*. New York: Anchor.

15. Kościński, K. (2007). Facial attractiveness: General patterns of facial preferences. *Anthropological Review*, 70(1), 45–79.

16. Law Smith, M. J., et al. (2006). Facial appearance is a cue to oestrogen levels in women. *Proceedings of the Royal Society B: Biological Sciences*, 273(1583), 135–40.

17. Little, A. C., et al. (2008). Symmetry is related to sexual dimorphism in faces: Data across culture and species. *PLoS ONE*, 3(5), e2106.

18. Thornhill, R., Gangestad, S. W. (1999). Facial attractiveness. *Trends in Cognitive Sciences,* 3(12), 452–60.

19. Ellison, P. T. (1998). Reproductive ecology and reproductive cancers. In Panter–Brick, & C., Worthman, C. (Eds.), *Hormones, Health and Behavior* (pp. 184–209). Cambridge: Cambridge University Press.

20. Thornhill, R., & Grammer, K. (1999). The body and face of woman: One ornament that signals quality? *Evolution and Human Behavior,* 20(2), 105–20.

21. Edwards, K. (1987). Effects of sex and glasses on attitudes toward intelligence and attractiveness. *Psychological Reports*, 60(2), 590.

22. Terry, R. L. (1993). How wearing eyeglasses affects facial recognition. *Current Psychology*, 12(2), 151–62.

23. Swami, V., Stieger, S., Pietschnig, J., Voracek, M., Furnham, A., & Tovée, M. J. (2011). The influence of facial piercings and observer personality on perceptions of physical attractiveness and intelligence. *European Psychologist*, 1(1), 1-9.

24. Thompson, L., Malmberg, J., Goodell, N., & Boring, R. (2004). The distribution of attention across a talker's face. *Discourse Process*, 38(1), 145–68.

25. Russell, R. (2009). A sex difference in facial contrast and its exaggeration by cosmetics. *Perception*, 38(8), 1211—19.

26. Russell, R. (2003). Sex, beauty, and the relative luminance of facial features. *Perception*, 32(9), 1093–107.

27. Gründl, M., Knoll, S., Eisenmann-Klein, M., & Prantl, L. (2012). The blue-eyes stereotype: Do eye color, pupil diameter, and scleral color affect attractiveness? *Aesthetic Plastic Surgery*, 36(2), 234–40.

28. Laeng, B., Mathisen, R., & Johnsen, J. A. (2007). Why do blue-eyed men prefer women with the same eye colour? *Behavioral Ecology and Sociobiology*, 61(3), 371–84.

29. Gunter, J. P., & Antrobus, S. D. (1997). Aesthetic analysis of the eyebrows. *Plastic and Reconstructive Surgery*, 99(7), 1808–16.

30. Wolfort, F. G., Gee, J., Pan, D., & Morris, D. (1997). Nuances of aesthetic blepharoplasty. *Annals of Plastic Surgery*, 38(3), 257–62.

31. Biller, J. A., & Kim, D. W. (2009). A contemporary assessment of facial aesthetic preferences. *Archives of Facial Plastic Surgery*, 11(2), 91–97.

32. Cohen, J. L. (2010). Enhancing the growth of natural eyelashes: The mechanism of bimatoprost-induced eyelash growth. *Dermatologic Surgery*, 36(9), 1361–71.

33. Jones, D. (2011). Enhanced eyelashes: Prescription and over-the-counter options. *Aesthetic Plastic Surgery*, 35(1), 116–21.

34. Johnstone, M. A., & Albert, D. M. (2002). Prostaglandin-induced hair growth. *Survey of Ophthalmology*, 47(Suppl 1), S185–202.

35. Tracy, J. L., & Beall, A. T. (2011). Happy guys finish last: The impact of emotion expressions on sexual attraction. *Emotion*, 11(6), 1379–87.

36. Dong, J. K., Jin, T. H., Cho, H. W., & Oh, S. C. (1999). The esthetics of the smile: A review of some recent studies. *The International Journal of Prosthodontics*, 12(1), 9–19.

37. Dunn, W. J., Murchison, D. F., & Broome, J. C. (1996). Esthetics: patients' perceptions of dental attractiveness. *Journal of Prosthodontics*, 5(3), 166–71.

38. Ong, E., Brown, R. A., & Richmond, S. (2006). Peer assessment of dental attractiveness. *American Journal of Orthodontics and Dentofacial Orthopedics*, 130(2), 163—69.

39. Nagel, R. (2009). *Cure tooth decay: Heal and prevent cavities with nutrition*. Los Gatos (CA): Golden Child Publishing.

40. Peters, M. C., Tallman, J. A., Braun, T. M., & Jacobson, J. J. (2010). Clinical reduction of *S. mutans* in pre-school children using a novel liquorice root extract lollipop: a pilot study. *European Archives of Paediatric Dentistry*, 11(6), 274—78.

41. Fink, B., Grammer, K., & Thornhill, R. (2001). Human (*Homo sapiens*) facial attractiveness in relation to skin texture and color. *Journal of Comparative Psychology*, 115(1), 92–99.

42. Ferriman, D., & Gallwey, J. D. (1961). Clinical assessment of body hair growth in women. *Journal of Clinical Endocrinology and Metabolism*, 21, 1440—47.

43. Graham, J. A., & Jouhar, A. J. (1981). The effects of cosmetics on person perception. *International Journal of Cosmetic Science*, 3(5), 199–210.

44. Cash, T. F., Dawson, K., Davis, P., Bowen, M., & Galumbeck, C. (1989). Effects of cosmetics use on the physical attractiveness and body image of American college women. *The Journal of Social Psychology*, 129(3), 349–55.

45. Workman, J. E., & Johnson, K. K. (1991). The role of cosmetics in impression formation. *Clothing and Textiles Research Journal*, 10(1), 63–67.

46. Mulhern, R., Fieldman, G., Hussey, T., Lévêque, J.-L. & Pineau, P. (2003). Do cosmetics enhance female Caucasian facial attractiveness? *International Journal of Cosmetic Science*, 25(4), 199–205.

47. Fink, B., & Neave, N. (2005). The biology of facial beauty. *International Journal of Cosmetic Science*, 27(6), 317–25.

48. Stephen, I. D., & McKeegan, A. M. (2010). Lip colour affects perceived sex typicality and attractiveness of human faces. *Perception*, 39(8), 1104–10.

49. Rogers, M. F. (1999). *Barbie culture*. London: Sage Publication.

CHAPTER 2: SKIN

1. Kościński, K. (2007). Facial attractiveness: General patterns of facial preferences. *Anthropological Review*, 70(1), 45–79.

2. Darbre, P. D., Aljarrah, A., Miller, W. R., Coldham, N. G., Sauer, M. J., & Pope, G. S. (2004). Concentrations of parabens in human breast tumours. *Journal of Applied Toxicology*, 24(1), 5–13.

3. Patil, S. M., Singh, P., & Maibach, H. I. (1994). Cumulative irritancy in man to sodium lauryl sulfate: The overlap phenomenon. *International Journal of Pharmaceutics*, 110(2), 147–54.

4. Cosmetic Ingredient Review. (1983). Final report on the safety assessment of sodium lauryl sulfate and ammonium lauryl sulfate. *Journal of the American College of Toxicology*, 2(7), 127–81.

5. Shi, J., Yu, J., Pohorly, J. E., & Kakuda, Y. (2003). Polyphenolics in grape seeds-biochemistry and functionality. *Journal of Medicinal Food*, 6(4), 291—99.

6. Kohno, Y., Egawa, Y., Itoh, S., Nagaoka, S., Takahashi, M., & Mukai, K. (1995). Kinetic study of quenching reaction of singlet oxygen and scavenging reaction of free radical by squalene in n-butanol. *Biochimica et Biophysica Acta*, 1256(1), 52–56.

7. Pareja B., & Kehl H. (1990). Contribution to the identification of the active principles of Rosa aff Rubiginosa L. *Anales de la Real Academia de Farmacia*, 56(2), 283–94.

8. Habashy, R. R., Abdel-Naim, A. B., Khalifa, A. E., & Al-Azizi, M. M. (2005). Anti-inflammatory effects of jojoba liquid wax in experimental models. *Pharmacological Research*, 51(2), 95–105.

9. Nissen, H. P., Blitz, H., & Muggli, R. (1995). The effects of gamma-linolenic acid on skin smoothness, humidity and TEWL: A clinical study. *INFORM*, 6(4), 519.

10. Swisher, H. E. (1988). Avocado oil: From food use to skin care. *Journal of the American Oil Chemists' Society*, 65(11), 1704–6.

11. Upadhyay, N. K., et al. (2009). Safety and healing efficacy of Sea buckthorn (*Hippophae rhamnoides L.*) seed oil on burn wounds in rats. *Food and Chemical Toxicology*, 47(6), 1146–53.

12. Cordain, L. (2005). Implications for the role of diet in acne. *Seminars In Cutaneous Medicine and Surgery*, 24(2), 84–91.

13. Smith, R. N., Mann, N. J., Braue, A., Mäkeläinen, H., & Varigos, G. (2007). A low glycemic load improves symptoms in acute vulgaris patients: A randomised controlled trial. *American Journal of Clinical Nutrition*, 86(1), 107–15.

14. Franks, S. (1995). Polycystic ovary syndrome. *New England Journal of Medicine*, 333(13), 853–61.

15. Armanini, D, et al. (2004) Licorice reduces serum testosterone in healthy women. *Steroids*, 69(11-12), 763—66.

16. Marks, L. S., Hess, D. L., Dorey, F. J., Luz Macairan, M., Cruz Santos, P. B., & Tyler, V. E. (2001). Tissue effects of saw palmetto and finasteride: Use of biopsy cores for in situ quantification of prostatic androgens. *Urology*, 57(5), 999-1005.

17. Amann, W. (1967). Improvement of acne vulgaris with Agnus castus (Agnolyt™). [Article in German] *Therapie der Gegenwart*, 106(1), 124—26.

18. Zaun, H. (1972). Gastric function in patients with skin diseases: Analysis of electrogastrographical findings in 1282 dermatologic patients. [Article in German] *Münchener Medizinische Wochenschrift*, 114(1), 33–37.

19. Henseler, T. (1995) Mucocutaneous candidiasis in patients with skin diseases. [Article in German] *Mycoses*, 38(Suppl 1), 7–13.

20. Enshaieh, S., Jooya, A., Siadat, A. H., & Iraji, F. (2007). The efficacy of 5% topical tea tree oil gel in mild to moderate acne vulgaris: A randomized, double-blind placebo-controlled study. *Indian Journal of Dermatology*, 73(1), 22–25.

21. Bassett, I. B., Pannowitz, D. L., & Barnetson, R. S. (1990). A comparative study of tea-tree oil versus benzoylperoxide in the treatment of acne. *Medical Journal of Australia*, 153(8), 455—58.

22. Webster, G., Cargill, D. I., Quiring, J., Vogelson, C. T., & Slade, H. B. (2009). A combined analysis of 2 randomized clinical studies of tretinoin gel 0.05% for the treatment of acne. *Cutis; Cutaneous Medicine for the Practitioner*, 83(3), 146–54.

23. Shalita, A., et al. (1996). A comparison of the efficacy and safety of adapalene gel 0.1% and tretinoin gel 0.025% in the treatment of acne vulgaris: A multicenter trial. *Journal of the American Academy of Dermatology*, 34(3), 482—85.

24. Callaway, J., et al. (2005). Efficacy of dietary hempseed oil in patients with atopic dermatitis. *Journal of Dermatological Treatment*, 16(2), 87–94.

25. Shalin-Karrila, M., Mattila, L., Jansen, C. T., & Uotila, P. (1987). Evening primrose oil in the treatment of atopic eczema: Effect on clinical status, plasma phospholipid fatty acids and circulating blood prostaglandins. *British Journal of Dermatology*, 117(1), 11–19.

26. Saeedi, M., Morteza-Semnani, K., & Ghoreishi, M. R. (2003). The treatment of atopic dermatitis with licorice gel. *Journal of Dermatological Treatment*, 14(3), 153—57.

27. Ditre, C. M., et al. (1996). Effects of alpha hydroxy-acids on photoaged skin: A pilot clinical, histologic and ultrastructural study. *Journal of the American Academy of Dermatology*, 34(2 pt. 1), 187–95.

28. Van Scott, E. J., Ditre, C. M., & Yu, R. J. (1996). Alpha-hydroxyacids in the treatment of signs of photoaging. *Clinics in Dermatology*, 14(2), 217–26.

29. Miller, S. J. (1989). . *Journal of the American Academy of Dermatology*, 21(1), 1–30.

30. Purba, M. B., et al. (2001). Skin wrinkling: can food make a difference? *Journal of the American College of Nutrition*, 20(1), 71–80.

31. Page, R. L. (2008). *Healthy Healing's Detoxification*. Healthy Healing LLC.

32. Stephen, I. D., Coetzee, V., Law Smith, M. J., & Perrett, D. I. (2009). Skin blood perfusion and oxygenation colour affect perceived human health. *PLoS ONE*, 4(4), e5083.

33. Axelsson, J., Sundelin, T., Ingre, M., Van Someren, E. J., Olsson, A., & Lekander, M. (2010). Beauty sleep: Experimental study on the perceived health and attractiveness of sleep deprived people. *British Medical Journal*, 341, c6614.

34. O'Donoghue, M. N. (1991). Cosmetics for the elderly. *Dermatologic Clinics*, 9(1), 29–34.

35. Gunn, D. A., et al. (2009). Why Some Women Look Young for Their Age. *PLoS ONE*, 4(12), e8021.

36. Hensley, K., & Floyd, R. A. (2002). Reactive oxygen species and protein oxidation in aging: A look back, a look ahead. *Archives of Biochemistry and Biophysics*, 397(2), 377–83.

37. Hanson, K. M., Gratton, E., & Bardeen, C. J. (2006). Sunscreen enhancement of UV-induced reactive oxygen species in the skin. *Free Radical Biology and Medicine*, 41(8), 1205–12.

38. Warner, W. G., Yin, J. J., & Wei, R. R. (1997). Oxidative damage to nucleic acids photosensitized by titanium dioxide. *Free Radical Biology and Medicine*, 23(6), 851—58.

39. Silverberg, N., Silverberg, L. (1989). Aging and the skin. *Postgraduate Medicine*, 86(1), 131–6, 141—44.

40. Baumann, L. (2007). Skin ageing and its treatment. *Journal of Pathology*, 211(2), 241–51.

41. Varani, J., et al. (2000). Vitamin A antagonizes decreased cell growth and elevated collagen-degrading matrix metalloproteinases and stimulates collagen accumulation in naturally aged human skin. *Journal of Investigative Dermatology*, 114(3), 480–86.

42. Nusgens, B. V., et al. (2001). Topically applied vitamin C enhances the mRNA level of collagens I and III, their processing enzymes and tissue inhibitor of matrix

metalloproteinase 1 in the human dermis. *Journal of Investigative Dermatology*, 116(6), 853–59.

43. Griffiths, C. E., Russman, A. N., Majmudar, G., Singer, R. S., Hamilton, T. A., & Voorhees, J. J. (1993). Restoration of collagen formation in photodamaged human skin by tretinoin (retinoic acid). *New England Journal of Medicine*, 329(8), 530—35.

44. Bhawan, J., et al. (1995). Reversible histologic effects of tretinoin on photodamaged skin. *Journal of Geriatric Dermatology*, 3, 62–67.

45. Kang, S., Fisher, & G. J., Voorhees, J. J. (2001). Photoaging: Pathogenesis, prevention, and treatment. *Clinics in Geriatric Medicine*, 17(4), 643–59.

46. Gilchrest, B. A. (1997). Treatment of photodamage with topical tretinoin: an overview. *Journal of the American Academy of Dermatology*, 36(3 pt. 2), S27–36.

47. Latriano, L., Tzimas, G., Wong, F., & Wills, R. J. (1997). The percutaneous absorption of topically applied tretinoin and its effect on endogenous plasma concentrations of tretinoin and its metabolites after single doses or long-term use. *Journal of the American Academy of Dermatology*, 36(3 pt. 2), S37–46.

48. Ellis, C. N., Weiss, J. S., Hamilton, T. A., Headington, J. T., Zelickson, A. S., & Voorhees, J. J. (1990). Sustained improvement with prolonged topical tretinoin (retinoic acid) for photoaged skin. *Journal of the American Academy of Dermatology*, 23(4 pt. 1), 629–37.

49. Kerscher, M., & Buntrock, H. (2011). Anti-aging creams. What really helps? [Article in German] *Hautarzt*, 62(8), 607–13.

50. Kafi, R., et al. (2007). Improvement of naturally aged skin with vitamin A (retinol). *Archives of Dermatology*, 143(5), 606–12.

51. Feinberg, C., Hawkins, S., Battaglia, A., & Weinkauf, R. (2004). Comparison of anti-aging efficacy from cosmetic ingredients on photoaged skin. *Journal of the American Academy of Dermatology*, 50(3), P27.

52. Draelos, Z. D. (2005). Novel approach to the treatment of hyperpigmented photodamaged skin: 4% hydroquinone/0.3% retinol versus tretinoin 0.05% emollient cream. *Dermatologic Surgery*, 31 (7 pt. 2), 799–804.

53. Seité, S., et al. (2005). Histological evaluation of a topically applied retinol-vitamin C combination. *Skin Pharmacology and Physiology*, 18(2),81–87.

54. Nusgens, B. V., Humbert, P., Rougier, A., Richard, A., & Lapière, C. M. (2002). Stimulation of collagen biosynthesis by topically applied vitamin C. *European Journal of Dermatology*, 12(4), XXXII–IV.

55. Burke, K. E. (2007). Interaction of vitamins C and E as better cosmeceuticals. *Dermatologic Therapy*, 20(5), 314–21.

56. Fitzpatrick, R. E., & Rostan, E. F. (2002). Double-blind, half-face study comparing topical vitamin C and vehicle for rejuvenation of photodamage. *Dermatologic Surgery*, 28(3), 231–36.

57. Humbert, P. G., et al. (2003). Topical ascorbic acid on photoaged skin. Clinical, topographical and ultrastructural evaluation: Double blind-study vs. placebo. *Experimental Dermatology*, 12(3), 237–44.

58. Darr, D., Combs, S., Dunston, S., Manning, T., & Pinnell, S. (1992). Topical vitamin C protects porcine skin from ultraviolet radiation-induced damage. *British Journal of Dermatology*, 127(3), 247–53.

59. Lin, F. H., et al. (2005). Ferulic acid stabilizes a solution of vitamins C and E and doubles its photoprotection of skin. *Journal of Investigative Dermatology*, 125(4), 826–32.

60. Chiu, P. C., Chan, C. C., Lin, H. M., & Chiu, H. C. (2007). The clinical antiaging effects of topical kinetin and niacinamide, in Asians: A randomized, double-blind, placebo-controlled, split-face comparative trial. *Journal of Cosmetic Dermatology*, 6(4), 243–49.

61. Weinstein, G. D., McCullough, J. L., Ali, N. N., Shull, T. F., & Moudy, D. (1997). A double blind vehicle-controlled study of kinetin lotions for improving the appearance of aging photodamaged facial skin with 24 weeks of twice daily topical application. In Photoaging: Latest Advances in Understanding, Treatment and Prevention. Short Hills, NJ.

62. McDaniel, D. H., Neudecker, B. A., DiNardo, J. C., Lewis II, J. A., & Maibach, H. I. (2005). Clinical efficacy assessment in photodamaged skin of 0.5% and 1.0% idebenone. *Journal of Cosmetic Dermatology*, 4(3), 167–73.

63. Danhof, I. E. (1993). Potential reversal of chronological and photo-aging of the skin by topical application of natural substances. *Phytotherapy Research*, 7(7), S53–56.

64. Aust, M. C., et al. (2008). Percutaneous collagen induction: Minimally invasive skin rejuvenation without risk of hyperpigmentation—fact or fiction? *Plastic and Reconstructive Surgery*, 122(5), 1553–63.

65. Weiss, R. A., McDaniel, D. H., Geronemus, R. G., & Weiss, M. A. (2005). Clinical trial of a novel non-thermal LED array for reversal of photoaging: clinical, histologic, and surface profilometric results. *Lasers in Surgery and Medicine*, 36(2), 85–91.

66. Weiss, R. A., Weiss, M. A., Geronemus, R. G., & McDaniel, D. H. (2004). A novel non-thermal non-ablative full panel LED photomodulation device for reversal of photoaging: digital microscopic and clinical results in various skin types. *Journal of Drugs in Dermatology*, 3(6), 605–10.

67. Burgess, C. M. (2006). Principles of soft tissue augmentation for the aging face. *Journal of Clinical Interventions in Aging*, 1(4), 349–55.

68. Kahn, D. M., & Shaw, R. B. (2010). Overview of current thoughts on facial volume and aging. *Facial Plastic Surgery*, 26(5), 350–55.

69. Rieger, M. (1998). Hyaluronic acid in cosmetics. *Cosmetics and Toiletries*, 113(3), 35–42.

70. Burke, K. E. (1990). Facial wrinkles: Prevention and nonsurgical correction. *Postgraduate Medicine*, 88(1), 207–10, 213–16, 219–22.

71. Wang, F. et al. (2007). In vivo stimulation of de novo collagen production caused by cross-linked hyaluronic acid dermal filler injections in photodamaged human skin. *Archives of Dermatology*, 143(2), 155–63.

72. Cho H. S., et al. (2007) Anti-wrinkling effects of the mixture of vitamin C, vitamin E, pycnogenol and evening primrose oil, and molecular mechanisms on hairless mouse skin caused by chronic ultraviolet B irradiation. *Photodermatology, Photoimmunology and Photomedicine*, 23(5), 155–62.

73. Kockaert, M., & Neumann, M. (2003). Systemic and topical drugs for aging skin. *Journal of Drugs in Dermatology*, 2(4), 435–41.

74. Shao, L., Li, Q. H., & Tan, Z. (2004). L-carnosine reduces telomere damage and shortening rate in cultured normal fibroblasts. *Biochemical and Biophysical Research Communications*, 324(2), 931–36.

75. Münch, G., et al. (1997). Influence of advanced glycation end-products and AGE-inhibitors on nucleation-dependent polymerization of beta-amyloid peptide. *Biochimica et Biophysica Acta*, 1360(1), 17–29.

76. Rattan, S. I., & Sodagam, L. (2005). Gerontomodulatory and youth-preserving effects of zeatin on human skin fibroblasts undergoing aging in vitro. *Rejuvenation Research*, 8(1), 46–57.

77. Stahl, W., & Sies, H. (2007). Carotenoids and flavonoids contribute to nutritional protection against skin damage from sunlight. *Molecular Biotechnology*, 37(1), 26–30.

78. Köpcke, W., Krutmann, J., (2008). Protection from Sunburn with beta-carotene—a meta-analysis. *Photochemistry and Photobiology*, 84(2), 284–88.

79. Cho, S., et al. (2010). Differential effects of low-dose and high-dose beta-carotene supplementation on the signs of photoaging and type I procollagen gene expression in human skin in vivo. *Dermatology*, 221(2), 160–71.

80. Middelkamp-Hup, M., et al. (2004). Oral Polypodium leucotomos extract decreases ultraviolet-induced damage of human skin. *Journal of the American Academy of Dermatology*, 51(6), 910–18.

81. González, S., Pathak, M. A., Cuevas, J., Villarrubia, V. G., & Fitzpatrick, T. B. (1997). Topical or oral administration with an extract of Polypodium leucotomos prevents acute sunburn and psoralen-induced phototoxic reactions as well as depletion of Langerhans cells in human skin. *Photodermatology, Photoimmunology and Photomedicine*, 13(1-2), 50–60.

82. Gonzalez, S., Gilaberte, Y., & Philips, N. (2010). Mechanistic insights in the use of a Polypodium leucotomos extract as an oral and topical photoprotective agent. *Photochemical and Photobiological Sciences*, 9(4), 559–63.

83. Camera, E., et al. (2009). Astaxanthin, canthaxanthin and beta-carotene differently affect UVA-induced oxidative damage and expression of oxidative stress-responsive enzymes. *Experimental Dermatology*, 18(3), 222-31.

84. Seki, T., Sueki, H., Kohno H., Suganuma, K., & Yamashita, E. (2001). Effects of astaxanthin from *Haematococcus pluvialis* on human skin. *Fragrance Journal*, 12, 98–103.

85. Yamashita, E. (2002). Cosmetic benefit of dietary supplements including astaxanthin and tocotrienol on human skin. *FOOD Style*, 6(6), 112–17.

86. Yamashita, E. (2006). The effects of a dietary supplement containing astaxanthin on skin condition. *Carotenoid Science*, 10, 91–95.

87. Zague, V., de Freitas, V., da Costa Rosa, M., de Castro, G. Á., Jaeger, R. G., & Machado-Santelli, G. M. (2011). Collagen hydrolysate intake increases skin collagen expression and suppresses matrix metalloproteinase 2 activity. *Journal of Medicinal Food*, 14(6), 618–24.

88. Liang, J., Pei, X., Zhang, Z., Wang, N., Wang, J., & Li, Y. (2010). The protective effects of long-term oral administration of marine collagen hydrolysate from chum salmon on collagen matrix homeostasis in the chronological aged skin of Sprague-Dawley male rats. *Journal of Food Science*, 75(8), H230–38.

89. Duan, L., Xiang, X., Dan, L., Jianguo, S., Peijun, W., & Jing, L. (1996). The antiaging effects of pearl-powder on mice aging model induced by D-glactose or ozone. *Pharmacology and Clinics of Chinese Materia Medica*, 5.

90. Chen, H. S., Chang, J. H., & Wu, J. S. (2008). Calcium bioavailability of nanonized pearl powder for adults. *Journal of Food Science*, 73(9), H246–51.

91. Guo, C. T., et al. (2006). Edible bird's nest extract inhibits influenza virus infection. *Antiviral Research*, 70(3), 140–46.

92. Wolff, E. F., Narayan, D., & Taylor, H. S. (2005). Long-term effects of hormone therapy on skin rigidity and wrinkles. *Fertility and Sterility*, 84(2), 285–88.

93. Dunn, L. B., Damesyn, M., Moore, A. A., Reuben, D. B., & Greendale, G. A. (1997). Does estrogen prevent skin aging? Results from the First National Health and Nutrition Examination Survey (NHANES I). *Archives of Dermatology*, 133(3), 339–42.

94. Schmidt, J. B., Binder, M., Demschik, G., Bieglmayer, C., & Reiner, A. (1996). Treatment of skin aging with topical estrogens. *International Journal of Dermatology*, 35(9), 669–74.

95. Holzer, G., Riegler, E., Hönigsmann, H., Farokhnia S., & Schmidt, J. B. (2005). Effects and side-effects of 2% progesterone cream on the skin of peri- and postmenopausal women: results from a double-blind, vehicle-controlled, randomized study. *British Journal of Dermatology*, 153(3), 626–34.

96. Rudman, D., et al. (1990). Effects of human growth hormone in men over 60 years old. *New England Journal of Medicine*, 323(1), 1–6.

97. Yoshikawa, I., et al. (1990). Scavenging effects of *Aspalathus linearis* (Rooibos tea) on active oxygen species. *Advances in Experimental Medicine and Biology*, 264, 171–74.

98. Joubert, E., Winterton, P., Britz, T. J., & Gelderblom, W. C. (2005). Antioxidant and pro-oxidant activities of aqueous extracts and crude polyphenolic fractions of rooibos (*Aspalathus linearis*). *Journal of Agricultural and Food Chemistry*, 53(26), 10260–67.

99. Von Gadow, A., Joubert, E., & Hansmann C. F. (1997). Comparison of the antioxidant activity of rooibos tea (Aspalathuslinearis) with green, oolong and black tea. *Food Chemistry*, 60(1), 737.

100. Hsu. S. (2005). Green tea and the skin. *Journal of the American Academy of Dermatology*, 52(6), 1049–59.

101. Cosgrove, M. C., Franco, O. H., Granger, S. P., Murray, P. G., & Mayes, A. E. (2007). Dietary nutrient intakes and skin-aging appearance among middle-aged American women. *American Journal of Clinical Nutrition*, 86(4), 1225–31.

102. Hipkiss, A. R. (2006). Does chronic glycolysis accelerate aging? Could this explain how dietary restriction works? *Annals of the New York Academy of Sciences*, 1067, 361–68.

103. Monnier, V. M. (1990). Nonenzymatic glycosylation, the Maillard reaction and the aging process. *Journal of Gerontology*, 45(4), B105–10.

104. Danby, F. W. (2010). Nutrition and aging skin: sugar and glycation. *Clinics in Dermatology*, 28(4), 409–11.

105. Purba, M. B., et al (2001). Skin wrinkling: can food make a difference? *Journal of the American College of Nutrition*, 20(1), 71–80.

106. Wu, D., & Cederbaum, A. I. (2003). Alcohol, oxidative stress, and free radical damage. *Alcohol Research and Health*, 27(4), 277–84.

107. Valavanidis, A., Vlachogianni, T., & Fiotakis, K. (2009). Tobacco smoke: involvement of reactive oxygen species and stable free radicals in mechanisms of oxidative damage, carcinogenesis and synergistic effects with other respirable particles. *International Journal of Environmental Research and Public Health*, 6(2), 445–62.

108. Ernster, V. L., Grady, D., Miike, R., Black, D., Selby, J., & Kerlikowske, K. (1995). Facial wrinkling in men and women, by smoking status. *American Journal of Public Health*, 85(1), 78–82.

109. Koh, J. S., Kang, H., Choi, S. W., & Kim, H. O. (2002). Cigarette smoking associated with premature facial wrinkling: Image analysis of facial skin replicas. *International Journal of Dermatology*, 41(1), 21–27.

110. Doshi, D. N., Hanneman, K. K., & Cooper, K. D. (2007). Smoking and skin aging in identical twins. *Archives of Dermatology*, 143(12), 1543–6.

111. Yin, L., Morita, A. & Tsuji, T. (2001). Skin aging induced by ultraviolet exposure and tobacco smoking: Evidence from epidemiological and molecular studies. *Photodermatology, Photoimmunology and Photomedicine*, 17(4), 178–83.

112. Stephen, I. D., Law Smith, M. J., Stirrat, M. R., & Perrett, D. I. (2009). Facial skin coloration affects perceived health of human faces. *International Journal of Primatology*, 30(6), 845–57.

113. Singer, M., & Baer, H. (2008). *Killer commodities: Public health and the corporate production of harm.* Lanham (MD): AltaMira Press.

114. Daniel, S., Reto, M., Fred, Z., & Mibelle AG Cosmetics. (2002). Collagen glycation and skin aging. *Cosmetics and Toiletries Manufacture Worldwide*, 118–24.

115. Postaire, E., Jungmann, H., Bejot, M., Heinrich, U., & Tronnier, H. (1997). Evidence for antioxidant nutrients-induced pigmentation in skin: Results of a clinical trial. *Biochemistry and Molecular Biology International*, 42(5), 1023–33.

CHAPTER 3: HAIR

1. Bereczkei, T., & Mesko, N. (2006). Hair length, facial attractiveness, personality attribution: A multiple fitness model of hairdressing. *Review of Psychology*, 13(1), 35–42.

2. Sorokowski, P. (2008) Attractiveness of blonde women in evolutionary perspective: Studies with two Polish samples. *Perceptual and Motor Skills*, 106(3), 737–44.

3. Lynn, M. (2009). Determinants and consequences of female attractiveness and sexiness: Realistic tests with restaurant waitresses. *Archives of Sexual Behavior*, 38(5), 737–45.

4. Price, M. (2008). Fund-raising success and a solicitor's beauty capital: Do blondes raise more funds? *Economics Letters*, 100(3), 351–54.

5. Mesko, N., & Bereczkei, T. (2004). Hairstyle as an adaptive means of displaying phenotypic quality. *Human Nature*, 15(3), 251–70.

6. Hinsz, V. B., Matz, D. C., & Patience, R. A. (2001). Does women's hair signal reproductive potential? *Journal of Experimental Social Psychology*, 37(2), 166–72.

7. Holick, M. (1996). Study on Skin Enhancement and Hair Growth. *Drug and Cosmetic Industry Magazine*.

8. Sherrie, S., & Lewis, S. (1996). *Emu Oil: Reexamining a Natural Remedy with Today's Technology.* Nardin (OK): Emu Today and Tomorrow LLC.

9. Hay, I. C., Jamieson, M., & Ormerod, A. D. (1998). Randomized trial of aromatherapy. Successful treatment for alopecia areata. *Archives of Dermatology*, 134(11), 1349–52.

10. Wagner, H., Bladt, S., & Zgainski, F. M. (1994). *Plant drug analysis.* Versa Berlin Publisher, 291–304.

11. Wolf, R., Matz, H., Zalish, M., Pollack, A., & Orion, E. (2003). Prostaglandin analogs for hair growth: Great expectations. *Dermatology Online Journal*, 9(3), 7.

12. Uno, H., Zimbrick, M., Albert, D., & Stjernschantz, J. (2002). Effect of latanoprost on hair growth in the bald scalp of the stump-tailed macaque: a pilot study. *Acta Dermato-Venereologica*, 82(1), 7–12.

13. Brooker, R.. (2005). Gene transcription and RNA modification. In *Genetics: Analysis and principles* (pp. 318–25). (2nd ed.). New York: McGraw-Hill. Chapter 12 .

14. Awe, E. O., & Makinde J. M., (2009). The hair growth promoting effect of *Russelia equisetiformis* (Schclect & Chan). *Journal of Natural Products*, 2, 70–73.

CHAPTER 4: BODY

1. Singh D. (2006). Universal allure of the hourglass figure: An evolutionary theory of female physical attractiveness. *Clinics In Plastic Surgery*, 33(3), 359–70.

2. Singh, D. (1993). Body shape and women's attractiveness: The critical role of waist-to-hip ratio. *Human Nature*, 4(3), 297–321.

3. Singh, D., & Young, R. (1995). Body weight, waist-to-hip ratio, breasts and hips: Role in judgments of female attractiveness and desirability for relationships. *Ethology and Sociobiology*, 16, 483–507.

4. Tovee, M., Hancock, P., Mahmoodi, S., Singleton, B., & Cornelissen, P. (2002). Human female attractiveness: Waveform analysis of body shape. *Proceedings of the Royal Society B: Biological Sciences*, 269(1506), 2205–13.

5. Confer, J. C., Perilloux, C., & Buss, D. M. (2010). More than just a pretty face: Men's priority shifts toward bodily attractiveness in short-term versus long-term mating contexts. *Evolution and Human Behavior*, 31(5), 348–53.

6. Singh, D. (1993). Adaptive significance of female physical attractiveness: Role of waist-to-hip ratio. *Journal of Personality and Social Psychology*, 65(2), 293–307.

7. Macro, A. (1997). Why Barbie is perceived as beautiful. *Perceptual and Motor Skills*, 85(1), 363–74.

8. DeRidder, C. M., et al. (1990). Body fat mass, body fat distribution and plasma hormones in early puberty in females. *Journal of Clinical and Endocrinological Metabolism*, 70(4), 888–93.

9. Marlowe, F., & Wetsman, A. (2001). Preferred waist-to-hip ratio and ecology. *Personality and individual differences*, 30(3), 481–9.

10. Zaadstra B. M., et al. (1993). Fat and female fecundity: Prospective study of effect of body fat distribution on conception rates. *British Medical Journal*, 306(6876), 484–87.

11. Wass, P., Waldenström, U., Rössner, S., & Hellberg, D. (1997). An android body fat distribution in females impairs pregnancy rate of in-vitro fertilization-embryo transfer. *Human Reproduction*, 12(9), 2057–60.

12. Kirschner, M. A., & Samojilik, E. (1991). Sex hormone metabolism in upper and lower body obesity. *International Journal of Obesity*, 15(Suppl 2), 101–8.

13. Bjorntorp, P. (1988). The associations between obesity, adipose tissue distribution and disease. *Acta Medica Scandinavica*, 723, 121–34.

14. Seidell, J. C. (1992). Regional obesity and health. *International Journal of Obesity*, 16(Suppl. 2), S31–34.

15. Singh, D. (1993). Adaptive significance of female physical attractiveness: Role of waist-to-hip ratio. *Journal of Personality and Social Psychology*, 65(2), 293–307.

16. Evans, D. J., Hoffmann, R. G., Kalkoff, R. K., & Kissebah, A. H. (1983). Relationship of androgenic activity to body fat topography, fat cell morphology and metabolic aberrations in premenopausal women. *Journal of Clinical Endocrinology and Metabolism*, 57(2), 304–10.

17. den Tonkelaar, I., Seidell, J. C., van Noord, P. A., Baanders-van Halewijn, E. A., & Ouwehand, I. J. (1990). Fat distributionin relation to age, degree of obesity, smoking habits, parity and estrogen use: A cross-sectional study in 11,825 Dutch women participating in the DOM-project. *International Journal of Obesity*, 14(9), 753–61.

18. Chandeying, V., & Sangthawan, M. (2007). Efficacy comparison of *Pueraria mirifica* (PM) against conjugated equine estrogen (CEE) with/without medroxyprogesterone acetate (MPA) in the treatment of climacteric symptoms in perimenopausal women: phase III study. *Journal of the Medical Association of Thailand*, 90(9), 1720–26.

19. Gholap, S., & Kar, A. (2004). Hypoglycemic effects of some plant extracts are possibly mediated through inhibition in corticosteroid concentration. *Pharmazie*, 59(11), 876–78.

20. Marlowe, F., Apicella, C., & Reed, D. (2005). Men's preferences for women's profile waist-to-hip ratio in two societies. *Evolution and Human Behavior*, 26(6), 458–68.

21. Cuenca-Guerra, R., & Quezada, J. (2004). What makes buttocks beautiful? A review and classification of the determinants of gluteal beauty and the surgical techniques to achieve them. *Aesthetic Plastic Surgery*, 28(5), 340–47.

22. Swami, V., Neto, F., Tovee, M, J., & Furnham, A. (2007). Preferences for female body weight and shape in three European countries. *European Psychologist*, 12(3), 220–28.

23. Tovée, M. J., Reinhardt, S., Emery, J. L., & Cornelissen, P. L. (1998). Optimum body-mass index and maximum sexual attractiveness. *Lancet*, 352(9127), 548.

24. Swami, V., Miller, R., Furnham, A., Penke, L., & Tovée, M. J. (2008). The influence of men's sexual strategies on perceptions of women's bodily attractiveness, health and fertility. *Personality and Individual Differences*, 44(1), 98–107.

25. Tovée, M. J., Maisey, D. S., Emery, J. L., & Cornelissen, P. L. (1999). Visual cues to female physical attractiveness. *Proceedings of the Royal Society B: Biological Sciences*, 266(1415), 211–18.

26. Tovée, M. J., & Cornelissen, P. L. (2001). Female and male perceptions of female physical attractiveness in front-view and profile. *British Journal of Psychology*, 92, 391–402.

27. Lake, J. K., Power, C., & Cole, T. J. (1997). Women's reproductive health: The role of body mass index in early and adult life. *International Journal of Obesity*, 21(6), 432–38.

28. Manson, J. E., et al. (1995). Body weight and mortality among women. *New England Journal of Medicine*, 333(11), 677–85.

29. Reid, R. L., & Van Vugt, D. A. (1987). Weight-related changes in reproductive function. *Fertility and Sterility*, 48(6), 905–13.

30. Kaplan, A. S. (1990). Biomedical variables in the eating disorders. *Canadian Journal of Psychiatry*, 35(9), 745–53.

31. Frisch, R. E. (1988). Fatness and fertility. *Scientific American*, 258(3), 88–95.

32. Smith, J. E., Waldorf, V. A., & Trembath, D. L. (1990). Single white male looking for thin, very attractive. *Sex Roles*, 23, 675–85.

33. Fallon, A. E., & Rozin, P. (1985). Sex differences in perceptions of desirable body shape. *Journal of Abnormal Psychology*, 94(1), 1025.

34. Singh, D. (1994). Is thin really beautiful and good? Relationship between waist-to-hip ratio (WHR) and female attractiveness. *Personality and Individual Differences*, 16(1), 123–32.

35. Rodin, J., Radke-Sharpe, N., Rebuffé-Scrive, M., & Greenwood, M. R. (1990). Weight cycling and fat distribution. *International Journal of Obesity*, 14(4), 303–10.

36. van der Kooy, K., Leenen, R., Seidell, J. C., Deurenberg, P., & Hautvast, J. G. (1993). Effect of a weight cycle on visceral fat accumulation. *American Journal of Clinical Nutrition*, 58(6), 853–57.

37. Beunza, J. J., et al. (2010). Adherence to the Mediterranean diet, long-term weight change, and incident overweight or obesity: the Seguimiento Universidad de Navarra (SUN) cohort. *American Journal of Clinical Nutrition*, 92(6), 1484-2493.

38. Romaguera, D., et al. (2010). Mediterranean dietary patterns and prospective weight change in participants of the EPIC-PANACEA project. *American Journal of Clinical Nutrition*, 92(4), 912–21.

39. Shai I., et al. (2008). Weight loss with a low-carbohydrate, Mediterranean, or low-fat diet. *New England Journal of Medicine*, 359(3), 229–41.

40. Knoops, K. T., et al. (2004). Mediterranean diet, lifestyle factors, and 10-year mortality in elderly European men and women: The HALE project. *Journal of the American Medical Association*, 292(12), 1433–39.

41. Murray, M., & Pizzorno, J. (1998). *Encyclopedia of Natural Medicine* (2nd ed.). New York: Three Rivers Press.

42. Haskell, C. F., Kennedy, D. O., Wesnes, K. A., Milne, A. L., & Scholey, A. B. (2007). A double-blind, placebo-controlled, multi-dose evaluation of the acute behavioural effects of guaraná in humans. *Journal of Psychopharmacology*, 21(1), 65–70.

43. Brooks, R., Shelly, J. P., Fan, J., Zhai, L., & Chau, D. K. (2010). Much more than a ratio: Multivariate selection on female bodies. *Journal of Evolutionary Biology*, 23(10), 2238–48.

44. Swami, V., Einon, D., & Furnham, A. (2006). The leg-to-body ratio as a human aesthetic criterion. *Body Image*, 3(4), 317–23.

45. Sorokowski, P., & Pawlowski, B. (2008). Adaptive preferences for leg length in a potential partner. *Evolution and Human Behavior*, 29(2), 86–91.

46. Saino, N., Romano, M., & Innocenti, P. (2006). Length of index and ring fingers differentially influence sexual attractiveness of men's and women's hands. *Behavioral Ecology and Sociobiology*, 60(3), 447–54.

47. Kościński, K. (2011). Determinants of hand attractiveness: A study involving digitally manipulated stimuli. *Perception*, 40(6), 682–94.

48. Voracek, M., Fisher, M. L., Rupp, B., Lucas, D., & Fessler, D. M. (2007). Sex differences in relative foot length and the perceived attractiveness of female feet: Relationships among anthropometry, physique, and preference ratings. *Perceptual and Motor Skills*, 104(3, pt. 2), 1123–38.

49. Schick, V. R., Rima, B. N., & Calabrese, S. K. (2011). Evulvalution: the portrayal of women's external genitalia and physique across time and the current Barbie doll ideals. *Journal of Sex Research*, 48(1), 74–81.

50. Fink, B., & Neave, N. (2005). The biology of facial beauty. *International Journal of Cosmetic Science*, 27(6), 317–25.

CHAPTER 5: BREASTS

1. Low, B. S., Alexander, R. D., & Noonan, K.M. (1987). Human hips, breast, and buttocks: Is fat deceptive? *Ethology and Sociobiology*, 8(4), 249–57.

2. Arieli, R. (2004). Breasts, buttocks, and the camel hump. *Israel Journal of Zoology*, 50(1), 87–91.

3. Jasieńka, G., Ziomkiewicz, A., Ellison, P. T., Lipson, S. F., & Thune, I. (2004). Large breasts and narrow waist indicate high reproductive potential in women. *Proceedings of the Royal Society B: Biological Sciences*, 271(1545), 1213–17.

4. Roumen, F. J., Doesburg, W. H., & Rolland, R. (1982). Hormonal patterns in infertile women with a deficient postcoital test. *Fertility and Sterility*, 38(1), 42–7.

5. Marlowe, F. (1997). The nubility hypothesis: The human breast as an honest signal of residual reproductive value. *Human Nature*, 9(3), 263–71.

6. Mazur, A. (1986). U.S. trends in feminine beauty and overadaptation. *Journal of Sex Research*, 22(3), 281–303.

7. Gitter, A. G., Lomranz, J., Saxe, L., & Bar-Tel, Y. (1983). Perceptions of female physique characteristics by American and Israeli students. *Journal of Social Psychology*, 121, 7–13.

8. Katch, V. L., Campaigne, B., Freedson, P., Sady, S., Katch, F. L., & Behnke, A. R. (1980). Contribution of breast volume and weight to body fat distribution in females. *American Journal of Physical Anthropology*, 53, 93–100.

9. Horvath, T. (1981). Physical attractiveness: The influence of selected torso parameters. *Archives of Sexual Behavior.* 10(1), 21–24.

10. Tantleff-Dunn, S. (2002). Biggest isn't always best: The effect of breast size on perceptions of women. *Journal of Applied Social Psychology*, 32(11), 2253–65.

11. Gueguen, N. (2007). Women's bust size and men's courtship solicitation. *Body Image*, 4(4), 386-390.

12. Zelazniewicz, A., & Pawlowski, B. (2011). Female breast size attractiveness for men as a function of sociosexual orientation (restricted vs. unrestricted). *Archives of Sexual Behavior*, 40(6), 1129–35.

13. Kleinke, C., & Staneski, R. (1980). First impressions of female bust size. *Journal of Social Psychology*, 110(1), 123–34.

14. Singh, D., & Young, R. K. (1995) Body weight, waist-to-hip ratio, breasts, and hips: Role in judgments of female attractiveness and desirability for relationships. *Ethology and Sociobiology*, 16(6), 483–507.

15. Furnham, A., Dias, M., & McClelland, A. (1998). The role of body weight, waist-to-hip ratio, and breast size in judgments of female attractiveness. *Sex Roles*, 39(3-4), 311–26.

16. Dixson, B. J., Grimshaw, G. M., Linklater, W. L., & Dixson, A. F. (2011). Eye-tracking of men's preferences for waist-to-hip ratio and breast size of women. *Archives of Sexual Behavior*, 40(1), 43–50.

17. Silberstein, G. B., Van Horn, K., Shyamala, G., & Daniel, C. W. (1994). Essential role of endogenous estrogen in directly stimulating mammary growth demonstrated by implants containing pure antiestrogens. *Endocrinology*, 134(1), 84–90.

18. Beral, V., et al. (2003). Breast cancer and hormone-replacement therapy in the Million Women Study. *Lancet*, 362(9382), 419–27.

19. Anderson, G. L., et al. (2003). Effects of estrogen plus progestin on gynecologic cancers and associated diagnostic procedures: The Women's Health Initiative randomized trial. *Journal of the American Medical Association*, 290(13), 1739–48.

20. Weiderpass, E., et al. (1999). Risk of endometrial cancer following estrogen replacement with and without progestins. *Journal of the National Cancer Institute*, 91(13), 1131–37.

21. Ohlsén, L., Ericsson, O., & Beausang-Linder, M. (1996). Rapid, massive and unphysiological breast enlargement. *European Journal of Plastic Surgery*, 19(6), 307–13.

22. Hartmann, B. W., Laml, T., Kirchengast, S., Albrecht, A. E., & Huber, J. C. (1998). Hormonal breast augmentation: Prognostic relevance of insulin-like growth factor-I. *Gynecological Endocrinology*, 12(2), 123–27.

23. Jernström, H., & Olsson, H. (1997). Breast size in relation to endogenous hormone levels, body constitution, and oral contraceptive use in healthy nulligravid women aged 19–25 years. *American Journal of Epidemiology*, 145(7), 571–80.

24. Ruan, W., Catanese, V., Wieczorek, R., Feldman, M., & Kleinberg, D. L. (1995). Estradiol enhances the stimulatory effect of insulin-like growth factor-I (IGF-I) on mammary development and growth hormone-induced IGF-I messenger ribonucleic acid. *Endocrinology*, 136(3), 1296–302.

25. Brown, D. J. (1994). Herbal research review: *Vitex agnus castus* clinical monograph. *Quarterly Review of Natural Medicine*, 111–21.

26. Milewicz, A., et al. (1993). *Vitex agnus castus* extract in the treatment of luteal phase defects due to latent hyperprolactinemia. Results of a randomized placebo-controlled double-blind study. [Article in German] *Arzneimittel-Forschung*, 43(7), 752–56.

27. Shyamala, G., Yang, X., Cardiff, R. D., & Dale, E. (2000). Impact of progesterone receptor on cell-fate decisions during mammary gland development. *Proceedings of the National Academy of Sciences*, 97(7), 3044–49.

28. Rinker, B., Veneracion, M., &Walsh., C. P. (2008). The Effect of Breastfeeding on Breast Aesthetics. *Aesthetic Surgery Journal*, 28(5), 534–37.

CHAPTER 6: HEALTH

1. Symons, D. (1979). *The evolution of human sexuality*. New York: Oxford University Press.

2. Hönekopp, J., Bartholomé, T., & Jansen, G. (2004). Facial attractiveness, symmetry, and physical fitness in young women. *Human Nature*, 15(2), 147–67.

3. Shackelford, T. K., & Larsen, R. J. (1999). Facial attractiveness and physical health. *Evolution and Human Behavior*, 20, 71–76.

4. Etcoff, N. (2000). *Survival of the prettiest: The science of beauty*. New York: Anchor.

5. Thornhill, R., & Gangestad, S. W. (1993). Human facial beauty: Averageness, symmetry and parasite resistance. *Human Nature*, 4(3), 237–69.

6. Null, Gary, PhD., et al. (2004). Death by medicine, *Life Extension Magazine*, 1–45.

7. Göbel, H., Schmidt, G., & Soyka, D. (1994). Effect of peppermint and eucalyptus oil preparations on neurophysiological and experimental algesimetric headache parameters. *Cephalalgia*, 14(3), 228–34.

8. Göbel, H., Fresenius, J., Heinze, A., & Dworschak, M., Soyka, D. (1996). Effectiveness of Oleum menthae piperitae and paracetamol in therapy of headache of the tension type [Article In German] *Nervenarzt*, 67(8), 672–81.

9. Ornish, D., et al. (1990). Can lifestyle changes reverse coronary heart disease? The Lifestyle Heart Trial. *The Lancet*, 336(8708), 129–33.

10. Katsouyanni, K., et al. (1986). Diet and breast cancer: A case-control study in Greece. *International Journal of Cancer*, 38(6), 815–20.

11. Blaylock, R. (1997). *Excitotoxins: The taste that kills.* Santa Fe: Health Press.

12. Alpert, M. E., Hutt, M. S., Wogan, G. N., & Davidson, C. S. (1971). Association between aflatoxin content of food and hepatoma frequency in Uganda. *Cancer*, 28(1), 253–60.

13. Carnaghan, R. B. (1967). Hepatic tumours and other chronic liver changes in rats following a single oral administration of aflatoxin. *British Journal of Cancer*, 21(4), 811–14.

14. Young, R. (2000). *Sick and tired? Reclaim your inner terrain.* Woodland Publishing.

15. Chen, F., Cole, P., Mi, Z., & Xing, L. Y. (1993). Corn and wheat-flour consumption and mortality from esophageal cancer in Shanxi, China. *International Journal of Cancer*, 53(6), 902–6.

16. La Vecchia, C., Negri, E., Decarli, A., D'Avanzo. B., & Franceschi, S. (1987). A case-control study of diet and gastric cancer in Northern Italy. *International Journal of Cancer*, 40(4), 484–89.

17. Toth, B., Patil, K., Pyysalo, H., Stessman, C., & Gannett, P. (1992). Cancer induction in mice by feeding the raw false morel mushroom *Gyromitra esculenta. Cancer Research*, 52(8), 2279–84.

18. Ghadirian P. (1987). Thermal irritation and esophageal cancer in northern Iran. *Cancer*, 60(8), 1909–14.

19. Ingram, D. M., Nottage, E., & Roberts, T. (1991). The Role of *Saccharomyces cerevisiae*—baker's, or brewer's, yeast—in the development of breast cancer: A case control study of patients with breast cancer, benign epithelial hyperplasia and fibrocystic disease of the breast. *British Journal of Cancer*, 64(1), 187–91.

20. Tombak, M. (2006). *Cure the incurable.* Blaine. (WA): Healthy Life Press Inc.

21. Room, R., Babor, T., & Rehm, J. (2005). Alcohol and public health. *The Lancet*, 365(9458), 519–30.

22. Pöschl, G., & Seitz, H. K. (2004). Alcohol and cancer. *Alcohol and Alcoholism*, 39(3), 155–65.

23. Allen, N. E., et al. (2009). Moderate alcohol intake and cancer incidence in women. *Journal of the National Cancer Institute*, 101(5), 296–305.

24. Mørch, L. S., et al. (2007). Alcohol drinking, consumption patterns and breast cancer among Danish nurses: A cohort study. *European Journal of Public Health*, 17(6), 624–29.

25. Erasmus, U. (1993). *Fats that heal, fats that kill: The omplete guide to fats, oils, cholesterol and human health*. Summertown (TN): Alive Books.

26. Cocoros, G., Cahn, P. H., & Siler, W. (1973). Mercury concentrations in fish, plankton and water from three Western Atlantic estuaries. *Journal of Fish Biology*, 5(6), 641–7.

27. Evans, E. C. (2002). FDA recommendations on fish intake during pregnancy. *Journal of Obstetric, Gynecologic, and Neonatal Nursing*, 31(6), 715–20.

28. Storelli, M. M., & Marcotrigiano, G. O. (2001). Total mercury levels in muscle tissue of swordfish (*Xiphias gladius*) and bluefin tuna (*Thunnus thynnus*) from the Mediterranean Sea (Italy). *Journal of Food Protection*, 64(7), 1058–61.

29. Jureʌɔa, D., & Blanuʌɔa, M. (2003). Mercury, arsenic, lead and cadmium in fish and shellfish from the Adriatic Sea. *Food Additives and Contaminants*, 20(3), 241–46.

30. Shaw, S. D., Brenner, D., Berger, M. L., Carpenter, D. O., Hong, C., & Kannan, K. (2006). PCBs, PCDD/Fs, and organochlorine pesticides in farmed atlantic salmon from maine, eastern canada, and norway, and wild salmon from alaska. *Environmental Science and Technology*, 40(17), 5347–54.

31. Easton, M. D., Luszniak, D., & Von der GE. (2002). Preliminary examination of contaminant loadings in farmed salmon, wild salmon and commercial salmon feed. *Chemosphere*, 46(7), 1053–74.

32. Hites, R. A., Foran, J. A., Carpenter, D. O., Hamilton, M. C., Knuth, B. A., & Schwager, S. J. (2004). Global assessment of organic contaminants in farmed salmon. *Science*, 303(5655), 226–29.

33. Hites, R. A., Foran, J. A., Schwager, S. J., Knuth, B. A., Hamilton, M. C., & Carpenter, D. O. (2004). Global assessment of polybrominated diphenyl ethers in farmed and wild salmon. *Environmental Science and Technology*, 38(19), 4945–49.

34. Airey, D. (1983). Total mercury concentrations in human hair from 13 countries in relation to fish consumption and location. *Science of the Total Environment*, 31(2), 157–80.

35. Mozaffarian, D., & Rimm, E. B. (2006). Fish intake, contaminants, and human health: evaluating the risks and the benefits. *Journal of the American Medical Association*, 296(15), 1885–99.

36. Lee, A. T., & Cerami, A. (1992). Role of glycation in aging. *Annals of the New York Academy of Science*, 663, 63–70.

37. Monnier, V. M. (1990). Nonenzymatic glycosylation, the Maillard reaction and the aging process. *Journal of Gerontology*, 45(4), B105–10.

38. Dyer, D. G., et al. (1993). Accumulation of Maillard reaction products in skin collagen in diabetes and aging. *Journal of Clinical Investigation*, 91(6), 2463–69.

39. Furth, A., & Harding, J. (1989). Why sugar is bad for you. *New Scientist*, 44.

40. Szanto, S., & Yudkin, J. (1969). The Effect of Dietary Sucrose on Blood Lipids, Serum Insulin, Platelet Adhesiveness and Body Weight in Human Volunteers. *Postgraduate Medicine Journal*, 45(527), 602–7.

41. Takahashi, E. (1982). Tohoku University School of Medicine. *Wholistic Health Digest*, 41.

42. Quillin, P. (2000). Cancer's Sweet Tooth. *Nutrition Science News*, .

43. Michaud, D., et al. (2002). Dietary sugar, glycemic load, and pancreatic cancer risk in a prospective study. *Journal of the National Cancer Institute*, 94(17), 1293–300.

44. Moerman, C. J., et al. (1993). Dietary sugar intake in the aetiology of biliary tract cancer. *International Journal of Epidemiology*, 2(2), 207–14.

45. De Stefani, E. (1998). Dietary sugar and lung cancer: A case–control study in Uruguay. *Nutrition and Cancer*, 31(2), 132–37.

46. Cornée, J., et al. (1995). A case-control study of gastric cancer and nutritional factors in Marseille, France. *European Journal of Epidemiology*, 11(1), 55–65.

47. Darlington, L., Ramsey, & N. W. Mansfield, J. R. (1986). Placebo-controlled, blind study of dietary manipulation therapy in rheumatoid arthritis. *The Lancet*, 8475(1), 236–38.

48. Erlander, S. (1979). *The Cause and Cure of Multiple Sclerosis, The Disease to End Disease*, 1(3), 59–63.

49. Beck, Nielsen H., Pedersen O., & Schwartz Sørenesen N. (1978). Effects of diet on the cellular insulin binding and the insulin sensitivity in young healthy subjects. *Diabetologia*, 15(4), 289-296.

50. Reiser, S., et al. (1986). Effects of sugars on indices on glucose tolerance in humans. *American Journal of Clinical Nutrition*. 43(1), 151–59.

51. Tjäderhane, L., & Larmas, M. (1998). A high sucrose diet decreases the mechanical strength of bones in growing rats. *Journal of Nutrition*, 128(10), 1807–10.

52. Frey, J. (2001). Is there sugar in the Alzheimer's disease? *Annales de Biologie Clinique*, 59(3), 253–57.

53. Veromann, S. et al. (2003). Dietary sugar and salt represent real risk factors for cataract development. *Ophthalmologica*, 217(4), 302–7.

54. Yudkin, J., Kang, S., & Bruckdorfer, K. (1980). Effects of high dietary sugar. *British Journal of Medicine*, 282(6259), 223–24.

55. Lechin, F., et al. (1992). Effects of an oral glucose load on plasma neurotransmitters in humans: Involvement of REM sleep? *Neurophychobiology*, 26(1-2), 4–11.

56. Soffritti, M., et al. (2010). Aspartame administered in feed, beginning prenatally through life span, induces cancers of the liver and lung in male Swiss mice. *American Journal of Industrial Medicine*, 53(12), 1197–206.

57. Inness-Brown, V. (2010). *My Aspartame Experiment: Report from a Private Citizen.* North Charleston (SC): BookSurge Publishing.

58. Potenza, D. P., & el-Mallakh, R. S. (1989). Aspartame: clinical update. Connecticut Medicine, 53(7), 395–400.

59. Goyal, S. K., Samsher. Goyal R. K. (2010). Stevia (*Stevia rebaudiana*) a bio-sweetener: a review. *International Journal of Food Sciences and Nutrition*, 61(1), 1–10.

60. Lailerd, N., Saengsirisuwan, V., Sloniger, J.A., Toskulkao, C., & Henriksen, E. J. (2004). Effects of stevioside on glucose transport activity in insulin-sensitive and insulin-resistant rat skeletal muscle. *Metabolism—Clinical and Experimental*, 53(1), 101–7.

61. Jeppesen, P. B., et al. (2003). Antihyperglycemic and blood pressure-reducing effects of stevioside in the diabetic Goto-Kakizaki rat. *Metabolism Clinical and Experimental*, 52(3), 372–78.

62. Dyrskog, S. E., Jeppesen, P. B., Colombo, M., Abudula, R., & Hermansen, K. (2005). Preventive effects of a soy-based diet supplemented with stevioside on the development of the metabolic syndrome and type 2 diabetes in Zucker diabetic fatty rats. *Metabolism Clinical and Experimental*, 54(9), 1181–88.

63. Jones, R. (2001). *Honey and healing through the ages. InP. Munn, & R. Jones(Eds.), Honey and Healing.* Cardiff: International Bee Research Association.

64. Marcucci M. C. (1995). Propolis: chemical composition, biological properties and therapeutical activity. *Apidologie*, 26(2), 83–99.

65. Castaldo, S., & Capasso, F. (2002). Propolis, an old remedy used in modern medicine. *Fitoterapia*, 73(Suppl 1), S1–6.

66. Molan, P. C. (1999). Why honey is effective as a medicine. 1. Its use in modern medicine. *Bee World*, 80(2), 80–92.

67. Manyi-Loh, C. E., Clarke, A. M., & Ndip, R. N. (2011). An overview of honey: Therapeutic properties and contribution in nutrition and human health. *African Journal of Microbiology Research*, 5(8), 844–52.

68. Buratti, S., Benedetti, S., & Cosio, M. S. (2007). Evaluation of the antioxidant power of honey, propolis and royal jelly by amperometric flow injection analysis. *Talanta*, 71(3), 1387–92.

69. Bogdanov, S. (2011). Functional and Biological Properties of the Bee Products: a Review. *Bee Product Science* online: *at www.bee-hexagon.net,* 1-12.

70. Tamura, T., Fujii, A., Kuboyama, N. (1987). Anti-tumor effects of royal jelly (RJ). *Nippon Yakurigaku Zasshi*, 89(2), 73–80.

71. Nakaya, M., Onda, H., Sasaki, K., Yukiyoshi, A., Tachibana, H., & Yamada, K.

(2007). Effect of royal jelly on bisphenol A-induced proliferation of human breast cancer cells. *Bioscience, Biotechnology and Biochemistry*, 71(1), 253–55.

72. Orᴧolić, N., Sacases, F., Percie du Sert, P., & Bašić, I. (2007). Antimetastatic ability of honey bee products, *Periodicum Biologorum*, 109(2), 173–80.

73. Mavric, E., Wittman, S., Barth, G., & Henle, T. (2008). Identification and quantification of methylglyoxal as the dominant antibacterial constituent of Manuka (*Leptospermum scoparium*) honeys from New Zealand. *Molecular Nutrition and Food Research*, 52(4), 483–89.

74. Nagai, T., Sakai, M., Inoue, R., Inoue, H., & Suzuki, N. (2001). Antioxidative activities of some commercially honeys, royal jelly, and propolis. *Food Chemistry*, 75(2), 237–40.

75. Kimura, M., & Itokawa, Y. (1990). Cooking losses of minerals in foods and its nutritional significance. *Journal of Nutritional Science and Vitaminology*, 36(Suppl 1) S25–32, S33.

76. Adzersen, K. H., Jess, P., Freivogel, K. W., Gerhard, I., & Bastert, G. (2003). Raw and cooked vegetables, fruits, selected micronutrients, and breast cancer risk: A case-control study in Germany. *Nutrition and Cancer*, 46(2), 131–37.

77. Yuan, G. F., Sun, B., Yuan, J., & Wang, Q. M. (2009). Effects of different cooking methods on health-promoting compounds of broccoli. *Journal of Zhejiang University Science. 10(8), 580–88.*

78. Jägerstad, M., & Skog, K. (2005). Genotoxicity of heat-processed foods. *Mutation Research*, 574(1-2), 156–72.

78. Cross, A, J., et al. (2010). A large prospective study of meat consumption and colorectal cancer risk: An investigation of potential mechanisms underlying this association. *Cancer Research*, 70(6), 2406–14.

79. Anderson, K, E., et al. (2002). Meat intake and cooking techniques: Associations with pancreatic cancer. *Mutation Research*, 506–7, 225–31.

80. Stolzenberg-Solomon, R. Z., et al. (2007). Meat and meat-mutagen intake and pancreatic cancer risk in the NIH-AARP cohort. *Cancer Epidemiology, Biomarkers, and Prevention*, 16(12), 2664–75.

81. Carlsen, M. H., et al. (2010). The total antioxidant content of more than 3100 foods, beverages, spices, herbs and supplements used worldwide. *Nutrition Journal*, 9.

82. Rupérez, P. (2002). Mineral content of edible marine seaweeds. *Food Chemistry*, 79(1), 23–26.

83. Teas, J. (1983). The dietary intake of Laminaria, a brown seaweed, and breast cancer prevention. *Nutrition and Cancer*, 4(3), 217–22.

84. Tokudome, S., Kuriki, K., & Moore, M. A. (2001). Seaweed and Cancer Prevention. *Japanese Journal of Cancer Research*, 92(9), 1008–10.

85. Yuan, Y. V., & Walsh, N. A. (2006). Antioxidant and antiproliferative activities of extracts from a variety of edible seaweeds. *Food and Chemical Toxicology*, 44(7), 1144–50.

86. Teas, J., Harbison, M. L., & Gelman, R. S. (1984). Dietary seaweed (Laminaria) and mammary carcinogenesis in rats. *Cancer Research*, 44(7), 2758–61.

87. Cho, E. J., Rhee, S. H., & Park, K. Y. (1998). Antimutagenic and cancer cell growth inhibitory effects of seaweeds. *Journal of Food Science and Nutrition*, 2(4), 348–53.

88. Funahashi, H., et al. (2001). Seaweed prevents breast cancer? *Japanese Journal of Cancer Research*, 92(5), 483–87.

89. Trichopoulou, A., Costacou, T., Bamia, C., & Trichopoulos, D. (2003). Adherence to a Mediterranean diet and survival in a Greek population. *The New England Journal of Medicine*, 348(26), 2599–608.

90. Trudeau, K. (2005). *Natural Cures "They" Don't Want You To Know About.* Elk Groove Village (IL): Alliance Publishing.

91. Di Renzo, L., et al. (2007). Is antioxidant plasma status in humans a consequence of the antioxidant food content influence? *European Review for Medical and Pharmacological Sciences*, 11(3), 185–92.

92. Benbrook, C., Zhao, X., Yáñez, J., Davies, N., & Andrews, P. (2008). New evidence confirms the nutritional superiority of plant-based organic foods. The Organic Center Publication.

93. Worthington, V. (2001). Nutritional quality of organic versus conventional fruits, vegetables and grains. *Journal of Alternative and Complementary Medicine*, 7(2), 161–73.

94. Woese, K., Lange, D., Boess, C., & Bögl, K. W. (1997). A comparison of organically and conventionally grown foods—results of a review of the relevant literature. *Journal of the Science of Food and Agriculture*, 74(3), 281–93.

95. Haenlein, G. F. W. (2004). Goat milk in human nutrition. *Small Ruminant Research*, 51(2), 155–63.

96. Morales, E., et al. (2005). Nutritional value of goat and cow milk protein, *Options Méditerranéennes*, Series A(67), 167–70.

97. Crewe, J. (1929). Raw milk cures many diseases. *Certified Milk Magazine*, 3–6.

98. Mattick, E., & Golding, J. (1931). Relative value of raw and heated milk in nutrition. *The Lancet*, 217(5612), 662–67.

99. Yang, C. S., & Landau, J. M. (2000). Effects of tea consumption on nutrition and health. *The Journal of Nutrition*, 130(10), 2409–12.

100. Vipin, K., Sharma, A., Bhattacharya, A., Kumar, Hitesh, & K. Sharma. (2007). Health benefits of tea Consumption. *Tropical Journal of Pharmaceutical Research*, 6(3), 785–92.

101. Rietveld, A., & Wiseman, S. (2003). Antioxidant effects of tea: Evidence from human clinical trials. *The Journal of Nutrition*, 133(10), 3285S–3292S.

102. Jankun, J., Selman, S. H., Swiercz, R., & Skrzypczak-Jankun, E. (1997). Why drinking green tea could prevent cancer. *Nature*, 387(6633), 561.

103. Katiyar, S. K., & Mukhtar, H. (1997). Tea antioxidants in cancer chemoprevention. *Journal of Cellular Biochemistry*, 27, S59–67.

104. Sinija, V. R., & Mishra, H. N. (2008). Green tea: Health benefits. *Journal of Nutritional and Environmental Medicine*, 17(4), 232–42.

105. Duh, P. D., Yen, G. C., Yen, W. J., Wang, B. S., & Chang, L. W. (2004). Effects of pu-erh tea on oxidative damage and nitric oxide scavenging. *Journal of Agricultural and Food Chemistry*, 52(26), 8169–76.

106. Gong, J. S., Peng, C. X., He, X., Li, J. H., Li, B. C., & Zhou, H. J. (2009). Antioxidant activity of extracts of pu-erh tea and its material. *Asian Journal of Agricultural Sciences*, 1(2), 48–54.

107. Santana-Rios, G., et al. (2001). Potent antimutagenic activity of white tea in comparison with green tea in the Salmonella assay. *Mutation Research*, 495(1-2), 61–74.

108. Campbell, T. C., & Campbell, T. M, II. (2005). *The China Study: startling implications for diet, weight loss, and long-term health*. Dallas (TX): BenBella Books, Inc.

109. Madhavan, T. V., & Gopalan, C. (1968). The effect of dietary protein on carcinogenesis of aflatoxin. *Archives of Pathology*, 85(2), 133–37.

110. Dunaif, G. E., & Campbell, T. C. (1987). Relative contribution of dietary protein level and aflatoxin B1 dose in generation of presumptive preneoplastic foci in rat liver. *Journal of the National Cancer Institute*, 78(2), 365–69.

111. Youngman, L. D., & Campbell, T. C. (1992). Inhibition of aflatoxin B1-induced gamma-glutamyltranspeptidase positive (GGT+) hepatic preneoplastic foci and tumors by low protein diets: Evidence that altered GGT+ foci indicate neoplastic potential. *Carcinogenesis*, 13(9), 1607–13.

112. Marion, J. *(1999). Anti-Aging manual: The encyclopedia of natural health*. Carrollton (MS): Information Pioneers Pub.

113. Diamond, H., & Diamond, M. (2010). *Fit for Life*. Wellness Central.

114. Cuthbert, S. C., & Goodheart, G. J. Jr. (2007). On the reliability and validity of manual muscle testing: A literature review. *Chiropractic and Osteopathy*, 15(4).

115. Andersson, I., et al. (1988). Mammographic screening and mortality from breast cancer: The Malmö mammographic screening trial. *British Medical Journal*, 297(6654), 943–48.

116. Cristofanilli, M., et al. (2004). Circulating tumor cells, disease progression, and survival in metastatic breast cancer. *The New England Journal of Medicine*, 351(8), 781–91.

117. Meletis C. D. (2001). Cleansing of the Human Body: A Daily Essential Process. *Alternative and Complementary Therapies*, 7(4), 196–202.

118. Gerson, C. (2001). *The Gerson therapy: The proven nutritional program for cancer and other illnesses*. New York: Kensington Publishing Corp.

119. Gerson, M. (1958). *A cancer therapy: Results of fifty cases and the cure of advanced cancer by diet therapy*. San Diego (CA): The Gerson Institute.

200. Schnare, D.W., Denk, G., Shields M., & Brunton S. (1982). Evaluation of a detoxification regimen for fat stored xenobiotics. *Medical Hypotheses*, 9(3), 265–82.

201. Schnare, D. W., Ben, M., & Shields M. G. (1984). Body burden reduction of PCBS, PBBs and chlorinated pesticides in human subjects. *AMBIO*, 13(5–6), 378–80.

203. Schnare, D. W., & Robinson, P. C. (1986). Reduction of the human body burdens of hexachlorobenzene and polychlorinated biphenyls. *IARC Scientific Publication*, (77), 597–603.

204. Root, D. E., & Lionelli, G. T. (1987). Excretion of a lipophilic toxicant through the sebaceous glands: A case report. *Journal of Toxicology—Cutaneous and Ocular Toxicology*, 6(1), 13–89.

205. Kilburn, K.H., Warsaw, R.H., & Shields, M.G. (1989). Neurobehavioral dysfunction in firemen exposed to polycholorinated biphenyls (PCBs): Possible improvement after detoxification. *Archives of Environmental Health*, 44(6), 345–50.

206. Inculet, R. I., Norton, J. A., Nichoalds, G. E., Maher, M. M., White, D. E., & Brennan, M. F. (1987). Water-soluble vitamins in cancer patients on parenteral nutrition: A prospective study. *Journal of Parenteral and Enteral Nutrition*, 11(3), 243–49.

207. Black, P.H., & Garbutt, L.D. (2002). Stress, inflammation, and cardiovascular disease. *Journal of Psychosomatic Research*, 52(1), 1–23.

208. Martin, R. A., & Dobbin, J. P. (1988). Sense of humor, hassles, and immunoglobulin A: Evidence for a stress-moderating effect of humor. *International Journal of Psychiatry In Medicine*, 18(2), 93–105.

209. Fairfield, K. M., & Fletcher, R. H. (2002). Vitamins for chronic disease prevention in adults: Scientific review. *Journal of the American Medical Association*, 287(23), 3116–26.

210. Liu, R. H. (2004). Potential synergy of phytochemicals in cancer prevention: Mechanism of action. *The Journal of Nutrition*, 134(12), 3479S–3485S.

211. Thiel, R. J. (2000). Natural vitamins may be superior to synthetic ones. *Medical Hypotheses*, 55(6), 461–69.

212. King, J. C, & Cousins, R. J. (2005). Zinc. In M. E. Shills, J. A. Olsen, M. Shike, & A. C. Ross (Eds.), *Modern Nutrition in Health and Disease* (10th ed.) (pp. 271–85). Philadelphia: Lipponcott, Williams and Wilkins,.

213. Hayat, M. J., Howlader, N., Reichman, M. E., & Edwards, B. K. (2007). Cancer statistics, trends, and multiple primary cancer analyses from the Surveillance, Epidemiology, and End Results (SEER) Program. *Oncologist*, 12(1), 20–37.

214. Gershwin, M. E., & Amha Belay. (Eds.). (2008). *Spirulina in human nutrition and health*. Boca Raton: CRC Press.

215. Ciferri, O. (1983). Spirulina, the edible microorganism. *Microbiological Reviews*, 47(4), 551–78.

216. Babadzhanov, A. S., Abdusamatova, N., Yusupova, F. M., Faizullaeva, N., Mezhlumyan, L. G., & Malikova, M. K. (2004). Chemical composition of *Spirulina platensis* cultivated in Uzbekistan. *Chemistry of Natural Compounds*, 40(3), 276–79.

217. Belay, A. (2002). The potential application of *Spirulina* (*Arthrospira*) as a nutritional and therapeutic supplement in health management. *Journal of the American Nutraceutical Association*. 5(2), 27-48.

218. Goodhart, S. R., & Shils, E. M. (1980). *Modern nutrition in health and disease*. (6th ed.). Lea and Febinger: Philadelphia, 134–38.

219. Simopoulos, A. P. (2002). Omega-3 fatty acids in inflammation and autoimmune diseases. *Journal of the American College of Nutrition*, 21(6), 495-505.

220. Francois, C. A., Connor, S. L., Bolewicz, L. C., & Connor, W. E. (2003). Supplementing lactating women with flaxseed oil does not increase docosahexaenoic acid in their milk. *American Journal of Clinical Nutrition*, 77(1), 226–33.

221. Rohdewald, P. (2002). A review of the French maritime pine bark extract (Pycnogenol), a herbal medication with a diverse clinical pharmacology. *International Journal of Clinical Pharmacology and Therapeutics*, 40(4), 158–68.

222. Wood, J. E., Senthilmohan, S. T., & Peskin, A. V. (2002). Antioxidant activity of procyanidin-containing plant extracts at different pHs. *Food Chemistry*, 77(2), 155–61.

223. Xiaoguang, C., et al. (1998). Cancer chemopreventive and therapeutic activities of red ginseng. *Journal of Ethnopharmacology*, 60(1), 71–78.

224. Nishino, H., et al. (2001). Cancer chemoprevention by ginseng in mouse liver and other organs. *Journal of Korean Medical Science*, 16(Suppl), S66–69.

225. Jeong, T. C., et al. (1997). Protective effects of red ginseng saponins against carbon tetrachloride-induced hepatotoxicity in Sprague Dawley rats. *Planta Medica*, 63(2), 136–40.

226. Kwon, Y. S., & Jang, K. H. (2004). The effect of Korean red ginseng on liver regeneration after 70% hepatectomy in rats. *The Journal of Veterinary Medical Science*, 66(2), 193–95.

227. Bilska, A., & Włodek, L. (2005). Lipoic acid—the drug of the future? *Pharmacological Reports*, 57(5), 570–77.

228. Berkson, B. M. (1998). Alpha-lipoic acid (thioctic acid): My experience with this outstanding therapeutic agent. *Journal of Orthomolecular Medicine*, 13(1), 44–48.

229. Rosenfeldt, F. L., et al. (2007). Coenzyme Q10 in the treatment of hypertension: A meta-analysis of the clinical trials. *Journal of Human Hypertension*, 21(4), 297–306.

230. Soja, A. M., & Mortensen, S. A. (1997). Treatment of congestive heart failure with coenzyme Q10 illuminated by meta-analyses of clinical trials. *Molecular Aspects of Medicine*, 18(Suppl), S159–68.

231. Jolliet P, et al. (1998). Plasma coenzyme Q10 concentrations in breast cancer: Prognosis and therapeutic consequences. *International Journal of Clinical Pharmacology and Therapeutics*, 36(9), 506–9.

232. Lockwood, K., Moesgaard, S., & Folkers, K. (1994). Partial and complete regression of breast cancer in patients in relation to dosage of coenzyme Q10. *Biochemical and Biophysical Research Communications*, 199(3), 1504–8.

233. Rosenfeldt, F., et al. (2004). Response of the senescent heart to stress: Clinical therapeutic strategies and quest for mitochondrial predictors of biological age. *Annals of the New York Academy of Sciences*, 1019, 78–84.

234. Narayanan, B. A., Geoffroy, O., Willingham, M. C., Re, G. G., & Nixon, D. W. (1999). p53/p21(WAF1/CIP1) expression and its possible role in G1 arrest and apoptosis in ellagic acid treated cancer cells. *Cancer Letters*, 136(2), 215–21.

235. Wang, N., et al. (2012). Ellagic acid, a phenolic compound, exerts anti-angiogenesis effects via VEGFR-2 signaling pathway in breast cancer. *Breast Cancer Research and Treatment*.

236. Amagase H, Petesch B. L., Matsuura H., Kasuga S., & Itakura Y. (2001). Intake of garlic and its bioactive components. *The Journal of Nutrition*, 131(3), 955S–962S.

237. Thomson, M., & Ali, M. (2003). Garlic [*Allium sativum*]: A review of its potential use as an anti-cancer agent. *Current Cancer Drug Targets*, 3(1), 67–81.

238. Ishikawa, H., et al. (2006). Aged garlic extract prevents a decline of NK cell number and activity in patients with advanced cancer. *The Journal of Nutrition*, 136(3 Suppl), 816S–820S.

239. Vucenik, I., & Shamsuddin, A. M. (2003). Cancer inhibition by inositol hexaphosphate (IP6) and inositol: from laboratory to clinic. *The Journal of Nutrition*, 133(11 Suppl 1), 3778S–3784S.

240. Tantivejkul, K., Vucenik, I., & Shamsuddin, A. M. (2003). Inositol hexaphosphate (IP6) inhibits key events of cancer metastasis: I. In vitro studies of adhesion, migration and invasion of MDA-MB 231 human breast cancer cells. *Anticancer Research*, 23(5A), 3671–79.

241. Saati, G. E., & Archer, M. C. (2011). Inhibition of fatty acid synthase and Sp1 expression by 3,3'-diindolylmethane in human breast cancer cells. *Nutrition and Cancer*, 63(5), 790–94.

242. Kandala, P. K., & Srivastava, S. K. (2012). Diindolylmethane suppresses ovarian cancer growth and potentiates the effect of cisplatin in tumor mouse model by targeting signal transducer and activator of transcription 3 (STAT3). *BMC Medicine*, 10(9).

243. Bhatnagar, N., Li, X., Chen, Y., Zhou, X., Garrett, S. H., & Guo, B. (2009). 3,3'-diindolylmethane enhances the efficacy of butyrate in colon cancer prevention through down-regulation of survivin. *Cancer Prevention Research*, 2(6), 581–89.

244. Goodman, S. (1988). Therapeutic effects of organic germanium. *Medical Hypotheses*, 26(3), 207–15.

245. Tao, S. H., & Bolger, P. M. (1997). Hazard assessment of germanium supplements. *Regulatory Toxicology and Pharmacology*, 25(3), 211–19.

246. Kidd, P. M. (1997). Glutathione: Systemic protectant against oxidative and free radical damage. *Alternative Medicine Review*, 2(3), 155–76.

247. Nuttall, S. L., Martin, U., Sinclair, A. J., & Kendall, M. J. (1998). Glutathione: In Sickness and in Health, *The Lancet*, 351(9103), 645–46.

248. Valenzuela, A., Aspillaga, M., Vial, S., & Guerra, R. (1989). Selectivity of silymarin on the increase of the glutathione content in different tissues of the rat. *Planta Medica*, 55(5), 420–22.

249. Wellington, K., & Jarvis, B. (2001). Silymarin: A review of its clinical properties in the management of hepatic disorders. *BioDrugs*, 15(7), 465–89.

250. Szilárd, S., Szentgyörgyi, D., & Demeter, I. (1988). Protective effect of Legalon in workers exposed to organic solvents. *Acta Medica Hungarica*, 45(2), 249–56.

251. Schütz, K., Carle, R., & Schieber, A. (2006). Taraxacum—A review on its phytochemical and pharmacological profile. *Journal of Ethnopharmacology*, 107(3), 313–23.

252. Sweeney, B., Vora, M., Ulbricht, C., & Basch, E. (2005). Evidence-based systematic review of dandelion (*Taraxacum officinale*) by natural standard research collaboration. *Journal of Herbal Pharmacotherapy*, 5(1), 79–93.

253. Chandan, B. K., Sharma, A. K., & Anand, K. K. (1991). *Boerhaavia diffusa*: A study of its hepatoprotective activity. *Journal of Ethnopharmacology*, 31(3), 299–307.

254. Olaleye, M. T., Akinmoladun, A. C., Ogunboye, A. A., & Akindahunsi, A. A. (2010). Antioxidant activity and hepatoprotective property of leaf extracts of *Boerhaavia diffusa* Linn against acetaminophen-induced liver damage in rats. *Food and Chemical Toxicology*, 48(8–9), 2200–5.

256. Thyagarajan, S., Jayaram, S., Gopalakrishnan, V., Hari, R., Jeyakumar, P., & Sripathi, M. J. (2002). Herbal medicines for liver diseases in India. *Journal of Gastroenterology and Hepatology*, 17(Suppl 3), S370–6.

257. Huseini, H. F., Alavian, S. M., Heshmat, R., Heydari, M. R., & Abolmaali, K. (2005). The efficacy of Liv-52 on liver cirrhotic patients: A randomized, double-blind, placebo-controlled first approach. *Phytomedicine*, 12(9), 619–24.

258. Girish, C., Koner, B. C., Jayanthi, S., Rao, K. R., Rajesh, B., & Pradhan, S. C. (2009). Hepatoprotective activity of six polyherbal formulations in paracetamol induced liver toxicity in mice. *The Indian Journal of Medical Research*, 129(5), 569–78.

259. Jagetia, G. C., Ganapathi, N. G., Venkatesh, P., Rao, N., & Baliga, M. S. (2006). Evaluation of the radioprotective effect of Liv 52 in mice. *Environmental and Molecular Mutagenesis*, 47(7), 490–502.

260. Ghosh, N., Ghosh, R., Mandal, V., & Mandal, S. C. (2011). Recent advances in herbal medicine for treatment of liver diseases. *Pharmaceutical Biology*, 49(9), 970–88.

261. Krishnaswami, K., & Raghuramulu, N. (1998). Bioactive phytochemicals with emphasis on dietary practices. *Indian Journal of Medical Research*, 108, 167–81.

262. Soni, K. B., Rajan, A., & Kuttan, R. (1992). Reversal of aflatoxin induced liver damage by turmeric and curcumin. *Cancer Letters*, 66(2), 115–21.

263. Madhuri, S., Pandey, G., & Verma, K. S. (2011). Antioxidant, Immunomodulatory and anticancer activities of *Emblica officinalis*: An overview. *International Research Journal of Pharmacy*, 2(8), 38–42.

264. Khan, K.H. (2009). Roles of *Emblica officinalis* in medicine—A review. *Botany Research International*, 2(4), 218–28.

265, Seeram, N. P. (2008). Berry fruits: Compositional elements, biochemical activities, and the impact of their intake on human health, performance, and disease. *Journal of Agricultural and Food Chemistry*, 56(3), 627–29.

266. Pedraza-Chaverri, J., Cárdenas-Rodríguez, N., Orozco-Ibarra, M., & Pérez-Rojas, J. M. (2008). Medicinal properties of mangosteen (Garcinia mangostana). *Food and Chemical Toxicology*, 46(10), 3227–39.

267. Moongkarndi, P., Kosem, N., Kaslungka, S., Luanratana, O., Pongpan, N., & Neungton, N. (2004). Antiproliferation, antioxidation and induction of apoptosis by *Garcinia mangostana* (mangosteen) on SKBR3 human breast cancer cell line. *Journal of Ethnopharmacology*, 90(1), 161–66.

268. Kang, T. H., Hur, J. Y., Kim, H. B., Ryu, J. H., & Kim, S. Y. (2006). Neuroprotective effects of the cyanidin-3-O-β-d-glucopyranoside isolated from mulberry fruit against cerebral ischemia. *Neuroscience Letters*, 391(3), 122–26.

269. Rocha-González, H. I., Ambriz-Tututi, M., & Granados-Soto, V. (2008). Resveratrol: A natural compound with pharmacological potential in neurodegenerative diseases. *CNS Neuroscience and Therapeutics*, 14(3), 234–47.

270. Chen, P. N., et al. (2006). Mulberry anthocyanins, cyanidin 3-rutinoside and cyanidin 3-glucoside, exhibited an inhibitory effect on the migration and invasion of a human lung cancer cell line. *Cancer Letters*, 235(2), 248–59.

280. Horsfall, A. U., Olabiyi, O., Aiyegbusi, A., Noronha, C. C., & Okanlawon, A. O. (2008). *Morinda citrifolia* fruit juice augments insulin action in Sprague-Dawley

rats with experimentally induced diabetes. Nigerian *Quarterly Journal of Hospital Medicine*, 18(3), 162–65.

281. Harada, S., Hamabe, W., Kamiya, K., Satake, T., & Tokuyama, S. (2009). Protective effect of *Morinda citrifolia* on the ischemic neuronal damage. *Yakugaku Zasshi*, 129(2), 203–7.

282. Amagase, H., Sun, B., & Borek, C. (2009). *Lycium barbarum* (goji) juice improves in vivo antioxidant biomarkers in serum of healthy adults. *Nutrition Research*, 29(1), 19–25.

283. Schauss, A. G., et al. (2006). Phytochemical and nutrient composition of the freeze-dried amazonian palmberry, *Euterpe oleraceae* Mart. (acai). *Journal of Agricultural and Food Chemistry*, 54(22), 8598–603.

284. Fife, B. (2001). *The detox book: How to detoxify your body to improve your health, stop disease and reverse aging.* Colorado Springs: Piccadilly Books.

285. Sweet F., Kao M. S., Lee S. C., Hagar W. L., & Sweet W. E. (1980). Ozone selectively inhibits growth of human cancer cells. *Science*, 209(4459), 931–33.

286. Zaky, S., et al. (2011). Preliminary results of ozone therapy as a possible treatment for patients with chronic hepatitis C. *Journal of Alternative and Complementary Medicine*, 17(3), 259–63.

287. McCabe, E. (2004). *Flood your body with oxygen.* Spring Lake (NC): Breath Of God Ministry.

288. Reid, D. (1995). *A handbook of Chinese healing herbs.* Boston: Shambhala Publishing, Inc.

289. Gulinuer, M., et al. (2004). Anti-aging function study on echinacoside. *Acta Biochimica et Biophysica Sinica*, 20(3), 183–87.

290. Ghosal, S. (1990). Chemistry of shilajit, an immunomodulatory Ayurvedic rasayan. *Pure and Applied Chemistry*, 62(7), 1285–88.

291. Parle, M., & Bansal, N. (2006). Traditional medicinal formulation, Chyawanprash—A review. *Indian Journal of Traditional Knowledge*, 5(4), 484–88.

292. Prilepskaya, V. N., Ledina, A. V., Tagiyeva, A. V, & Revazova, F. S. (2006). *Vitex agnus castus*: Successful treatment of moderate to severe premenstrual syndrome. *Maturitas*, 55(1), S55–S63.

293. Bedi, M. K., & Shenefelt, P. D. (2002) Herbal therapy in dermatology. *Archives of Dermatology*, 138(2), 232–42.

294. Sağlam, H., Pabuçcuoğlu, A., & Kıvçak, B. (2007). Antioxidant Activity of *Vitex agnus-castus* L. Extracts. *Phytotherapy Research*, 21(11), 1059–60.

295. Dittmar, F. W., et al. (1992). Premenstrual syndrome: Treatment with a phytopharmaceutical. *Therapiwoche Gynäkol*, 5, 60–68.

296. Loch, E. G., Selle, H., & Boblitz, N. (2000). Treatment of premenstrual

syndrome with a phytopharmaceutical formulation containing *Vitex agnus castus*. *Journal of Women's Health and Gender-Based Medicine*, 9(3), 315–20.

297. Schellenberg, R. (2001). Treatment for the premenstrual syndrome with ag-nus castus fruit extract: Prospective, randomized, placebo controlled study. *British Medical Journal*, 322(7279), 134–37.

298. Ma, L., Lin, S., Chen, R., Zhang, Y., Chen, F., & Wang, X. (2010). Evaluating therapeutic effect in symptoms of moderate-to-severe premenstrual syndrome with *Vitex agnus castus* (BNO 1095) in Chinese women. *The Australian and New Zealand Journal of Obstetrics*, 50(2), 189–93.

299. Mayo, J. (1997). A healthy menstrual cycle. *Clinical Nutrition Insights*, 5(9).

300. Darby, S. B. (2009). Traditional Chinese medicine: A complement to conven-tional. *Nursing for Women's Health*, 13(3), 198–206.

301. Muangman, V., & Cherdshewasart, W. (2001). Clinical trial of the phytoe-strogen-rich herb, *Pueraria mirifica* as a crude drug in the treatment of symptoms in menopausal women. *Siriraj Hospital Gazete*, 200(53), 300–309.

302. Mahadevan, S., & Park, Y. (2008). Multifaceted therapeutic benefits of Gink-go biloba L.: Chemistry, efficacy, safety, and uses. *Journal of Food Science*, 73(1), R14–9.

303. Weinmann, S., Roll, S., Schwarzbach, C., Vauth, C., & Willich, S. N. (2010). Effects of Ginkgo biloba in dementia: Systematic review and meta-analysis. *BMC Geriatrics*, 10, 14.

304. Guyton, Arthur C. (1976). *Textbook of Medical Physiology (5th ed.)*. Philadel-phia: W.B. Saunders. p. 424.

305. The Nader report—Troubled waters on tap, Duff Conacher and Assc. Center For Study of Responsive Law, 1988.

306. Duff Conacher, Center for Study of Responsive Law (1988). Troubled waters on tap: Organic chemicals in public drinking ater systems and the failure of regu-lation. Washington (DC): *Center for Study of Responsive Law*.

307. Ali, M. (2003). *Oxygen and aging*. New York: Canary 21 Press.

308. Richardson, S. D., et al. (2010). What's in the pool? A comprehensive identi-fication of disinfection by-products and assessment of mutagenicity of chlorinated and brominated swimming pool water. *Environmental Health Perspectives*, 118(11), 1523–30.

309. Zwiener, C., Richardson, S. D., DeMarini, D. M, Grummt, T., Glauner, T., & Frimmel, F. H. (2007). Drowning in disinfection byproducts? Assessing swimming pool water. *Environmental Science and Technology*. 41(2), 363–72.

310. Raloff, J. (1986). Toxic showers And baths, *Science News*, 130, 190.

311. Anderson, I. (1986). Showers Pose a Risk to Health. *New Scientist*, 18.

312. Cherry, N. (2001). Evidence that electromagnetic fields from high voltage powerlines and in buildings are hazardous to human health, especially to young children. *Human Sciences Division, Lincoln University*, NZ.

313. Floderus, B., et al. (1993). Occupational exposure to electromagnetic fields in relation to leukemia and brain tumors: A case-control study in Sweden. *Cancer Causes Control,* 4(5), 465–76.

314. Tynes, T., Andersen, A., & Langmark, F. (1992). Incidence of cancer in Norwegian workers potentially exposed to electromagnetic fields. *American Journal of Epidemiology*, 136(1), 81–88.

315. Zamanian, A. & Hardiman, C. (2005). Electromagnetic Radiation and Human Health: A Review of Sources and Effects. *High Frequency Electronics*, 16–26.

316. Vallejo, F., Tomás-Barberán, F. A., & Garcia-Viguera, C. (2003). Phenolic compound contents in edible parts of broccoli inflorescences after domestic cooking. *Journal of the Science of Food and Agriculture*, 83(14), 1511–16.

317. Gursatej Gandhi, A. (2005). Genetic Damage in Mobile Phone Users: Some Preliminary Findings. *Indian Journal of Human Genetics*, 11(2), 99–104.

318. Ruediger, H. W. (2009). Genotoxic effects of radiofrequency electromagnetic fields. *Pathophysiology*, 16(2–3), 89–102.

319. REFLEX: Risk Evaluation of Potential Environmental Hazards from Low Energy Electromagnetic Field Exposure Using Sensitive in vitro Methods. A project funded by the EU under the programme "Quality of Life and Management of Living Resources", Key Action 4 "Environment and Health": QLK4-CT-1999-01574.

320. Hardell, L., & Carlberg, M. (2009). Mobile phones, cordless phones and the risk for brain tumours. *International Journal of Oncology*, 35(1), 5–17.

321. Lönn, S., Ahlbom, A., Hall, P., & Feychting, M. (2004). Mobile phone use and the risk of acoustic neuroma. *Epidemiology*, 15(6), 653–59.

323. Baan, R., et al. (2011). Carcinogenicity of radiofrequency electromagnetic fields. *The Lancet Oncology*, 12(7), 624–26.

324. Schwentner, I., et al. (2006). Distant metastasis of parotid gland tumors. *Acta Oto-Laryngologica*, 126(4), 340–45.

325. Sadetzki, S., et al. (2008). Cellular phone use and risk of benign and malignant parotid gland tumors—A nationwide case-control study. *American Journal of Epidemiology*, 167(4), 457–67.

326. Salford, L. G., Brun, A. E., Eberhardt, J. L., Malmgren, L., & Persson, B. R. (2003). Nerve cell damage in mammalian brain after exposure to microwaves from GSM mobile phones. *Environmental Health Perspectives*, 111(7), 881–83.

327. Tombak, M. (2005). *Can we live 150 years? Your body maintenance handbook.* Point Roberts (WA): Healthy Life Press Inc.

328. Colbert, A. P., et al. (1999). Magnetic mattress pad use in patients with fibromyalgia: A randomized double-blind pilot study. *Journal of Back and Musculoskeletal Rehabilitation*, 13, 19–31.

329. Eccles, N. K. (2005). A critical review of randomized controlled trials of static magnets for pain relief. *The Journal of Alternative and Complementary Medicine*, 11(3), 495–509.

340. Budiansky, S. (1980). Indoor air quality. *Environmental Science and Technology*, 14(9), 1023–27.

341. Shaughnessy, R. J., et al. (1994). Effectiveness of portable indoor air cleaners: Sensory testing results. *Indoor Air*, 4(3), 179–88.

342. Lohr, V. I., Pearson-Mims C. H. (1996). Particulate matter accumulation on horizontal surfaces in interiors: Influence of foliage plants. *Atmospheric Environment*, 30(14), 2565–68.

343. Wolverton, B. C., Johnson, A., & Bounds, K. (1989). Interior landscape plants for indoor air pollution abatement. National Aeronautics and Space Administration, John C. Stennis Space Center. MS 39529-6000.

344. Wolverton B.C., McDonald R.C., & Watkins Jr. E.A. (1984). Foliage plants for removing air pollutants from energy-efficient homes. *Economic Botany*, 38(2), 224–28.

345. Nilsson, E., et al. (2000). Electrochemical treatment of tumours. *Bioelectrochemistry*, 51(1), 1–11.

346. Chen, B., Xie, Z., & Zhu, F. (1994). Experimental study on electrochemical treatment of cancer in mice. *European Journal of Surgery—Supplement*, (574), 75–77.

347. Miklavcic, D., An, D., Belehradek Jr., J., & Mir, L. M. (1997) Host's immune response in electrotherapy of murine tumors by direct current. *European Cytokine Network*, 8(3), 275–79.

348. Mercola, J. M., & Kirsch, D. L. (1995). The basis for microcurrent electrical therapy (MET) in conventional medical practice. *Journal of Advancement in Medicine*, 8(2), 107–20.

349. Xiong, H., et al. (2006). Semi-conductor laser for coronary heart disease of blood-stasis syndrome: A randomized, blind and parallel control study. *Chinese Journal of Clinical Rehabilitation*, 10(39), 36–38.

350. Jiang, M., & Yang, A. (2001). Observation of endonasal low energy He-Ne laser treatment of 105 cases of brain disease. [Article in Chinese] *Laser Journal*, 22(4), 17.

351. Brosseau, L., et al. (2000). Low level laser therapy for osteoarthritis and rheumatoid arthritis: A metaanalysis. *The Journal of Rheumatology*, 27(8), 1961–69.

352. Turner, J. G., Clark, A. J., Gauthier, D. K., & Williams, M. (1998). The effect of therapeutic touch on pain and anxiety in burn patients. *Journal of Advanced Nursing*, 28(1), 10–20.

353. Keller, E., & Bzdek, V. M. (1986). Effects of therapeutic touch on tension headache pain. *Nursing Research*, 35(2), 1016.

354. Eckes Peck, S. D. (1997). The effectiveness of therapeutic touch for decreasing pain in elders with degenerative arthritis. *Journal of Holistic Nursing*, 15(2), 176–98.

355. Bronfort, G., Haas, M., Evans, R., Leininger, B., & Triano, J. (2010). Effectiveness of manual therapies: The UK evidence report. *Chiropractic and Osteopathy*, 18(3), 3.

356. Robertshawe, P. (2007). Massage for osteoarthritis of the knee. *Journal of the Australian Traditional-Medicine Society*, 13(2), 87.

357. Robinson, N., Lorenc, A., & Liao, X. (2011). The evidence for Shiatsu: a systematic review of Shiatsu and acupressure. *BMC Complementary and Alternative Medicine*, 11, 88.

358. Ernst, E., Pittler, M. H., Wider, B., Boddy, K. (2007). Acupuncture: its evidence-base is changing. *American Journal of Chinese Medicine*, 35(1), 21–25.

359. Lee, M. S., & Ernst, E. (2011). Acupuncture for pain: An overview of Cochrane reviews. *Chinese Journal of Integrative Medicine*, 17(3), 187–89.

360. Long, A. F. (2008). The effectiveness of shiatsu: Findings from a cross-European, prospective observational study. *Journal of Alternative and Complementary Medicine*, 14(8), 921–30.

361. Marr, M., Baker, J., Lambon, N., & Perry, J. (2011). The effects of the Bowen technique on hamstring flexibility over time: A randomised controlled trial. *Journal of Bodywork and Movement Therapies*, 15(3), 281–90.

362. Benford, M. S., Talnagi, J., Burr-Doss, D., Boosey, S., & Arnold, L. E. (1999). Gamma radiation fluctuations during alternative healing therapy. *Alternative Therapies in Health and Medicine*, 5(4), 51–56.

363. Terwee, C. B. (2008). Successful treatment of food allergy with Nambudripad's Allergy Elimination Techniques (NAET) in a 3-year old: A case report. *Cases Journal*, 1(1).

364. Shang A., et al. (2005). Are the clinical effects of homoeopathy placebo effects? Comparative study of placebo-controlled trials of homoeopathy and allopathy. *The Lancet*, 366(9487), 726–32.

365. Ernst, E. (2002). A systematic review of systematic reviews of homeopathy. *British Journal of Clinical Pharmacology*, 54(6), 577–82.

366. Linde, K., Hondras, M., Vickers, A., ter Riet, G., & Melchart, D. (2001). Systematic reviews of complementary therapies—an annotated bibliography. Part 3: homeopathy. *BMC Complementary and Alternative Medicine*, 1, 4.

367. Kim, L. S., et al. (2005). Treatment of seasonal allergic rhinitis using homeopathic preparation of common allergens in the southwest region of the US: A randomized, controlled clinical trial. *The Annals of Pharmacotherapy*, 39(4), 617–24.

368. Colin, P. (2006). Homeopathy and respiratory allergies: A series of 147 cases. *Homeopathy*, 95(2), 68–72.

367. Riley, D., Fischer, M., Singh, B., Haidvogl, M., & Heger, M. (2001). Homeopathy and conventional medicine: An outcomes study comparing effectiveness in a primary care setting. *Journal of Alternative and Complementary Medicine*, 7(2), 149–59.

368. Barrager, E., Veltmann, J. R. Jr., Schauss, A. G., & Schiller, R. N. (2002). A multicentered, open-label trial on the safety and efficacy of methylsulfonylmethane in the treatment of seasonal allergic rhinitis. *Journal of Alternative and Complementary Medicine*, 8(2), 167–73.

367. Radulovic, S., Wilson, D., Calderon, M., & Durham, S. (2011). Systematic reviews of sublingual immunotherapy (SLIT). *Allergy*, 66(6), 740–52.

368. Di Rienzo, V., et al. (2003). Long-lasting effect of sublingual immunotherapy in children with asthma due to house dust mite: A 10-year prospective study. *Clinical and Experimental Allergy*, 33(2), 206–10.

369. Grant, W. B. (2004). Breast cance—risk and risk reduction factors. SUNARC.

370. Holick, M. F. (2004). Sunlight and vitamin D for bone health and prevention of autoimmune diseases, cancers, and cardiovascular disease. *American Journal of Clinical Nutrition*, 80(6 Suppl), 1678S–1688S.

371. Zittermann, A. (2003). Vitamin D in preventive medicine: are we ignoring the evidence? *British Journal of Nutrition*, 89(5), 552–72.

372. Jensen, J. D., Wing, G. J., & Dellavalle, R. P. (2010). Nutrition and melanoma prevention. *Clinics in Dermatology*, 28(6), 644–49.

373. Kushi, L. H., et al. (1997). Physical activity and mortality in postmenopausal women. *Journal of the American Medical Association*, 277(16), 1287–92.

374. Sherman, S. E., D'Agostino, R. B., Cobb, J. L., & Kannel, W. B. (1994). Physical activity and mortality in women in the Framingham Heart Study. *American Heart Journal*, 128(5), 879–84.

375. Blair, S. N., Kohl, H. W III, Barlow, C. E., Paffenbarger Jr., R. S., Gibbons L. W., & Macera, C. A. (1995). Changes in physical fitness and all-cause mortality. A prospective study of healthy and unhealthy men. *Journal of the American Medical Association*, 273(14), 1093–98.

376. Warburton, D. E., Nicol, C. W., & Bredin, S. S. (2006). Health benefits of physical activity: The evidence. *Canadian Medical Association Journal*, 174(6), 801–9.

377. Rockhill, B., Willett, W. C., Hunter, D, J., Manson, J. E., Hankinson, S. E., & Colditz, G. A. (1999). A prospective study of recreational physical activity and breast cancer risk. *Archives of Internal Medicine*, 159(19), 2290–96.

378. Holmes, M. D., et al. (2005). Physical activity and survival after breast cancer diagnosis. *Journal of the American Medical Association*, 293(20), 2479–86.

379. Radak, Z., Chung, H. Y., Goto, S. (2005). Exercise and hormesis: Oxidative stress-related adaptation for successful aging. *Biogerontology*, 6(1), 71–75.

380. Castillo-Garzón, M. J., Ruiz, J. R., Ortega, F. B., & Gutiérrez, Á. (2006). Anti-aging therapy through fitness enhancement. *Journal of Clinical Interventions in Aging*, 1(3), 213–20.

381. Puterman, E., Lin, J., Blackburn, E., O'Donovan, A., Adler, N., & Epel, E. (2010). The power of exercise: buffering the effect of chronic stress on telomere length. *PLoS One*, 5(5), e10837.

382. Carter, A. E. (1979). *The Miracles of Rebound Exercise*. Washington: The National institute of Reboundology and Health, Inc.

383. McGlone, C., L. Kravitz, J. J., & Janot J. (2002). Rebounding exercise versus treadmill jogging: A cardiorespiratory comparison. *Medicine and Science In Sports and Exercise,* 34(5).

384. McGlone, C., L. Kravitz, & Janot J. (2002). Rebounding: A low-impact exercise alternative. *ACSM's Health & Fitness Journal*, 6(2), 11–15.

385. Larkey, L., Jahnke, R., Etnier, J., & Gonzalez, J. (2009). Meditative movement as a category of exercise: Implications for research. *Journal of Physical Activity and Health*, 6(2), 230–38.

386. Hefen, X., Huining, X., Meiguang, B., Chengming, Z., & Shuying, Z. (1993). Clinical study of the anti-aging effect of qigong. *Proceedings, Second World Conference for Academic Exchange of Medical Qigong*. Beijing, China, 137.

387. Kuang, A., Wang, C., Xu, D., & Qian, Y. (1991). Research on the anti-aging effect of qigong. *Journal of Traditional Chinese Medicine*, 11(2), 153–58.

388. Sancier, K. M., & Holman, D. (2004). Multifaceted health benefits of medical qigong. *Journal of Alternative and Complementary Medicine*, 10(1), 163–65.

389. Jahnke, R., Larkey, L., Rogers, C., Etnier, J., & Lin, F. (2010). A comprehensive review of health benefits of qigong and tai chi. *American Journal of Health Promotion*, 24(6), e1–e25.

390. Ross, A., & Thomas, S. (2010). The health benefits of yoga and exercise: a review of comparison studies. *Journal of Alternative and Complementary Medicine*, 16(1), 3–12.

391. Woodyard, C. (2011). Exploring the therapeutic effects of yoga and its ability to increase quality of life. *International Journal of Yoga*, 4(2), 49–54.

392. Manchanda, S. C., et al. (2000). Retardation of coronary atherosclerosis with yoga lifestyle intervention. *Journal of Association of Physicians of India*, 48(7), 687–94.

393. Michalsen, A., et al. (2005). Rapid stress reduction and anxiolysis among distressed women as a consequence of a three-month intensive yoga program. *Medical Science Monitor*, 11(12), CR555–61.

394. Hamblin, H. T. (1923). *Dynamic Thought*. Chicago: Yogi Publication Society.

395. Amen, D. G. (1999). *Change your brain, change your life: The breakthrough program for conquering anxiety, depression, obsessiveness, anger, and impulsiveness.* New York: Three Rivers Press.

396. Tugade, M. M., Fredrickson, B. L., & Barrett, L. F. (2004). Psychological resilience and positive emotional granularity: Examining the benefits of positive emotions on coping and health. *Journal of Personality,* 72(6), 1161–90.

397. Fredrickson, B. L. (2000). Cultivating positive emotions to optimize health and well-being. *Prevention and Treatment,* 3(1).

398. Wahbeh, H., Haywood, A., Kaufman, K., Harling, N., & Zwickey, H. (2009). Mind-body medicine and immune system outcomes: A systematic review. *The Open Complementary Medicine Journal,* 1, 25–34.

399. Ellison, C. G., & Levin, J. S. (1998). The religion-health connection: Evidence, theory, and future directions. *Health Education and Behavior,* 25(6), 700–20.

400. Mueller, P. S., Plevak, D. J., & Rummans, T. A. (2001). Religious involvement, spirituality, and medicine: implications for clinical practice. *Mayo Clinic Proceedings,* 76(12), 1225–35.

401. Green, M., & Elliott, M. (2010). Religion, health, and psychological well-being. *Journal of Religion and Health,* 49(2), 149–63.

402. McCullough, M. E., Hoyt, W. T., Larson, D. B., Koenig, H. G., & Thoresen, C. (2000). Religious involvement and mortality: A meta-analytic review. *Health Psychology,* 19(3), 211–22.

403. Aukst-Margetić, B., & Margetić, B. (2005). Religiosity and health outcomes: Review of literature. *Collegium Antropologicum,* 29(1), 365–71.

404. Appleton, N. (2002). *Lick the Sugar Habit.* New York: Avery Trade.

405. Nawrot, P., Jordan, S., Eastwood, J., Rotstein, J., Hugenholtz, A., & Feeley, M. (2003). Effects of caffeine on human health. *Food Additives and Contaminants,* 20(1), 1–30.

406. Kerrigan, S., Lindsey, T. (2005). Fatal caffeine overdose: Two case reports. *Forensic Science International,* 153(1), 67–69.

407. Vartanian, L. R., Schwartz, M. B., & Brownell, K. D. (2007). Effects of soft drink consumption on nutrition and health: A systematic review and meta-analysis. *American Journal of Public Health,* 97(4), 667–75.

408. Seifert, S. M., Schaechter, J. L., Hershorin, E. R., & Lipshultz, S. E. (2011). Health effects of energy drinks on children, adolescents, and young adults. *Pediatrics,* 127(3), 511–28.

409. Steinke, L., Lanfear, D. E., Dhanapal, V., & Kalus, J. S. (2009). Effect of "energy drink" consumption on hemodynamic and electrocardiographic parameters in healthy young adults. *The Annals of Pharmacotherapy,* 43(4), 596–602.

410. Worthley, M. I., Prabhu, A., De Sciscio, P., Schultz, C., Sanders, P., & Willoughby, S. R. (2010). Detrimental effects of energy drink consumption on platelet and endothelial function. *The American Journal of Medicine*, 123(2), 184–87.

411. Mets, M. A., et al. (2011). Positive effects of Red Bull® Energy Drink on driving performance during prolonged driving. *Psychopharmacology*, 214(3), 737–45.

412. Horne, J. A., Reyner, L. A. (2001). Beneficial effects of an "energy drink" given to sleepy drivers. *Amino Acids*, 20(1), 83–89.

413. Seidl, R., Peyrl, A., Nicham, R., & Hauser, E. (2000). A taurine and caffeine-containing drink stimulates cognitive performance and well-being. *Amino Acids*, 19(3-4), 635–42.

414. Alford, C., Cox, H., & Wescott, R. (2001). The effects of red bull energy drink on human performance and mood. *Amino Acids*, 21(2), 139–50.

415. Duchan, E., Patel, N. D., & Feucht, C. (2010). Energy drinks: a review of use and safety for athletes. *The Physician and Sportsmedicine*, 38(2), 171–9.

416. Mandel, P., et al. (1985). Effects of taurine and taurine analogues on aggressive behavior. *Progress in Clinical and Biological Research*, 179, 449–58.

417. Geiß, K. R., Jester, I., Falke, W., Hamm, M., & Waag, K. -L. (1994). The effect of a taurine-containing drink on performance in 10 endurance-athletes. *Amino Acids*, 7(1), 45–56.

418. Beyranvand, M. R., Khalafi, M. K., Roshan, V. D., Choobineh, S., Parsa, S. A., & Piranfar, M. A. (2011). Effect of taurine supplementation on exercise capacity of patients with heart failure. *Journal of Cardiology*, 57(3), 333–37.

419. Rahman, M. M., et al. (2011). Taurine prevents hypertension and increases exercise capacity in rats with fructose-induced hypertension. *American Journal of Hypertension*, 24(5), 574–81.

420. Acharya, M., & Lau-Cam, C. A. (2010). Comparison of the protective actions of N-acetylcysteine, hypotaurine and taurine against acetaminophen-induced hepatotoxicity in the rat. *Journal of Biomedical Science*, 17(Suppl 1), S35.

421. Ahrens R. A., Douglass, L. W., Flynn, M. M., & Ward, G. M. (1987). Lack of effect of dietary supplements of glucuronic acid and glucuronolactone on longevity of the rat. *Nutrition Research*, 7(6), 683–88.

422. Teitelbaum, J. E., Johnson, C., & St. Cyr, J. (2006). The use of D-ribose in chronic fatigue syndrome and fibromyalgia: a pilot study. *Journal of Alternative and Complementary Medicine*, 12(9), 857–62.

423. Wall, B. T., Stephens, F. B., Constantin-Teodosiu, D., Marimuthu, K., Macdonald, I. A., Greenhaff, P. L. (2011). Chronic oral ingestion of L-carnitine and carbohydrate increases muscle carnitine content and alters muscle fuel metabolism during exercise in humans. *The Journal of Physiology*, 589(Pt 4), 963–73.

424. Malaguarnera, M. (2012). Carnitine derivatives: clinical usefulness. *Current Opinion in Gastroenterology*, 28(2), 166–76.

425. Haskell, C. F., Kennedy, D. O., Wesnes, K. A., Milne, A. L., & Scholey, A. B. (2006). A double-blind, placebo-controlled, multi-dose evaluation of the acute behavioural effects of guarana in humans. *Journal of Psychopharmacology*, 21(1), 65–70.

426. de Oliveira Campos, M. P., Riechelmann, R., Martins, L. C., Hassan, B. J., Casa, F. B., & Del Giglio, A. (2011). Guarana (*Paullinia cupana*) improves fatigue in breast cancer patients undergoing systemic chemotherapy. *Journal of Alternative and Complementary Medicine*, 17(6), 505–12.

427. Espinola, E. B., Dias, R. F., Mattei, R., & Carlini, E. A. (1997). Pharmacological activity of Guarana (*Paullinia cupana* Mart.) in laboratory animals. *Journal of Ethnopharmacology*, 55(3), 223–9.

428. Heck, C. I., & de Mejia, E. G. (2007). Yerba Mate Tea (*Ilex paraguariensis*): A comprehensive review on chemistry, health implications, and technological considerations. *Journal of Food Science*, 72(9), R138–51.

429. Forsyth, L. M., Preuss, H. G., MacDowell, A. L., Chiazze Jr., L., Birkmayer, G. D., & Bellanti, J. A. (1999). Therapeutic effects of oral NADH on the symptoms of patients with chronic fatigue syndrome. *Annals of Allergy, Asthma, and Immunology*, 82(2), 185–91.

430. Demarin, V., Podobnik, S. S., Storga-Tomic, D., & Kay, G. (2004). Treatment of Alzheimer's disease with stabilized oral nicotinamide adenine dinucleotide: A randomized, double-blind study. *Drugs Under Experimental and Clinical Research*, 30(1), 27–33.

431. Blomstrand, E. (2006). A role for branched-chain amino acids in reducing central fatigue. *The Journal of Nutrition*, 136(2), 544S–547S.

432. Ratamess, N. A., et al. (2007). Effects of an amino acid/creatine energy supplement on the acute hormonal response to resistance exercise. *International Journal of Sport Nutrition and Exercise Metabolism*, 17(6), 608–23.

433. Smith, A. (2002). Effects of caffeine on human behavior. *Food and Chemical Toxicology*, 40(9), 1243–55.

434. Lorist, M. M., Snel, J., Kok, A., & Mulder, G. (1994). Influence of caffeine on selective attention in well-rested and fatigued subjects. *Psychophysiology*, 31(6), 525-534.

435. Higdon, J. V., & Frei, B. (2006). Coffee and health: A review of recent human research. *Critical Reviews In Food Science and Nutrition*, 46(2), 101–23.

436. Butt, M. S., & Sultan, M. T. (2011). Coffee and its consumption: Benefits and risks. *Critical Reviews in Food Science and Nutrition*, 51(4), 363–73.

437. Klatsky, A.L., Morton, C., Udaltsova, N., & Friedman, G.D. (2006). Coffee, cirrhosis, and transaminase enzymes. *Archives of Internal Medicine*, 166(11), 1190–95.

438. Corrao, G., Zambon, A., Bagnardi, V., D'Amicis, A., & Klatsky, A. (2001). Coffee, caffeine, and the risk of liver cirrhosis. *Annals of Epidemiology*, 11(7), 458–65.

439. Zhang, Y., Lee, E. T., Cowan, L. D., Fabsitz, R. R., & Howard, B. V. (2011). Coffee consumption and the incidence of type 2 diabetes in men and women with normal glucose tolerance: The Strong Heart Study. *Nutrition, Metabolism and Cardiovascular Diseases*, 21(6), 418–23.

440. Shimazu, T., et al. (2005). Coffee consumption and the risk of primary liver cancer: Pooled analysis of two prospective studies in Japan. *International Journal of Cancer*, 116(1), 150–54.

441. Li, J., Seibold, P., et al. (2011). Coffee consumption modifies risk of estrogen-receptor negative breast cancer. *Breast Cancer Research*, 13(3), R49.

442. Yu, X., Bao, Z., Zou, J., & Dong, J. (2011). Coffee consumption and risk of cancers: A meta-analysis of cohort studies. *BMC Cancer*, 11, 96.

443. Je, Y., & Giovannucci, E. (2011). Coffee consumption and risk of endometrial cancer: Findings from a large up-to-date meta-analysis. *International Journal of Cancer*.

444. Je, Y., Hankinson, S. E., Tworoger, S. S., Devivo, I., & Giovannucci, E. (2011). A prospective cohort study of coffee consumption and risk of endometrial cancer over a 26-year follow-up. *Cancer Epidemiology, Biomarkers and Prevention*, 20(12), 2487–95.

445. Hamer, M. (2006). Coffee and health: Explaining conflicting results in hypertension. *Journal of Human Hypertension*, 20(12), 909–12.

446. Andersen, L. F., Jacobs Jr., D. R., Carlsen, M. H., & Blomhoff, R. (2006). Consumption of coffee is associated with reduced risk of death attributed to inflammatory and cardiovascular diseases in the Iowa Women's Health Study. *The American Journal of Clinical Nutrition*, 83(5), 1039–46.

447. Floegel, A., Pischon, T., Bergmann, M. M., Teucher, B., Kaaks, R., & Boeing, H. (2012). Coffee consumption and risk of chronic disease in the European Prospective Investigation into Cancer and Nutrition (EPIC)—Germany study. *The American Journal of Clinical Nutrition*, 95(4), 901–8.

448. Ames, B. N., & Gold, L. S. (1998). The causes and prevention of cancer: the role of environment. *Biotherapy*, 11(2–3), 205–20.

449. Mason, R. (2001). 200 mg of Zen; L-theanine boosts alpha waves, promotes alert relaxation. *Alternative & Complementary Therapies*, 7(2), 91–95.

450. Nakachi, K., Matsuyama, S., Miyake, S., Suganuma, M., & Imai, K. (2000). Preventive effects of drinking green tea on cancer and cardiovascular disease: Epidemiological evidence for multiple targeting prevention. *Biofactors*, 13(1–4), 49–54.

451. Sanchez, A., et al. (1973). Role of sugars in human neutrophilic phagocytosis. *The American Journal of Clinical Nutrition*, 26(11), 1180–84.

452. Bernstein, J., et al. (1997). Depression of lymphocyte transformation following oral glucose ingestion. *American Journal of Clinical Nutrition*, 30, 613.

453. Ringsdorf Jr., W., Cheraskin, E., Ramsay Jr., R. (1976). Sucrose, Neutrophilic Phagocytosis and Resistance to Disease. *Dental Survey*, 52(12), 46–48.

454. Banerjee, D., & Kaul, D. (2010). Combined inhalational and oral supplementation of ascorbic acid may prevent influenza pandemic emergency: A hypothesis. *Nutrition*, 26(1), 128–32.

455. Roxas, M., & Jurenka, J. (2007). Colds and influenza: A review of diagnosis and conventional, botanical, and nutritional considerations. *Alternative Medicine Review*, 12(1), 25–48.

456. Shah, S. A., Sander, S., White, C. M., Rinaldi, M., & Coleman, C. I. (2007). Evaluation of echinacea for the prevention and treatment of the common cold: A meta-analysis. *The Lancet Infectious Diseases*, 7(7), 473–80.

457. Hudson, J. B. (2012). Applications of the phytomedicine *Echinacea purpurea* (Purple Coneflower) in infectious diseases. *Journal of Biomedicine and Biotechnology*, 2012, 769896.

458. Clement-Kruzel, S., Hwang, S. A., Kruzel, M. C., Dasgupta, A, & Actor, J. K. (2008). Immune modulation of macrophage pro-inflammatory response by goldenseal and Astragalus extracts. *Journal of Medicinal Food*, 11(3), 493–98.

459. Steinberg, P. N. (1995). Cat's Claw: An herb from the Peruvian Amazon. [Article in Spanish] *Sidahora*, 35-36.

460. Reis, S. R., et al. (2008). Immunomodulating and antiviral activities of *Uncaria tomentosa* on human monocytes infected with Dengue Virus-2. *International Immunopharmacology*, 8(3), 468–76.

461. Barak, V., Halperin, T., & Kalickman, I. (2001). The effect of Sambucol, a black elderberry-based, natural product, on the production of human cytokines: I. Inflammatory cytokines. *European Cytokine Network*, 12(2), 290–96.

462. Krawitz, C., et al. (2011). Inhibitory activity of a standardized elderberry liquid extract against clinically-relevant human respiratory bacterial pathogens and influenza A and B viruses. *BMC Complementary and Alternative Medicine*, 11, 16.

463. Zakay-Rones, Z., Thom, E., Wollan, T., & Wadstein, J. (2004). Randomized study of the efficacy and safety of oral elderberry extract in the treatment of influenza A and B virus infections. *The Journal of International Medical Research*, 32(2), 132–40.

464. Tan, B. K., & Vanitha, J. (2004). Immunomodulatory and antimicrobial effects of some traditional Chinese medicinal herbs: A review. *Current Medicinal Chemistry*, 11(11), 1423–30.

465. Liu, H., & Zhu, Y. (2002). Effect of alcohol extract of Zingben officinale rose on immunologic function of mice with tumor. [Article in Chinese] *Journal of Hygiene Research*, 31(3), 208–9.

466. Pereira, M. M., Haniadka, R., Chacko, P. P., Palatty, P. L., & Baliga, M. S. (2011). *Zingiber officinale* Roscoe (ginger) as an adjuvant in cancer treatment: A review. *Journal of BUON*, 16(3), 414–24.

467. Utsunomiya, T., Kobayashi, M., Pollard, R. B., & Suzuki, F. (1997). Glycyrrhizin, an active component of licorice roots, reduces morbidity and mortality of mice infected with lethal doses of influenza virus. *Antimicrobial Agents and Chemotherapy*, 41(3), 551–56.

468. Wolkerstorfer, A., Kurz, H., Bachhofner, N., & Szolar, O. H. (2009). Glycyrrhizin inhibits influenza A virus uptake into the cell. *Antiviral Research*, 83(2), 171–78.

469. Michaelis M, et al. (2010). Glycyrrhizin inhibits highly pathogenic H5N1 influenza A virus-induced pro-inflammatory cytokine and chemokine expression in human macrophages. *Medical Microbiology and Immunology*, 199(4), 29197.

470. Cinatl, J., Morgenstern, B., Bauer, G., Chandra, P., Rabenau, H., & Doerr, H. W. (2003). Glycyrrhizin, an active component of liquorice roots, and replication of SARS-associated coronavirus. *Lancet*, 361(9374), 2045–46.

471. Lin, R. D., Mao, Y. W., Leu, S. J., Huang, C. Y., & Lee, M. H. (2011). The immuno-regulatory effects of *Schisandra chinensis* and its constituents on human monocytic leukemia cells. *Molecules*, 16(6), 4836–49.

472. Panossian, A., & Wikman, G. (2008). Pharmacology of Schisandra chinensis Bail.: An overview of Russian research and uses in medicine. *Journal of Ethnopharmacology*, 118(2), 183–212.

473. Gupta, A, et al. (2006). Immunomodulatory activity of biopolymeric fraction RLJ-NE-205 from *Picrorhiza kurroa*. *International Immunopharmacology*, 6(10), 1543–9.

474. Sharma, M. L., Rao, C. S., & Duda, P. L. (1994). Immunostimulatory activity of *Picrorhiza kurroa* leaf extract. *Journal of Ethnopharmacology*, 41(3), 185–92.

475. Khajuria A, et al. (2007). RLJ-NE-299A: A new plant based vaccine adjuvant. *Vaccine*, 25(14), 2706–15.

476. Watanabe, T., Watanabe, M., Watanabe, Y., & Hotta, C. (2000). Effects of oral administration of *Pfaffia paniculata* (Brazilian ginseng) on incidence of spontaneous leukemia in AKR/J mice. *Cancer Detection and Prevention*, 24(2), 173–78.

477. Park, B. S., et al. (2006). Antibacterial activity of *Tabebuia impetiginosa* Martius ex DC (Taheebo) against *Helicobacter pylori*. *Journal of Ethnopharmacology*, 105(1–2), 255–62.

478. Xu, G., Dou, J., Zhang, L., Guo, Q., & Zhou, C. (2010). Inhibitory effects of baicalein on the influenza virus in vivo is determined by baicalin in the serum. *Biological and Pharmaceutical Bulletin*, 33(2), 238–43.

479. Chen, L., et al. (2011). Synergistic activity of baicalein with ribavirin against influenza A (H1N1) virus infections in cell culture and in mice. *Antiviral Research*, 91(3), 314–20.

480. Naik, S. R., & Hule, A. (2009). Evaluation of immunomodulatory activity of an extract of andrographolides from *Andographis paniculata*. *Planta Medica*, 75(8), 785–91.

481. Rajagopal, S., Kumar, R. A., Deevi, D. S., Satyanarayana, C., & Rajagopalan, R. (2003). Andrographolide, a potential cancer therapeutic agent isolated from *Andrographis paniculata*. *Journal of Experimental Therapeutics and Oncology*, 3(3), 147–58.

482. Coon, J. T., & Ernst, E. (2004). Andrographis paniculata in the treatment of upper respiratory tract infections: A systematic review of safety and efficacy. *Planta Medica*, 70(4), 293–98.

483. Grossarth-Maticek, R., Kiene, H., Baumgartner, S. M., & Ziegler, R. (2001). Use of Iscador, an extract of European mistletoe (*Viscum album*), in cancer treatment: Prospective nonrandomized and randomized matched-pair studies nested within a cohort study. *Alternative Therapies in Health and Medicine*, 7(3), 5766, 68–72, 74–76.

484. Gardin, N. E. (2009). Immunological response to mistletoe (Viscum album L.) in cancer patients: A four-case series. *Phytotherapy Research*, 23(3), 407-11.

485. Karagöz, A., Onay, E., Arda, N., & Kuru, A. (2003). Antiviral potency of mistletoe (*Viscum album* ssp. album) extracts against human parainfluenza virus type 2 in Vero cells. *Phytotherapy Research*, 17(5), 560–62.

486. Murphy, E. A., Davis, J. M., & Carmichael, M. D. (2010). Immune modulating effects of β-glucan. *Current Opinion in Clinical Nutrition and Metabolic Care*, 13(6), 656–61.

487. Rondanelli, M., Opizzi, A., & Monteferrario, F. (2009). The biological activity of beta-glucans. [Article in Italian] *Minerva Medica*, 100(3), 237–45.

488. Vetvicka, V. (2011). Glucan-immunostimulant, adjuvant, potential drug. *World Journal of Clinical Oncology*, 2(2), 115–19.

489. Vetvicka, V., & Vetvickova, J. (2009). Effects of glucan on immunosuppressive actions of mercury. *Journal of Medicinal Food*, 12(5), 1098–104.

490. Lee, O. H., & Lee, B. Y. (2010). Antioxidant and antimicrobial activities of individual and combined phenolics in *Olea europaea* leaf extract. *Bioresource Technology*, 101(10), 3751–54.

491. Sudjana AN, et al. (2009). Antimicrobial activity of commercial *Olea europaea* (olive) leaf extract. *International Journal of Antimicrobial Agents*, 33(5), 461–63.

492. Faleiro, L., et al. (2005). Antibacterial and antioxidant activities of essential oils isolated from *Thymbra capitata* L. (Cav.) and *Origanum vulgare* L. *Journal of Agricultural and Food Chemistry*, 53(21), 8162–68.

493. Saeed, S., & Tariq, P. (2009). Antibacterial activity of oregano (*Origanum vulgare* Linn.) against gram positive bacteria. *Pakistan Journal of Pharmaceutical Sciences*, 22(4), 421–24.

494. Cueva C, et al. (2012). Antibacterial activity of wine phenolic compounds and oenological extracts against potential respiratory pathogens. *Letters In Applied Microbiology,* 54(6), 557–63.

495. Su, X., D'Souza, D. H. (2011). Grape seed extract for control of human enteric viruses. *Applied and Environmental Microbiology*, 77(12), 3982–87.

496. Amagase, H. (2006). Clarifying the real bioactive constituents of garlic. *The Journal of Nutrition*, 136(3 Suppl), 716S–725S.

497. Chandrashekar, P. M., Prashanth, K. V., & Venkatesh, Y. P. (2011). Isolation, structural elucidation and immunomodulatory activity of fructans from aged garlic extract. *Phytochemistry*, 72(2–3), 255–64.

498. Nantz, M. P., Rowe, C. A., Muller, C. E., Creasy, R. A., Stanilka, J. M., & Percival, S. S. (2012). Supplementation with aged garlic extract improves both NK and $\gamma\delta$-T cell function and reduces the severity of cold and flu symptoms: A randomized, double-blind, placebo-controlled nutrition intervention. *Clinical Nutrition, 31(3), 337–44.*

499. Josling, P. (2001). Preventing the common cold with a garlic supplement: A double-blind, placebo-controlled survey. *Advances in Therapy*, 18(4), 189–93.

500. Vickers, A. J., & Smith, C. (2000). Homoeopathic Oscillococcinum for preventing and treating influenza and influenza-like syndromes. *Cochrane Database of Systematic Reviews*, (2), CD001957.

501. Coulamy, A. (1998). Survey of the prescription habits of homeopathic doctors on the subject of a single medication: Influenzinum. *French Society of Homeopathy Conference Notes*, 1-16.

502. Uhm, Han S., Lee, Kwang H., & Seong, Baik L. (2009). Inactivation of H1N1 viruses exposed to acidic ozone water. *Applied Physics Letters*, 95(17), 173704.

503. Sukhinin, V. P., Zarubaev, V. V., Platonov, V. G., & Avtushenko, S. S. (1999) Effect of liposomal beta-carotene on experimentally lethal influenza infection. [Article in Russian] *Voprosy Virusologii*, 44(4), 163–67.

504. Puertollano, M. A., Puertollano, E., de Cienfuegos, G. Á., & de Pablo, M. A. (2011). Dietary antioxidants: immunity and host defense. *Current Topics In Medicinal Chemistry*, 11(14), 1752–66.

505. Chew, B. P., & Park, J. S. (2004). Carotenoid action on the immune response. *The Journal of Nutrition*, 134(1), 257S–261S.

506. Sur, T. K., et al. (2004). Effect of Sonachandi Chyawanprash and Chyawanprash Plus—two herbal formulations on immunomodulation. *Nepal Medical College Journal*, 6(2), 126–28.

507. Reap, E. A., & Lawson, J. W. (1990) Stimulation of the immune response by dimethylglycine, a nontoxic metabolite. *Journal of Laboratory and Clinical Medicine*, 115(4), 481–86.

509. Graber, C. D., Goust, J. M., Glassman, A. D., Kendall, R., & Loadholt, C. B. (1981). Immunomodulating properties of dimethylglycine in humans. *The Journal of Infectious Diseases*, 143(1), 101–5.

509. Wintergerst, E. S., Maggini, S., & Hornig, D. H. (2006). Immune-enhancing role of vitamin C and zinc and effect on clinical conditions. *Annals of Nutrition and Metabolism*, 50(2), 85–94.

510. Douglas, R. M., Hemila, H., D'Souza, R., Chalker, E. B., & Treacy B. (2004). Vitamin C for preventing and treating the common cold. *Cochrane Database of Systematic Reviews*, 4, CD000980.

511. Hemila, H. (2004). Vitamin C supplementation and respiratory infections: A systematic review. *Military Medicine*, 169(11), 920–25.

512. Gorton, H. C., Jarvis, K., Gorton, H. C., & Jarvis, K. (1999). The effectiveness of vitamin C in preventing and relieving the symptoms of virus-induced respiratory infections. *Journal of Manipulative and Physiological Therapeutics*, 22(8), 530–33.

513. Wong, C. P., & Ho, E. (2012). Zinc and its role in age-related inflammation and immune dysfunction. *Molecular Nutrition and Food Research*, 56(1), 77–87.

514. Garland, M. L., & Hagmeyer, K. O. (1998). The role of zinc lozenges in treatment of the common cold. *The Annals of Pharmacotherapy*, 32(1), 63–69.

515. Eby, G. A. (2004). Zinc lozenges: Cold cure or candy? Solution chemistry determinations. *Bioscience Reports*, 24(1), 23–39.

516. Hemilä, H. (2011). Zinc lozenges may shorten the duration of colds: A systematic review. *The Open Respiratory Medicine Journal*, 5, 51–58.

517. Singh, M., & Das, R. R. (2011). Zinc for the common cold. *Cochrane Database of Systematic Reviews*, 2(2), CD001364.

518. Eby III, G. A. (2010). Zinc lozenges as cure for the common cold—a review and hypothesis. *Medical Hypotheses*, 74(3), 482–92.

519. De Flora, S., Grassi, C., & Carati, L. (1997). Attenuation of influenza-like symptomatology and improvement of cell-mediated immunity with long-term N-acetylcysteine treatment. *European Respiratory Journal*, 10(7), 1535–41.

520. Axelrod, A. E. (1981). Role of the B vitamins in the immune response. *Advances in Experimental Medicine and Biology*, 135, 93–106.

521. Khani, S., Hosseini, H. M., Taheri, M., Nourani, M. R., & Imani Fooladi, A. A. (2012). Probiotics as an alternative strategy for prevention and treatment of human diseases: A review. *Inflammation and Allergy Drug Targets*, 11(2), 79–89.

522. Yan, F., & Polk, D. B. (2011). Probiotics and immune health. *Current Opinion In Gastroenterology*, 27(6), 496–501.

523. Rai, M. K., Deshmukh, S. D., Ingle, A. P., & Gade, A. K. (2012). Silver nanoparticles: The powerful nanoweapon against multidrug-resistant bacteria. *Journal of Applied Microbiology*, 112(5), 841–52.

524. Galdiero, S., Falanga, A., Vitiello, M., Cantisani, M., Marra, V., & Galdiero, M. (2011). Silver nanoparticles as potential antiviral agents. *Molecules*, 16(10), 8894–918.

525. Wasser, S. P. (2011). Current findings, future trends, and unsolved problems in studies of medicinal mushrooms. *Applied Microbiology and Biotechnology*, 89(5), 1323–32.

526. Skotnicki, A. B. (1989). Therapeutic application of calf thymus extract (TFX). *Medical Oncology and Tumor Pharmacotherapy*, 6(1), 31–43.

527. Vettori, G., Lazzaro, A., Mazzanti, P., & Cazzola, P. (1987). Prevention of recurrent respiratory infections in adults. *Minerva Medica*, 78(17), 1281–89.

528. Shing C. M., et al. (2007). Effects of bovine colostrum supplementation on immune variables in highly trained cyclists. *Journal of Applied Physiology*, 102(3), 1113–22.

529. Struff, W. G., & Sprotte, G. (2008). Bovine colostrum as a biologic in clinical medicine: A review—Part II: Clinical studies. *International Journal of Clinical Pharmacology and Therapeutics*, 46(5), 211–25.

530. Wang, G. L., & Lin, Z. B. (1996). The immunomodulatory effect of lentinan. [Article in Chinese] *Yao Xue Xue Bao*, 31(2), 86–90.

531. Bisen, P. S., Baghel, R. K., Sanodiya, B. S., Thakur, G. S., & Prasad, G. B. (2010). Lentinus edodes: A macrofungus with pharmacological activities. *Current Medicinal Chemistry*, 17(22), 2419–30.

532. Kupfahl, C., Geginat, G., & Hof, H. (2006). Lentinan has a stimulatory effect on innate and adaptive immunity against murine *Listeria monocytogenes* infection. *International Immunopharmacology*, 6(4), 686–96.

533. Dillon, K. M., Minchoff, B., & Baker, K. H. (1985–86). Positive emotional states and enhancement of the immune system. *International Journal of Psychiatry in Medicine*, 15(1), 13–18.

534. Berk, L. S, Felten, D. L., Tan, S. A., Bittman, B. B., & Westengard, J. (2001). Modulation of neuroimmune parameters during the eustress of humor-associated mirthful laughter. *Alternative Therapies In Health and Medicine*, 7(2), 62–72, 74–76.

535. Cousins, N. (1976). Anatomy of an illness (as perceived by the patient). *The New England Journal of Medicine*, 295(26), 1458–63.

536. Mroninski, C. R. L., Adriano, E. J., & Mattos, G. (2001). Meningococcinum: Its protective effect against meningococcal disease. *Homoeopathic Links Winter*, 14(4), 230–34.

537. Bracho, G., et al. (2010). Large-scale application of highly-diluted bacteria for Leptospirosis epidemic control. *Homeopathy*, 99(3), 156–66.

538. Rudnick, S. N., McDevitt, J. J., First, M. W., & Spengler, J. D. (2009). Inactivating influenza viruses on surfaces using hydrogen peroxide or triethylene glycol at low vapor concentrations. *American Journal of Infection Control*, 37(10), 813–19.

539. Tiralongo, E., Lea, R. A., Wee, S. S., Hanna, M. M., & Griffiths, L. R. (2012). Randomised, double blind, placebo-controlled trial of echinacea supplementation in air travellers. *Evidence-based Complementary and Alternative Medicine*, 417267.

540. Wolvers, D., Antoine, J. M., Myllyluoma, E., Schrezenmeir, J., Szajewska, H., & Rijkers, G. T. (2010). Guidance for substantiating the evidence for beneficial effects of probiotics: prevention and management of infections by probiotics. *The Journal of Nutrition*, 140(3), 698S-712S.

541. McFarland, L. V. (2007). Meta-analysis of probiotics for the prevention of traveler's diarrhea. *Travel Medicine and Infectious Disease*, 5(2), 97–105.

542. DuPont, H. L., et al. (2009). Expert review of the evidence base for self-therapy of travelers' diarrhea. *Journal of Travel Medicine*, 16(3), 161–71.

544. Juckett, G. (1999). Prevention and treatment of traveler's diarrhea. *American Family Physician*, 60(1), 119–24.

544. DuPont, H. L. (2008). Systematic review: Prevention of travellers' diarrhoea. *Alimentary Pharmacology and Therapeutics*, 27(9), 741–51.

545. Michael, M., et al. (2004). Phase II study of activated charcoal to prevent irinotecan-induced diarrhea. *Journal of Clinical Oncology*, 22(21), 4410–17.

546. Scazzocchio, F., Cometa, M. F., Tomassini, L., & Palmery, M. (2001). Antibacterial activity of *Hydrastis canadensis* extract and its major isolated alkaloids. *Planta Medica*, 67(6), 561–64.

547. Goncagul, G., & Ayaz, E. (2010). Antimicrobial effect of garlic (*Allium sativum*). *Recent Patents on Anti-Infective Drug Discovery*, 5(1), 91–93.

548. Hannan, A., Ikram, U., M., Usman, M., Hussain, S., Absar, M., & Javed, K. (2011). Anti-mycobacterial activity of garlic (*Allium sativum*) against multi-drug resistant and non-multi-drug resistant mycobacterium tuberculosis. *Pakistan Journal of Pharmaceutical Sciences*, 24(1), 81–85.

549. Sasaki, J., Kita, T., Ishita, K., Uchisawa, H., & Matsue, H. (1999) Antibacterial activity of garlic powder against *Escherichia coli* O-157. *Journal of Nutritional Science and Vitaminology*, 45(6), 785–90.

550. Wentworth Jr., P., et al. (2002). Evidence for antibody-catalyzed ozone formation in bacterial killing and inflammation. *Science*, 298(5601), 2195–99.

551. Mentel', R., Shirrmakher, R., Kevich, A., Dreĭzin, R. S., & Shmidt I. (1977). Virus inactivation by hydrogen peroxide. [Article in Russian] *Voprosy Virusologii*, (6), 731–33.

CHAPTER 7: STYLE

1. Whitman, B. (2004). *The hard truth about what men want*. Bloomington (IN): 1st Book Library.

2. Lennon, S. J. (1990). Effects of clothing attractiveness on perceptions. *Home Economics Research Journal*, 18(4), 303–10.

3. Blasberg, D. (2011). *Very classy: Even more exceptional advice for the extremely modern lady.* New York: Razorbill.

4. Martin, J. (2009). *Fashion for dummies.* Indianapolis (IN): For Dummies.

5. Radeloff, D. J. (1990). Role of color in perception of attractiveness. *Perceptual and Motor Skills*, 71(1), 151–60.

6. Roberts, S. C., Owen, R. C., & Havlicek, J. (2010). Distinguishing between perceiver and wearer effects in clothing color-associated attributions. *Evolutionary Psychology*, 8(3), 350–64.

7. Elliot, A. J., Niesta, D. (2008). Romantic red: Red enhances men's attraction to women. *Journal of Personality and Social Psychology*, 95(5), 1150–64.

8. Guéguen. N. (2010). Color and Women Hitchhikers' Attractiveness: Gentlemen Drivers Prefer Red. *Color Research and Application*, 37(1), 76–78.

9. Kayser, D., N., Elliot, A. J., & Feltman, R. (2010). Red and romantic behavior in men viewing women. *European Journal of Social Psychology*, 40(6), 901–8.

10. Lõhmus, M., Sundström, L. F., & Björklund, M. (2009). Dress for success: even unseen clothing increases female facial attractiveness. *Annales Zoologici Fennici*, 46, 75–80.

11. Stillman, J. W., & Hensley, W. E. (1980). She wore a flower in her hair: The effect of ornamentation on nonverbal communication. *Journal of Applied Communication Research*, 8(1), 31–39.

12. Cashman, M. W., & Sloan, S. B. (2010). Nutrition and nail disease. *Clinics in Dermatology.* 28(4), 420–25.

13. Drews, D. R., Allison, C. K., & Probst, J. R. (2000). Behavioral and self-concept differences in tattooed and nontattooed college students. *Psychological Reports*, 86(2), 475–81.

14. Degelman, D., & Price, N. D. (2002). Tattoos and ratings of personal characteristics. *Psychological Reports*, 90(2), 507–14.

15. Seiter, J. S., & Hatch, S. (2005). Effect of tattoos on perceptions of credibility and attractiveness. *Psychological Reports*, 96(3, pt. 2), 1113–20.

16. Bekhor, P. S., Bekhor, L, & Gandrabur, M. (1995). Employer attitudes towards persons with visible tattoos. *Australian Journal of Dermatology*, 36(2), 75–77.

17. Seiter, J. S., & Sandry, A. (2003). Pierced for success? The effects of ear and nose piercing on perceptions of job candidates' credibility, attractiveness, and hirability. *Communication Research Reports*, 20(4), 287–98.

18. Hirsch, A. R., & Gruss, J. J. (1999). Human male sexual response to olfactory stimuli. *Journal of Neurological and Orthopaedic Medicine and Surgery*, 19, 14–19.

19. Bridges, B. (2002). Fragrance: Emerging health and environmental concerns. *Flavour and Fragrance Journal*, 17(5), 361–71.

20. Liebl, B., & Ehrenstorfer, S. (1993). Nitro-musk compounds in breast milk. [Article in German] *Gesundheitswesen*, 55(10), 527–32.

21. Miller, S. L., & Maner, J. K. (2010). Scent of a woman: Men's testosterone responses to olfactory ovulation cues. *Psychological Science*, 21(2), 276–83.

CHAPTER 8: ELEGANCE

1. Zuckerman, M., & Driver, R. E. (1989). What sounds beautiful is good: The vocal attractiveness stereotype. *Journal of Nonverbal Behavior*, 13(2), 67-82.

CHAPTER 9: PERSONALITY

1. Kniffin, K., & Wilson, D. (2004). The effect of nonphysical traits on the perception of physical attractiveness: Three naturalistic studies. *Evolution and Human Behavior*, 25(2), 88–101.

2. Swami, V., et al. (2010). More than just skin deep? Personality information influences men's ratings of the attractiveness of women's body sizes. *Journal of Social Psychology*, 150(6), 628–74.

3. Li, N., & Kenrick, D. (2006). Sex similarities and differences in preferences for short-term mates: What, whether, and why. *Journal of Personality and Social Psychology*, 90(3), 468–89.

4. Regan, P. C. (1998). What if you can't get what you want? Willingness to compromise ideal mate selection standards as a function of sex, mate value, and relationship context. *Personality and Social Psychology Bulletin*, 24(12), 1294–303.

5. Brase, G., & Walker, G. (2004). Male sexual strategies modify ratings of female models with specific waist-to-hip ratios. *Human Nature*, 15(2), 209–24.

6. Simpson, J., & Gangestad, S. (1992). Sociosexuality and romantic partner choice. *Journal of Personality*, 60(1), 31–51.

7. Kenrick, D., Sadalla, E., Groth, G., & Trost, M. (1990). Evolution, traits, and the stages of human courtship: Qualifying the parental investment model. *Journal of Personality*, 58(1), 97–116.

8. Lewandowski, G. W., Aron, A., & Gee, J. (2007). Personality goes a long way: The malleability of opposite-sex physical attractiveness. *Personal Relationships*, 14(4), 571–85.

9. Alessandra, T. (2000). *Charisma: Seven keys to developing the magnetism that leads to success.* New York: Business Plus.

10. Tracy, B., & Arden, R. (2006). *The power of charm: How to win anyone over in any situation.* New York: Amacom.

11. Mehrabian, A., & Wiener, M. (1967). Decoding of Inconsistent Communications. *Journal of Personality and Social Psychology*, 6(1), 109–14.

12 Mehrabian, A., & Ferris, S. R. (1967). Inference of attitudes from nonverbal communication in two channels. *Journal of Consulting Psychology*, 31(3), 248–52.

13. Mueser, K. T., Grau, B. W., Sussman, S., & Rosen, A. J. (1984). You're only as pretty as you feel: Facial expression as a determinant of physical attractiveness. *Journal of Personality and Social Psychology*, 46(2), 469–78.

14. Jones, B. C., Debruine, L. M., Little, A. C., Conway, C. A. & Feinberg, D. A. (2006). Integrating gaze direction and expression in preference for attractive faces. *Psychological Science*, 17(7), 588–91.

15. Otta, E., Folladore E Abrosio, A., & Hoshino, R. L. (1996). Reading a smiling face: Messages conveyed by various forms of smiling. *Perceptual and Motor Skills*, 82(3 pt. 2), 1111–21.

16. Moore, M. M. (1985). Nonverbal courtship patterns in women: Context and consequences. *Ethology and Sociobiology*, 6(4), 237–47.

17. Surakka, V., & Hietanen, J. K. (1998). Facial and emotional reactions to Duchenne and non-Duchenne smiles. *International Journal of Psychophysiology*, 29(1), 23–33.

18. Lee, H. J., Macbeth, A. H., Pagani, J. H., & Young III, W. S. (2009). Oxytocin: The great facilitator of life. *Progress in Neurobiology*, 88(2), 127-51.

19. Wood, D., & Brumbaugh, C. C. (2009). Using revealed mate preferences to evaluate market force and differential preference explanations for mate selection. *Journal of Personality and Social Psychology*, 96(6), 1226-44.

20. Seidl, R., Peyrl, A., Nicham, R., & Hauser, E. (2000). A taurine and caffeine-containing drink stimulates cognitive performance and well-being. *Amino Acids*, 19(3–4), 635-42.

21. McCreadie, K. (2010). *Robert Collier's The secret of the ages: A modern-day interpretation of a self-help classic.* Oxford (UK): Infinite Ideas.

22. Gray, J. (2004). *Men are from Mars, women are from Venus: The classic guide to understanding the opposite sex.* New York: Harper Paperbacks.

23. Argov, S. (2002). *Why men love bitches: From doormat to dreamgirl—a woman's guide to holding her own in a relationship.* Avon (MA): Adams Media.

24. Fein, E., & Schneider, S. (1996). *The rules: Time-tested secrets for capturing the heart of Mr. Right.* New York: Grand Central Publishing.

25. Greene, R. (2003). *The art of seduction.* New York: Penguin.

26. Cialdini, R. B. (2008). *Influence: Science and practice (5th ed.).* Englewood Cliffs (NJ): Prentice Hall.

27. Waugh, C. E., & Fredrickson, B. L. (2006). Nice to know you: Positive emotions, self-other overlap, and complex understanding in the formation of a new relationship. *Journal of Positive Psychology*, 1(2), 93–106.

28. Abramowitz, J. S., Tolin, D. F., & Street, G. P. (2001). Paradoxical effects of thought suppression: A Meta-analysis of controlled studies. *Clinical Psychology Review*, 21(5), 683–703.

29. Petrie, K. J., Booth, R. J., & Pennebaker, J. W. (1998). The immunological effects of thought suppression. *Journal of Personality and Social Psychology*, 75(5), 1264–72.

30. Ritvo, R. Z., & Papilsky, S. B. (1999). Effectiveness of psychotherapy. *Current Opinion In Pediatrics*, 11(4), 323–27.

31. Kemp, A. H., Quintana, D. S., Felmingham, K. L., Matthews, S., & Jelinek, H. F. (2012). Depression, comorbid anxiety disorders, and heart rate variability in physically healthy, unmedicated patients: Implications for cardiovascular risk. *PLoS One*, 7(2), e30777.

32. Kemp, A. H., Quintana, D. S., Gray, M. A., Felmingham, K. L., Brown, K., & Gatt, J. M. (2010). Impact of depression and antidepressant treatment on heart rate variability: A review and meta-analysis. *Biological Psychiatry*, 67(11), 1067–74.

33. Butler, A. C., Chapman, J. E., Forman, E. M., & Beck, A. T. (2006). The empirical status of cognitive-behavioral therapy: A review of meta-analyses. *Clinical Psychology Review*, 26(1), 17–31.

34. Leichsenring, F. (2005). Are psychodynamic and psychoanalytic therapies effective: A review of empirical data. *International Journal of Psychoanalysis*, 86(pt. 3), 841–68.

35. Shedler, J. (2010). The efficacy of psychodynamic psychotherapy. *American Psychologist*, 65(2), 98–109.

36. Flammer, E., & Alladin, A. (2007). The efficacy of hypnotherapy in the treatment of psychosomatic disorders: Meta-analytical evidence. *International Journal of Clinical and Experimental Hypnosis*, 55(3), 251–74.

37. Staicu, M. L., & Cuȯv, M. (2010). Anger and health risk behaviors. *Journal of Medicine and Life*, 3(4), 372–75.

38. Reed, G. L., & Enright, R. D. (2006). The effects of forgiveness therapy on depression, anxiety, and posttraumatic stress for women after spousal emotional abuse. *Journal of Consulting and Clinical Psychology*, 74(5), 920–29.

39. Hirsch, J. K., Webb, J. R., & Jeglic, E. L. (2011). Forgiveness, depression, and suicidal behavior among a diverse sample of college students. *Journal of Clinical Psychology*, 67(9), 896–906.

40. Levine, P. (1997). *Waking the tiger: Healing trauma*. Berkeley (CA): North Atlantic Books.

41. Descilo, T., Greenwald, R., Schmitt, T. A., & Reslan, S. (2010). Traumatic incident reduction for urban at-risk youth and unaccompanied minor refugees: Two open trials. *Journal of Child & Adolescent Trauma*, 3(3), 181–91.

42. Bisson, J., & Andrew, M. (2007). Psychological treatment of post-traumatic stress disorder (PTSD). *Cochrane Database of Systematic Reviews*, 18(3), CD003388.

43. Leitch, M. L., Vanslyke, J., & Allen, M. (2009). Somatic experiencing treatment with social service workers following Hurricanes Katrina and Rita. *Social Work*, 54(1), 9–18.

44. Ventling, C. D., Bertschi, H., & Gerhard, U. (2008). Efficacy of bioenergetic psychotherapy with patients of known ICD-10 diagnosis: A retrospective evaluation. *USABP Journal*, 7(2), 26–32.

45. Gudat, U. (1997). The efficiency of bioenergetic analysis an outpatient psychotherapy. *Psychotherapie Forum*, 5, 28–37

46. Gudat, U. (2002). Efficacy of bioenergetic therapies as a method of psychotherapy. *Bioenergetic Analysis*, 13 (1), 21–56.

47. Nickel, M., et al. (2006). Bioenergetic exercises in inpatient treatment of Turkish immigrants with chronic somatoform disorders: A randomized, controlled study. *Journal of Psychosomatic Research*, 61(4), 507–3.

48. Baer, R. A. (2003). Mindfulness training as a clinical intervention: A conceptual and empirical review. *Clinical Psychology: Science and Practice*, 10(2), 125–43.

49. Hofmann, S. G., Sawyer, A. T., Witt, A. A., & Oh, D. (2010). The effect of mindfulness-based therapy on anxiety and depression: A meta-analytic review. *Journal of Consulting and Clinical Psychology*, 78(2), 169–83.

50. Carson, J. W., et al. (2004). Mindfulness-based relationship enhancement. *Behavior Therapy*, 35, 471–94.

51. Barnes, S., et al. (2007). The role of mindfulness in romantic relationship satisfaction and responses to relationship stress. *Journal of Marital and Family Therapy*, 33(4), 482–500.

52. Grossman, P., Niemann, L., Schmidt, S., & Walach, H. (2004). Mindfulness-based stress reduction and health benefits: A meta-analysis. *Journal of Psychosomatic Research*, 57(1), 35–43.

53. Chiesa, A., & Serretti, A. (2009). Mindfulness-based stress reduction for stress management in healthy people: A review and meta-analysis. *Journal of Alternative and Complementary Medicine*, 15(5), 593–600.

54. Sipe, W. E., & Eisendrath, S. J. (2012). Mindfulness-based cognitive therapy: Theory and practice. *Canadian Journal of Psychiatry*, 57(2), 63–69.

55. Teasdale, J. et al. (2000) Prevention of relapse/recurrence in major depression by mindfulness-based cognitive therapy. *Journal of Consulting and Clinical Psychology*, 68(4), 615–23.

56. Chapman, A. L. (2006). Dialectical behavior therapy: Current indications and unique elements. *Psychiatry*, 3(9), 62–68.

57. Verheul, R., Van Den Bosch, L. M., Koeter, M. W., De Ridder, M. A., Stijnen, T., & Van Den Brink, W. (2003). Dialectical behaviour therapy for women with borderline personality disorder: 12-month, randomised clinical trial in The Netherlands. *British Journal of Psychiatry*, 182, 135–40.

58. Koons, C. R., et al. (2001). Efficacy of dialectical behavior therapy in women veterans with borderline personality disorder. *Behavior Therapy*, 32(2), 371–90.

59. Linehan, M. M., et al. (2006). Two-year randomized controlled trial and follow-up of dialectical behavior therapy vs therapy by experts for suicidal behaviors and borderline personality disorder. *Archives of General Psychiatry*, 63(7), 757–66.

60. Linehan, M. M., Heard, H. L., & Armstrong, H. E. (1993). Naturalistic follow-up of a behavioral treatment for chronically parasuicidal borderline patients. *Archives of General Psychiatry*, 50(12), 971–74.

61. Bretz, H. J., Heekerens, H. P., & Schmitz, B. (1994). A meta-analysis of the effectiveness of gestalt therapy. [Article in German] *Zeitschrift für klinische Psychologie, Psychopathologie und Psychotherapie*, 42(3), 241–60.

62. Suzuki, T., & Suzuki, R. (1981). The effectiveness of in-patient Morita therapy. *The Psychiatric Quarterly*, 53(3), 201–13.

63. Fredrickson, B. L. et al. (2008). Open hearts build lives: Positive emotions, induced through loving-kindness meditation, build consequential personal resources. *Journal of Personality and Social Psychology*, 95(5), 1045–62.

64. Hutcherson, C., et al. (2008). Loving-kindness meditation increases social connectedness. *Emotion*, 8(5), 720–24.

65. Salas, M. M., Brooks, A. J., & Rowe, J. E. (2011). The immediate effect of a brief energy psychology intervention (Emotional Freedom Techniques) on specific phobias: A pilot study. *Explore* (NY), 7(3), 155–61.

66. Karatzias, T., et al. (2011) A controlled comparison of the effectiveness and efficiency of two psychological therapies for posttraumatic stress disorder: Eye movement desensitization and reprocessing vs. emotional freedom techniques. *The Journal of Nervous and Mental Disease*, 199(6), 372–78.

67. Callahan, R.J. (1985). *Five-minute phobia cure*. Wilmington: Enterprise.

68. Pignotti, M., & Steinberg, M. (2001). Heart rate variability as an outcome measure for Thought Field Therapy in clinical practice. *Journal of Clinical Psychology*, 57(10), 1193–206.

69. Callahan, R. J. (2001). The impact of Thought Field Therapy on heart rate variability. *Journal of Clinical Psychology*, 57(10), 1153–70.

70. Sakai, C., et al. (2001). Thought Field Therapy clinical applications: Utilization in an HMO in behavioral medicine and behavioral health services. *Journal of Clinical Psychology*, 57(10), 1215–27.

71. Benor, D. J. (2005). Self-healing interventions for clinical practice: Brief psychotherapy with WHEE—the wholistic hybrid of EMDR and EFT. *Complementary Therapies In Clinical Practice*, 11(4), 270–74.

72. Benor, D. J., Ledger, K., Toussaint, L., Hett, G., & Zaccaro, D. (2009). Pilot study of emotional freedom techniques, wholistic hybrid derived from eye movement desensitization and reprocessing and emotional freedom technique, and cognitive behavioral therapy for treatment of test anxiety in university students. *Explore* (NY), 5(6), 338–40.

73. Monti, D. A., Stoner, M. E., Zivin, G., & Schlesinger, M. (2007). Short term correlates of the Neuro Emotional Technique for cancer-related traumatic stress symptoms: a pilot case series. *Journal of Cancer Survivorship*, 1(2), 161–66.

74. Karpouzis, F. Pollard, H., & Benello, R. (2008). Separation anxiety disorder in a 13-year–old boy managed by the Neuro Emotional Technique as a biopsychosocial intervention. *Journal of Chiropractic Medicine*, 7(3), 101–6.

75. Bablis, P., & Pollard, H. (2009). Anxiety and depression profile of 188 consecutive new patients presenting to a Neuro-Emotional Technique practitioner. *Journal of Alternative and Complementary Medicine*, 15(2), 121–27.

76. Jensen, A. M., & Ramasamy, A. (2009). Treating spider phobia using Neuro Emotional Technique: Findings from a pilot study. *Journal of Alternative and Complementary Medicine*, 15(12), 1363–74.

77. Anderson, J. G., & Taylor, A. G. (2011). Effects of healing touch in clinical practice: A systematic review of randomized clinical trials. *Journal of Holistic Nursing*, 29(3), 221-28.

78. Feinstein, D. (2008). Energy psychology: A review of the preliminary evidence. *Psychotherapy*, 45(2), 199–213.

79. Stipancic M., Renner, W., Schütz, P., & Dond, R. (2010). Effects of Neuro-Linguistic Psychotherapy on psychological difficulties and perceived quality of life. *Counselling and Psychotherapy Research*, 10(1), 39–49.

80. Oliveros, J. C., Selman, A. M., Ortiz, T., & Arrigain, S. (1994). Silva's Method of mental control and changes in the EEG alpha rhythm. [Article in Spanish] *Actas luso-españolas de neurología, psiquiatría y ciencias afines*, 22(6), 290–91.

81. Rein, G. (October, 1996). Effect of conscious intention on human DNA. *Proceeds of the International Forum on New Science*, Denver, CO.

82. Lipton, B. (2008). *The biology of belief: Unleashing the power of consciousness, matter, and miracles*. USA: Hay House.

83. Bradt, J., Dileo, C., Grocke, D., & Magill, L. (2011). Music interventions for improving psychological and physical outcomes in cancer patients. *Cochrane Database of Systematic Reviews*, (8), CD006911.

84. Chan, M. F., Wong, Z. Y., & Thayala, N. V. (2011). The effectiveness of music listening in reducing depressive symptoms in adults: A systematic review. *Complementary Therapies In Medicine*, 19(6), 332–48.

85. Korhan, E. A., Khorshid, L., & Uyar, M. (2011). The effect of music therapy on physiological signs of anxiety in patients receiving mechanical ventilatory support. *Journal of Clinical Nursing*, 20(7–8), 1026–34.

86. Hughes, E. G., & da Silva, A. M. (2011). A pilot study assessing art therapy as a mental health intervention for subfertile women. *Human Reproduction*, 26(3), 611–15.

87. Strassel, J. K., Cherkin, D. C., Steuten, L., Sherman, K. J., & Vrijhoef, H. J. (2011). A systematic review of the evidence for the effectiveness of dance therapy. *Alternative Therapies in Health and Medicine*, 17(3), 50–59.

88. Akandere, M., & Demir, B. (2011). The effect of dance over depression. *Collegium Antropologicum*, 35(3), 651–56.

89. Matuszek, S. (2010). Animal-facilitated therapy in various patient populations: Systematic literature review. *Holistic Nursing Practice*, 24(4), 187–203.

90. Willis, D. A. (1997). Animal therapy. *Rehabilitation Nursing*, 22(2), 78–81.

91. Holford, P. (2004). *Optimum nutrition for the mind.* Laguna Beach (CA): Basic Health Publications.

92. Amen, D. G. (1999). *Change your brain, change your life: The breakthrough program for conquering anxiety, depression, obsessiveness, anger, and impulsiveness.* New York: Three Rivers Press.

93. Lakhan, S. E., & Vieira, K. F. (2008). Nutritional therapies for mental disorders. *Nutrition Journal*, 7, 2.

94. Bell, I. R. et al. (1991). B complex vitamin patterns in geriatric and young adult inpatients with major depression. *Journal of the American Geriatric Society*, 39(3), 252–57.

95. Stough, C., Scholey, A., Lloyd, J., Spong, J., Myers, S., & Downey, L. A. (2011). The effect of 90 day administration of a high dose vitamin B-complex on work stress. *Human Psychopharmacology*, 26(7), 470–76.

96. Gesch, B. (1990). The SCASO project. *International Journal of Biosocial Medical Research*, 12(1), 41–68.

97. Virkkunen M. (1986). Reactive hypoglycemic tendency among habitually violent offenders. *Nutrition Reviews*, 44(Suppl s3), 94–103.

98. Schoenthaler, S. J. (1983). Northern California Diet-Behavior Program: An empirical examination of 3,000 incarcerated juveniles in Stanislaus County Juvenile Hall. *International Journal of Biosocial Research*, 5(2), 99–106.

99. Schoenthaler, S. J. (1983). The Los Angeles Probation Department Diet Behavior Program: An empirical analysis of six institutional settings. *International Journal of Biosocial Research*, 5(2), 88–98.

100. Bateson-Koch, C. (1994). *Allergies: Disease in disguise.* Burnaby (BC): Alive Books.

101. Rosato, A., Vitali, C., Piarulli, M., Mazzotta, M., Argentieri, M. P., & Mallamaci, R. (2009). In vitro synergic efficacy of the combination of Nystatin with the essential oils of *Origanum vulgare* and *Pelargonium graveolens* against some Candida species. *Phytomedicine*, 16(10), 972–75.

102. Lee, Y. L., Wu, Y., Tsang, H. W., Leung, A. Y., & Cheung, W. M. (2011). A systematic review on the anxiolytic effects of aromatherapy in people with anxiety symptoms. *Journal of Alternative and Complementary Medicine*, 17(2), 101–8.

103. Yim, V. W., Ng, A. K., Tsang, H. W., & Leung, A. Y. (2009). A review on the effects of aromatherapy for patients with depressive symptoms. *Journal of Alternative and Complementary Medicine*, 15(2), 187–95.

104. Farmer. M. E., Locke, B. Z, Mościcki, E. K., Dannenberg, A. L., Larson, D. B., & Radloff, L. S. (1988). Physical activity and depressive symptoms: The NHANES I Epidemiologic Follow-up Study. *American Journal of Epidemiology*, 128(6), 1340–51.

105. De Moor, M. H. M., Beem, A. L., Stubbe, J. H., Boomsma, D. I., & De Geus, E. J. C. (2006). Regular exercise, anxiety, depression and personality: A population-based study. *Preventive Medicine*, 42(4), 273-79.

106. Stephens, T. (1988). Physical activity and mental health in the United States and Canada: Evidence from four population surveys. *Preventive Medicine*, 17(1), 35–47.

107. Arai, Y., Hisamichi, S. (1998). Self-reported exercise frequency and personality: a population-based study in Japan. *Perceptual and Motor Skills,* 87(3 pt. 2), 1371–75.

108. Blumenthal. J. A., et al. (1999). Effects of exercise training on older adults with major depression. *Archives of Internal Medicine*, 159(19), 2349–56.

109. Babyak, M. A., et al. (2000). Exercise treatment for major depression: Maintenance of therapeutic benefit at 10 months. *Psychosomatic Medicine*, 62(5), 633-38.

110. North, T. C., McCullagh, P., & Tran, Z. V. (1990). Effect of exercise on depression. *Exercise and Sport Sciences Reviews*, 18, 379–415.

111. Yeung, W. J., & Chan Y. (2007). The positive effects of religiousness on mental health in physically vulnerable populations: A review on recent empirical studies and related theories. *International Journal of Psychosocial Rehabilitation*, 11(2), 37–52

112. Seybold, K. S., & Hill, P. C. (2001). The role of religion and spirituality in mental and physical health. *Current Directions in Psychological Science*, 10(1), 21–24.

113. Koenig, H. G. (2009). Research on religion, spirituality, and mental health: A review. *Canadian Journal of Psychiatry*, 54(5), 283–91.

114. Ellison, C. G. (1992). Are religious people nice people? Evidence from the National Survey of Black Americans. *Social Forces*, 71(2), 411–30.

115. Genia, V. (1997). The Spiritual Experience Index: Revision and reformulation. *Review of Religious Research*, 38(4), 344–61.

116. Reinert, D. F., & Bloomingdale, J. R. (1999). Spiritual maturity and mental health: Implications for counseling. *Counseling & Values*, 43(3), 211–23.

117. McCullough, M. E., & Larson, D. B. (1999). Religion and depression: A review of the literature. *Twin Research*, 2(2), 126–36.

118. Shaw, A., Joseph S., & Linley, P. A. (2005). Religion, spirituality, and post-traumatic growth: A systematic review. *Mental Health, Religion and Culture*, 8(1), 1-11.

119. Francis, L. J., Robbins, M., Lewis C., A., & Barnes, L. P. (2008). Prayer and psychological health: A study among sixth-form pupils attending Catholic and Protestant schools in Northern Ireland. *Mental Health, Religion and Culture*, 11(1), 85–92.

120. Meisenhelder, J. B., & Chandler, E. N. (2000). Prayer and health outcomes in church members. *Alternative Therapies In Health and Medicine*, 6(4), 56–60.

121. Levine, M. (2008). Prayer as coping: A psychological analysis. *Journal of Health Care Chaplaincy*, 15(2), 80–98.

122. Bormann, J. E. et al. (2005). Efficacy of frequent mantram repetition on stress, quality of life, and spiritual well-being in veterans: A pilot study. *Journal of Holistic Nursing*, 23(4), 395–414.

123. Hamblin, H, T. (1921). *Dynamic Thought*. Chicago: Yogi Publication Society.

124. Ventegodt, S., Andersen, N.J., & Merrick, J. (2003). The life mission theory III. Theory of talent. *ScientificWorldJournal*, 3, 1286–1293.

125. Ventegodt, S. (2003). The life mission theory: A theory for a consciousness-based medicine. *International Journal of Adolescent Medicine and Health*, 15(1), 89–91.

126. Ring, K. (2006). *Lessons from the light: What we can learn from the near-death experience*. Needham (MA): Moment Point Press.

127. Griffin, A. M., & Langlois, J. H. (2006). Stereotype directionality and attractiveness stereotyping: Is beauty good or is ugly bad? *Social Cognition*, 24(2), 187–206.

128. Ybarra, O., et al. (2008). Mental exercising through simple socializing: Social interaction promotes general cognitive functioning. *Personality and Social Psychology Bulletin*, 34(2), 248–59.

129. Zeidan, F., Johnson, S. K., Diamond, B. J., David, Z., & Goolkasian, P. (2010). Mindfulness meditation improves cognition: Evidence of brief mental training. *Consciousness and Cognition*, 19(2), 597–605.

130. van Vugt, M. K., & Jha, A.P. (2011). Investigating the impact of mindfulness meditation training on working memory: A mathematical modeling approach. *Cognitive, Affective, and Behavioral Neuroscience*, 11(3), 344–53.

131. Jain, S., et al. (2007). A randomized controlled trial of mindfulness meditation versus relaxation training: Effects on distress, positive states of mind, rumination, and distraction. *Annals of Behavioral Medicine*, 33(1), 11–21.

132. Sifft, J. M., & Khalsa, G. C. (1991). Effect of educational kinesiology upon simple response times and choice response times. *Perceptual and Motor Skills*, 73(3 pt. 1), 1011–15.

133. Eilander, A., et al. (2010). Multiple micronutrient supplementation for improving cognitive performance in children: Systematic review of randomized controlled trials. *American Journal of Clinical Nutrition*, 91(1), 115–30.

134. Muldoon, M. F., Ryan, C. M., Sheu, L., Yao, J. K., Conklin, S. M., & Manuck, S. B. (2011). Serum phospholipid docosahexaenonic acid is associated with cognitive functioning during middle adulthood. *Journal of Nutrition Health and Aging*, 140(4), 848–53.

135. Aberg, M. A., Aberg, N., Brisman, J., Sundberg, R., Winkvist, A., & Torén, K. (2009). Fish intake of Swedish male adolescents is a predictor of cognitive performance. *Acta Paediatrica*, 98(3), 555–60.

136. Kesse-Guyot, E., et al. (2011). Thirteen-year prospective study between fish consumption, long-chain n-3 fatty acids intakes and cognitive function. *Journal of Nutrition Health and Aging*, 15(2), 115–20.

137. Hasselmo, M. E. (2006). The role of acetylcholine in learning and memory. *Current Opinion In Neurobiology*, 16(6), 710–15.

138. Mishra, L. C., Singh, B. B., & Dagenais, S. (2000). Scientific basis for the therapeutic use of *Withania somnifera* (ashwagandha): A review. *Alternative Medicine Review*, 5(4), 334–46.

139. Vinutha, B., et al. (2007). Screening of selected Indian medicinal plants for acetylcholinesterase inhibitory activity. *Journal of Ethnopharmacology*, 109(2), 359–63.

140. Roodenrys, S., Booth, D., Bulzomi, S., Phipps, A., Micallef, C., & Smoker, J. (2002). Chronic effects of Brahmi (*Bacopa monnieri*) on human memory. *Neuropsychopharmacology*, 27(2), 279–81.

141. Stough, C., et al. (2001). The chronic effects of an extract of *Bacopa monniera* (Brahmi) on cognitive function in healthy human subjects. *Psychopharmacology*, 156(4), 481–84.

142. Shinomol, G. K., Muralidhara, & Bharath, M. M. (2011). Exploring the role of "Brahmi" (*Bocopa monnieri* and *Centella asiatica*) in brain function and therapy. *Recent Patents on Endocrine, Metabolic and Immune Drug Discovery*, 5(1), 33–49.

143. Rao, M. K., Rao, M. S., & Rao, G. S. (2007). Treatment with Centalla asiatica (Linn) fresh leaf extract enhances learning ability and memory retention power in rats. *Neurosciences*, 12(3), 236–41.

144. Kennedy, D. O., Scholey, A. B., & Wesnes, K. A. (2001). Dose dependent changes in cognitive performance and mood following acute administration of Ginseng to healthy young volunteers. *Nutritional Neuroscience*, 4(4), 295–310.

145. Rai, D., Bhatia, G., Sen, T., & Palit, G. (2003). Anti-stress effects of Ginkgo biloba and Panax ginseng: A comparative study. *Journal of Pharmacological Sciences*, 93(4), 458–64.

146. Rocher, M. N., et al. (2011). Long-term treatment with standardized Ginkgo biloba extract (EGb 761) attenuates cognitive deficits and hippocampal neuron loss in a gerbil model of vascular dementia. *Fitoterapia*, 82(7), 1075–80.

147. Wesnes, K. A., Ward, T., McGinty, A., & Petrini, O. (2000). The memory enhancing effects of a Ginkgo biloba/Panax ginseng combination in healthy middle-aged volunteers. *Psychopharmacology*, 152(4), 353–61.

CHAPTER 10: CHARACTER

1. Peterson, C., & Seligman, M. E. P. (2004). *Character strengths and virtues: A handbook and classification*. Washington (DC): APA Press and Oxford University Press.

2. Fletcher J., Matschek C., Tycer G., & Siebert A. (2003). *Gathering wisdom: How to acquire wisdom from others while developing your own*. Portland (OR): Practical Psychology Press.

3. Scott, K. S. (2006). *The richest man who ever lived: King Solomon's secrets to success, wealth, and happiness*. New York: Crown Business.

4. Johnstone, B., & Glass, B., A. (2008). Support for a neuropsychological model of spirituality in persons with traumatic brain injury. *Zygon*, 43(4), 861-874.

5. Heinze, T. F. (2002). *How life began*. Ontario (CA): Chick Publications.

6. Schlehofer, M. M., Omoto, A. M., & Adelman, J. R. (2008). How do "Religion" and "Spirituality" differ? Lay definitions among older adults. *Journal for the Scientific Study of Religion*, 47(3), 411–25.

7. Sheldrake, P. (2007). *A brief history of spirituality*. Oxford: Wiley-Blackwell.

8. Teresa, M. (2010). *Where there is love, there is God: A path to closer union with God and greater love for others*. Doubleday Religion.

9. Moorjani, A. (2012). *Dying to be me: My journey from cancer, to near death, to true healing*. Carlsbad (CA): Hay House.

10. Dr. Ross, H. (2003, August 8). Fulfilled prophecy: Evidence for the reliability of the Bible. *Reasons to believe*. Retrieved January 24, 2011. Retrieved from http://www.reasons.org/fulfilled-prophecy-evidence-reliability-bible

11. Vivekananda, S. (1982). *Karma-Yoga*. New York: Ramakrishna Vivekanada Center.

12. Warren, R. (2002). *The Purpose Driven Life: What On Earth Am I Here For?* Grand Rapids (MI): Zondervan Publishing House.

13. Atwater, P. (2011). *Near-death experiences, the rest of the story: What they teach us about living and dying and our true purpose*. Charlottesville (VA): Hampton Roads.

14. Frankl, V. (2006). *Man's search for meaning*. Boston (MA): Beacon Press.

15. Ventegodt, S., Andersen, N.J., & Merrick, J. (2003). The life mission theory II. The structure of the life purpose and the ego. *TheScientificWorldJournal*, 3, 1277–85.

Appendix A

1. Slaney, R. B., Rice, K. G., Mobley, M., Trippi, J., & Ashby, J. S. (2001), The Revised Almost Perfect Scale, *Measurement and Evaluation in Counseling and Development*, 34(3), 130–45.

2. Rice, K. G., Leever, B. A., Christopher, J., & Porter, J. D. (2006). Perfectionism, stress and social (dis)connection: A short-term study of hopelessness, depression, and academic adjustment among honors students. *Journal of Counseling Psychology*, 53(4), 524–34.

3. Delegard, D. K. (2004). *The role of perfectionism in anxiety, depression, self-esteem, and internalized shame* (Unpublished doctoral dissertation). Marquette University, Milwaukee, WI.

4. Sassaroli, S., Lauro, L, J., Ruggiero, G. M., Mauri, M. C., Vinai, P., & Frost, R. (2008). Perfectionism in depression, obsessive-compulsive disorder and eating disorders. *Behaviour Research and Therapy*, 46(6), 757–65.

5. Park, L. E., DiRaddo, A. M., Calogero, R. M. (2009). Sociocultural influence and appearance-based rejection sensitivity among college students. *Psychology of Women Quarterly*, 33(1), 108–19.

Resources

BEAUTY

Cosmetic Procedures
www.realself.com

Cosmetics Safety Database
www.ewg.org/skindeep/

Skin Care Talk
www.skincaretalk.com

Natural Breast Enhancement
Forums
www.breastnexus.com

Body Mass Index Calculator
www.nhlbisupport.com/bmi/

HEALTH

World Health Organization
www.who.int

National Library of Medicine
www.ncbi.nlm.nih.gov/pubmed

Wiley Online Library
www.onlinelibrary.wiley.com

Peer-Reviewed Medical Journals
www.biomedcentral.com

Evidence-Based Natural
Therapies
www.naturalstandard.com

Disease Control and Prevention
www.cdc.gov

MD Travel Health
www.mdtravelhealth.com

Travel Health Online
www.tripprep.com

Lab Tests Database
www.labtestsonline.org

Complementary and Alternative Medicine
www.nccam.nih.gov

Natural Health News
www.naturalnews.com

Natural Health Topics
www.mercola.com

Health Sciences Institute
www.hsionline.com

Cutting Edge Health Information
www.healthsalon.org

Alternative Healing Therapies
www.educate-yourself.org

Holistic Health Care
www.shirleys-wellness-cafe.com

Herb Scientific Database
www.herbmed.org

Herb Profiles
www.herbwisdom.com

Cancer Cure Foundation
www.cancure.org

Independent Cancer Research Foundation
www.new-cancer-treatments.org

Healing Cancer Naturally
www.healingcancernaturally.com

Natural Cancer Treatments
www.cancertutor.com

Mind-Body Cancer Healing
www.alternative-cancer-care.com

Cancer Treatment Options
www.self-helpcancer.org

DCA Cancer Therapy Research
www.thedcasite.com

STYLE

Fashion Forecasting
www.fashiontrendsetter.com

Style and Fashion
www.stylebistro.com

Sample Sales
www.topbutton.com

ELEGANCE
www.elegantwoman.org

PERSONALITY
Behavior and Mental Health
www.psychologytoday.com

Social Psychology
www.socialpsychology.org

Psychology Information
www.allpsych.com

Mental Health and Psychology
Network
www.psychcentral.com

Orthomolecular Psychiatry
www.orthomolecular.org

IQ Test
www.iqtest.com

VARK Learning Styles
www.vark-learn.com

CHARACTER

Sacred Ancient Texts
www.sacred-texts.com

Quotations Database
www.brainyquote.com

Inspirational Quotes
www.sapphyr.net

Self-Improvement Resources
www.selfgrowth.com

Charity Evaluator
www.charitynavigator.org

Orphanages Worldwide
www.orphanage.org

Creation Evidence
www.creationevidence.org

Institute for Creation Research
www.icr.org

Faith and Inspiration
www.beliefnet.com

Religion Facts
www.religionfacts.com

Religion and Spirituality
www.patheos.com

Near-Death Studies
www.iands.org

Near-Death Research
www.nderf.org

Near-Death Experiences
www.near-death.com

Bible Search and Study
www.biblos.com

Bible Passage Search
www.biblegateway.com

Index

C

methods, 273

sophistication, key to, 247–248

Lecithin, 194

LED light therapy, 70

Lee, John R., 26

Lee, Kang, 21

Legs, 118–119

Lemons

daily cleansings, 162

hair rinse, 101

Lentinan, 204

Letterman, Elmer G., 280

Lewis, C.S., 271

Licorice root, 199

Lincoln, Abraham, 250

Lip gloss/lipstick, 39, 41

Liposuction, 118

facial, 19

Lips

color, 39, 41

cosmetic procedures, 30

Listening to others, 251

Liv 52, 172

Liver

cleanse, 164–165

supplements, 171–172

Lodewick, Peter A., 176

Long face shape, 15, 17, 18

Long hair, 94–95

Longan fruit, 77–78

Longfellow, Henry Wadsworth, 212

Lookism, 6

Loren, Sophia, 238

Louboutin, Christian, 213–214

Loving others, 286–287

Low-level laser therapy (LLLT), 182

Luther, Martin, 85

Lymphatic system cleansing, 163

M

Ma huang, 193

Maca root, 112, 196

Macaulay, Thomas B., 281

MacDonald, Kai, 253

Machado, Alicia, 272

Magnetic mattress pad, 179–180

Magnetic power of beauty, 6

Makeup, 38–41

attractiveness to men, 38

blush, 41

cheeks, contouring and highlighting, 40

eyes, 40–41

fashion dolls', 40–41

foundation, 44–45

lip color, 39, 41

natural look, 38–39

neutral and flesh tones, 39

too much makeup, 38–39

Male attraction to women

age of women, 10

arms and legs, 118–119

assertiveness, 256

beauty, 10

blondes, 89

body shape, 107–108, 113

breasts, 121

buttocks size and shape, 111–112

childlike facial features, 25

classiness, 245

color of clothing, 226–227

confident manner, 254

facial appearance and, 13

Q

R

www.ingramcontent.com/pod-product-compliance
Lightning Source LLC
Chambersburg PA
CBHW071829270326
41929CB00013B/1940